Prevention

LIVE TO
100
AND
LOVE IT!

An Easy Road Map to Longevity

Stacey Colino & the editors of Prevention

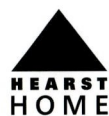

HEARST
HOME

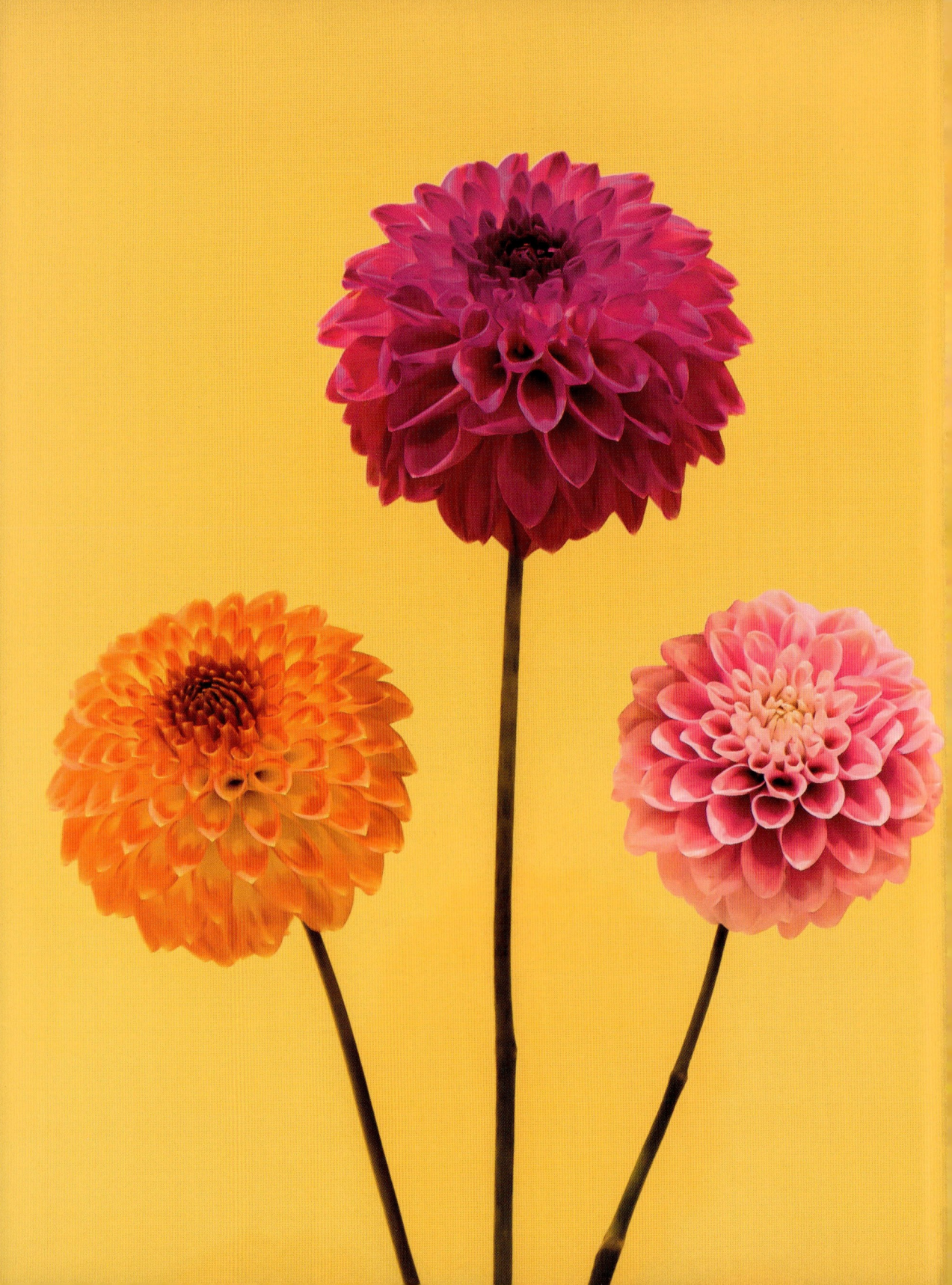

Contents

Welcome to Your Future—Upgraded 4

Chapter One
Rethink Aging 8

Chapter Two
Focus On Your Mind 31

Chapter Three
Care for Your Body 60

Chapter Four
Shift Your Lifestyle 111

Your Three-Week Longevity Challenge 166

Index 170

Credits 176

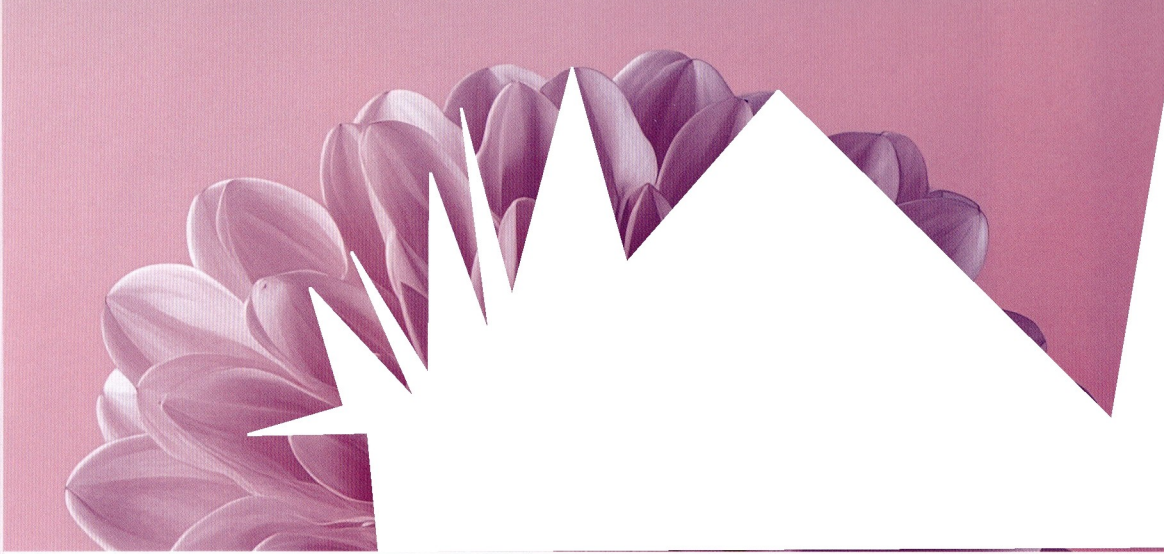

Welcome to Your Future—Upgraded

WHAT IF WE TOLD YOU THAT YOU COULD FEEL 10 to 20 years younger than you do right now? Or that you could continue to feel like your current age in 10, 20, or even 30 years?

It's actually possible, based on the many medical and technological advances that address diseases associated with aging, as well as the increased understanding of how lifestyle factors (such as excess stress, a poor diet, sedentary habits, and insufficient sleep) contribute to premature aging. The most exciting news: You have the power to harness the available insights and medical advances and even your own outlook to achieve optimum

health tomorrow—and today!

The reality is, people are living longer than they did a generation or two ago. In the U.S., the current life expectancy for men is 74.8 and for women it's 80.2; by comparison, in 1960 life expectancy for men was 66.6 years and for women, 73.1 years. And by the year 2060, average life expectancy in the U.S. is projected to reach a record high of 85.6 years for the total population, according to the U.S. Census Bureau. Meanwhile, with improvements in health care, lifestyle, and preventive medicine, there's also been a compression of morbidity—that is, a shorter period of illness and disability people can expect to experience at the end of their

lives. This means people today live longer and healthier lives with less time suffering from old age–related diseases or disorders.

THE NEW OLD AGE

With advances in the field of aging as well as breakthrough medical treatments and health-care technology, your aging experience is likely to be quite different from your grandparents' or even your parents'. Thanks to technology and treatments such as regenerative procedures (like stem cell therapy), immunotherapy for cancer, wearable medical devices, and implantation of artificial organs, among others, there's now a greater potential to prevent or reverse life-threatening diseases. We now know a lot more about the lifestyle changes that promote longevity. All of which means you can take steps to increase your health span—the length of time you live in good health—as well as your lifespan. The bottom line? You have more influence over aging processes than you may think you do. The potential to live to 100 while loving life has never been closer.

FUTURE-PROOF YOUR HEALTH TODAY

The best time to start making positive changes that could enhance your health and extend your life is right now. As Becca Levy, Ph.D., an expert on the psychology of successful aging, writes in *Breaking the Age Code*, "For those of us who aren't yet old, instead of viewing ourselves as fundamentally different from older people, it's helpful to think of ourselves as older people in training. If all goes well, we will become old."

Consider this book your training guide to aging well, a reliable source for the information you need to future-proof your health and live your longest, best life. This guide will help you discover strategies that can help you stay sharp and vibrant into your later years. It addresses your biggest concerns about aging and offers tools to address them,

with practical approaches to optimize your health and well-being well into your later years.

There are plenty of upsides to getting older—deeper wisdom, better decision-making, a broader understanding of the world, more self-confidence, greater self-acceptance, and even increased contentment—and it's important to appreciate each and every one. As professor of psychology at Stanford University and founding director of the Stanford Center on Longevity Laura Carstensen told *Prevention*, "I have so much fun telling my young students, 'When people tell you these are the best years of your lives, they're wrong!'"

How to Use This Book

▶ Throughout these pages, you'll discover the latest science and solutions behind aging well, including actions you can take to extend your health span and your lifespan.

CHAPTER ONE Discover the latest on the science of aging and envision your best future, starting now.

CHAPTER TWO Read about how the mind ages (yes, there's good news!) and find ways to connect with others to make your life richer.

CHAPTER THREE Find out about common age-related diseases and how to preserve your physical functionality.

CHAPTER FOUR Learn about lifestyle changes you can make—such as tweaks to your diet, exercise routine, stress management, and sleep—to help you feel your best every day.

PLUS In every section, read about folks just like you in the "You're in Good Company" stories. At the end of the book, you'll also find Your Three-Week Longevity Challenge to start increasing your longevity today.

You'll notice that key health-boosting strategies come up again and again. That's because what's good for your physical health is usually good for your mood too, and the interactions between better physical and mental health can lead to an upward spiral in well-being.

Pay attention to the positive changes you make and their benefits—this will motivate you to move forward into future vitality. Your best years are both now and ahead of you! Let's get started.

Expert Advice for a Long and Healthy Life

Prevention Medical Review Board Members share their science-backed advice (spoiler alert: you'll need sneakers) to live your most energized and happiest life.

"If you can **walk or take the stairs**, do it. You don't have to go to the gym for things to count as exercise."

—**Rekha B. Kumar, M.D., M.S.,** Associate Professor of Clinical Medicine, Weill Cornell Medicine Iris Cantor Women's Health Center, Endocrinology & Internal Medicine

"My single most important tip is to follow our motto from the UCLA Women's Cardiovascular Center: **'Move frequently... eat thoughtfully...connect deeply.'**"

—**Karol Watson, M.D., Ph.D.,** Professor of Medicine/Cardiology; Co-director, UCLA Program in Preventive Cardiology; Director, UCLA Barbra Streisand Women's Heart Health Program; David Geffen School of Medicine at UCLA; John Mazziotta, M.D., Ph.D., Endowed Chair in Medicine

"Here is my key to longevity: **Practice gratitude**. We don't always get to control our circumstances, but we can acknowledge the goodness that is here. Even if we have physical ailments, be grateful for the ways we can move our body! In times of stress, what is something you can appreciate?"

—**Jessica Hui, M.D.,** Allergy & Immunology physician

"Don't just count your years—**make your years count**. Stay engaged, curious, and socially active. The longest-living people aren't just eating kale and jogging; they're laughing, learning, and finding purpose every day."

—**Mona A. Gohara, M.D.,** Associate Clinical Professor of Dermatology, Yale School of Medicine

"My most important tip is to **be physically active**. According to a 2025 research paper in the *British Journal of Sports Medicine*, physical activity (defined as walking) can add years to your life. Most notably, if people over the age of 40 were as active as the top 25% of the active population, they could live an extra 5.3 years! The good news is that it is never too late to start, so grab a friend and get moving."

—**Dr. Karen Litzy, P.T., D.P.T.**

"From ancient Greece through modern times, wise people have quoted the maxim **'Everything in moderation, nothing in excess.'** For me this means a healthy, well-balanced diet—allowing for the occasional special treat or glass of wine; staying physically active with a mixed routine of strength training, cardio fitness, and stretching with relaxation; feeling fulfilled by work and engaged intellectually; and having fun— enjoying downtime with hobbies and creative pursuits. Finding balance and moderation in these pursuits is the key to a long and healthy life."

—**Ruth Oratz, M.D.,** Professor of Medicine, NYU Grossman School of Medicine

"Keep a strong and active social network."

—**Hiroshi Mashimo, M.D., Ph.D.,** Gastroenterologist, VA Boston Healthcare/Harvard Medical School

"Prioritize and protect your sleep, but don't live in fear of not getting enough."

—**W. Christopher Winter, M.D., D-ABSM, D-ABPN, F-AASM,** Sleep Specialist/Neurologist, Author of *The Rested Child* and *The Sleep Solution*

"**Move your body**—every day, in any way you can. Exercise is one of the most powerful and well-proven ways to prevent and even treat cardiovascular disease, and it's available to almost everyone. It strengthens the heart, improves circulation, and enhances overall physical and mental well-being. Whether it's walking, dancing, or lifting weights, find what you enjoy and make it a habit. Your heart and the rest of your body will thank you!"

—**Rigved V. Tadwalkar, M.D., M.S., F.A.C.C., F.A.C.P.,** Consultative Cardiologist & Partner, Pacific Heart Institute, Cedars-Sinai; Director of Cardiac Rehabilitation, Providence St. John's Health Center

"Long-term stress may impact your hormones and many aspects of your health. Once you have identified that you are stressed, find ways to reduce it right away through **mindfulness,** positive affirmations, deep breathing, and doing things you enjoy!"

—**Deena Adimoolam, M.D.,** Specialist in Endocrinology, Diabetes, and Metabolism

"**Preventive care** is the foundation of longevity and vitality— prioritize regular check-ups, healthy nutrition, and daily movement to thrive for years to come."

—**Brooke Williams, D.O., M.S., DipABOM**

"**Creating community** is beneficial for your mind, body, and spirit. Keep up with your old friends, but make new ones, too. There is a loneliness epidemic in our country, but the people who are thriving are the ones who have a robust sense of community. You can make community through your neighborhood, your school, your job, and your hobbies. Reach out, stay in touch!"

—**Oona Metz, L.I.C.S.W.,** is a psychotherapist and writer specializing in treating women navigating divorce.

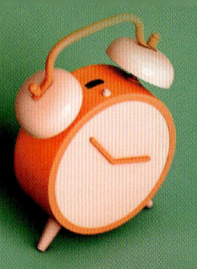
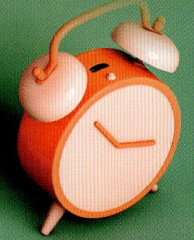
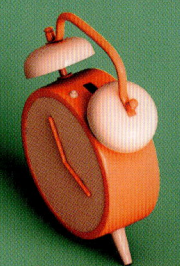
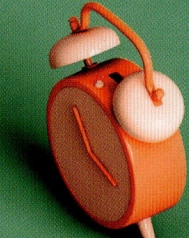
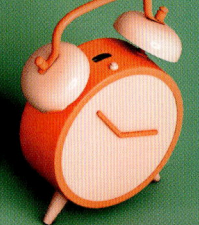

chapter one
RETHINK
AGING

With people experiencing longer lifespans and, as important, longer health spans, aging can be viewed like every new phase: an exciting opportunity for growth, change, and possibilities.

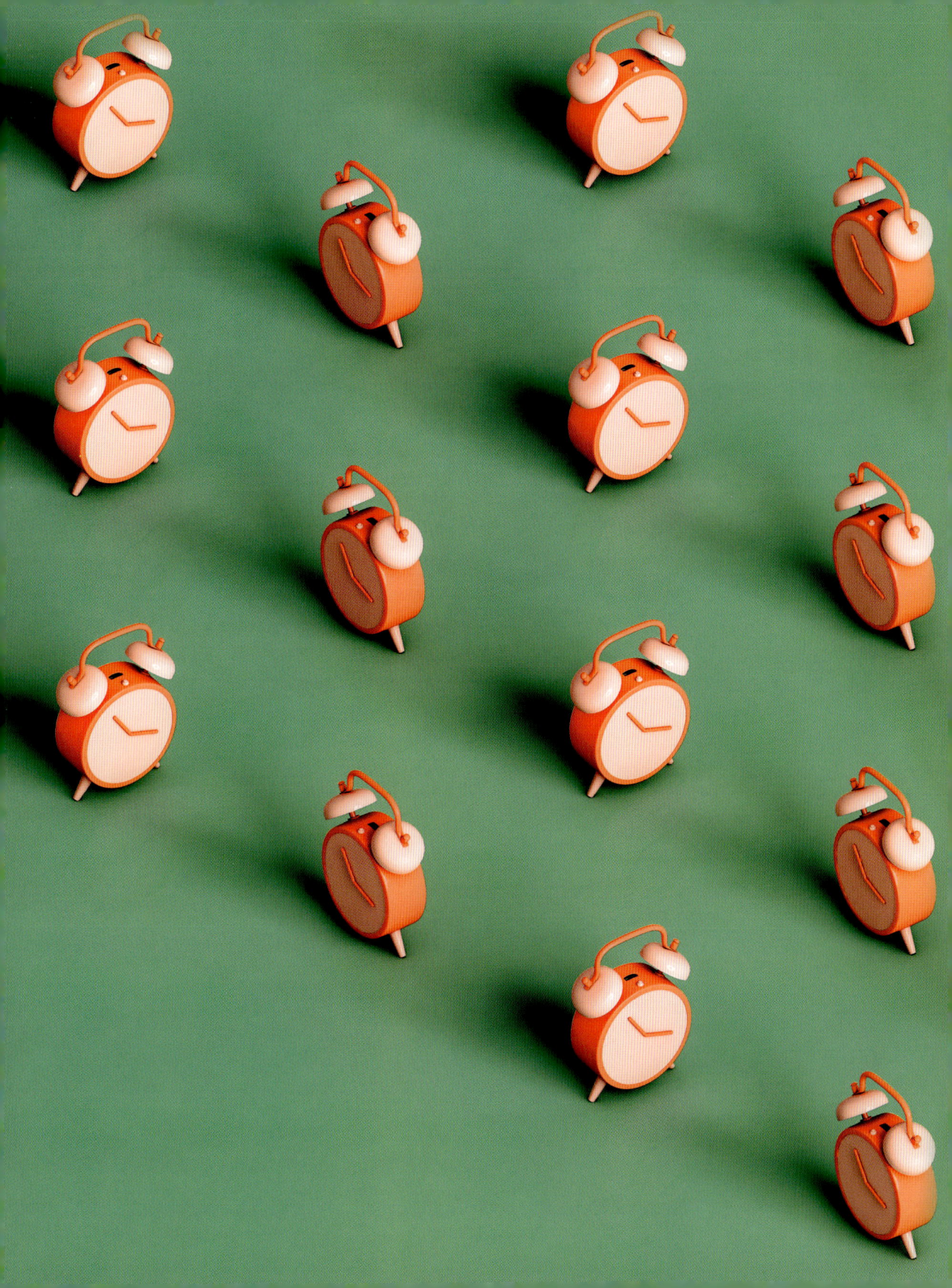

Feel Better, Longer

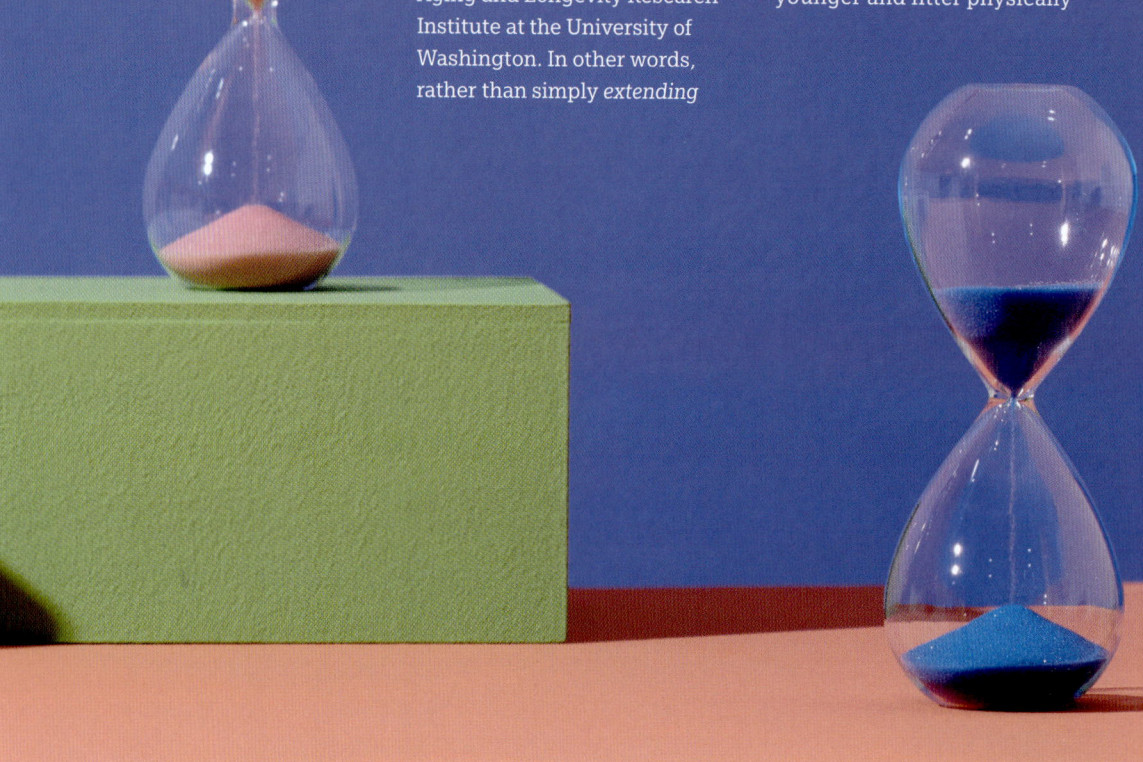

ASK PEOPLE IF THEY WANT TO LIVE TO 100 AND many will say no, because they don't want to be a burden to their kids or to become sick or disabled. They worry about what the future may look like for them. But what if you could reach very old age and remain fit enough to run a 10K or hike steep trails—and, as we all would like to do, live independently and keep pace with your great-grandkids or rescue puppy as they tear around your home? You can.

Scientists are shifting their attention from simply helping people celebrate many birthdays to making those older years great ones, says Matt Kaeberlein, Ph.D., CEO of Optispan and former director of the Healthy Aging and Longevity Research Institute at the University of Washington. In other words, rather than simply *extending* your lifespan, they want to *boost* your health span—meaning the number of years you go about your life alert, engaged, and active, says Stephen Kopecky, M.D., a cardiologist at the Mayo Clinic and author of *Live Younger Longer*.

In addition to scientists working to optimize your later years through medications and treatments, research suggests you can do a lot to affect your health span. We have the power to make changes to positively affect our longevity and our long-term health, to feel younger and fitter physically and mentally than your biological age. We *can* live to 100 and love it!

THE SCIENCE OF AGING

Most of the conditions we associate with aging start in our cells and tissues before they become visible as, say, heart disease. To counter these processes, health-span scientists are trying to figure out what exactly disrupts these cells and tissues. The list so far includes dysfunctions of mitochondria, the engines of cells; shortening of telomeres, substances at the ends of DNA that act like shoelace tips to keep chromosomes from fraying; and glitches in information within a cell.

Lifestyle and our environment are part of the picture of our cellular aging process, as are our genes. Researchers know this in part from studying lab animals—and, more recently, pets. Kaeberlein started the Dog Aging Project a few years ago because our furry friends are in many ways like people—subject to the effects of stress, environmental toxins, and less-than-ideal diets. But since they age more quickly, we can learn a lot from what they go through.

It's become clear that things we know are bad for us, like high blood sugar and lack of exercise, do their dirty work by causing cellular dysfunction. This means that the same strategies that can prevent conditions like diabetes and heart disease are also effective at targeting the biology of aging, Kaeberlein says.

How to Lower Your Biological Age

WHILE YOU CAN'T CHANGE YOUR PHYSICAL AGE, new research suggests you can do a few things to feel younger than your actual chronological age and slow the aging of your cells.

A study presented at the American Heart Association Scientific Sessions 2023 analyzed data from more than 6,500 adults who participated in the 2015–2018 National Health and Nutrition Examination Survey (NHANES). For the study, researchers from Columbia University's Mailman School of Public Health calculated participants' phenotypic age (a measure of a slew of biological factors) as well as the increasing phenotypic age of the participants.

The researchers discovered that people who had good cardiovascular health had a negative phenotypic age acceleration—meaning their biological health markers were

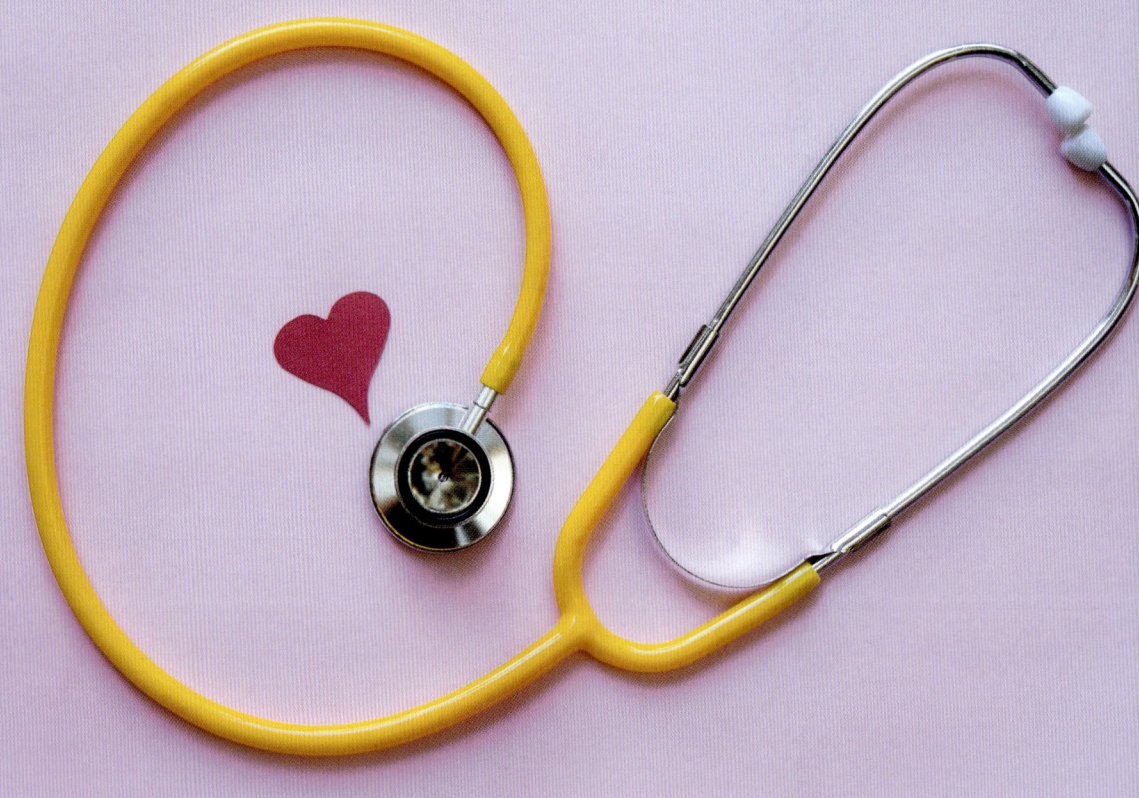

younger than their physical age. At the same time, people with worse cardiovascular health were biologically older than what would be expected for their age.

An example: The average actual age of people with good cardiovascular health was 41, but their average biological age was 36. By comparison, the average actual age of people with poor cardiovascular health was 53, while their biological age was 57.

The researchers found that people who scored high in the American Heart Association's Life's Essential 8 were more likely to have a biological age that was, on average, six years younger than their actual age.

So, what are Life's Essential 8? There are a lot of factors that go into your biological age, including underlying health conditions you have and your genetic makeup, says Cheng-Han Chen, M.D., board-certified interventional cardiologist and medical director of the Structural Heart Program at MemorialCare Saddleback Medical Center in Laguna Hills, California. The Essential 8, however, are lifestyle factors that you *can* control and that have a real impact on health and longevity.

"It's so logical," says Nicole Weinberg, M.D., a board-certified cardiologist at Pacific Heart Institute in Santa Monica, California. "I see people who lead long, healthy lives who eat well and are active—it doesn't need to be that hard. Just go for a walk after dinner, eat healthy, and get your blood pressure, cholesterol, and blood sugar checked."

Dr. Weinberg points out that while Life's Essential 8 focus on heart health, they are helpful for overall health. These are also good for brain, digestive, and immune health, she says.

That's why you will see the themes of the Essential 8 again and again in this book: practical, logical, and doable ways for you to affect your health, happiness, and longevity.

The Essential 8

1 Eat well
(see page 112)

2 Be active
(see page 124)

3 Don't use tobacco

4 Get plenty of sleep
(see page 158)

5 Manage your weight

6 Control your cholesterol

7 Manage your blood sugar

8 Manage your blood pressure
(for 6–8, page 64)

You're in Good Company

Moving to a new home is often considered a major stressor, but sometimes it involves a change for the better. Ed and Vicki started to feel isolated in their countryside home once they reached their 70s. They no longer felt comfortable driving but didn't want to burden their adult children or grandchildren with transportation requests or insist that friends always come to them. So they decided to move. After many months of hunting for a new home, they found a spacious condo in town that was a block away from a public library, a grocery store, a pharmacy, and public transportation. "The move transformed our lives," says Vicki. "We can go to museums and restaurants easily and see friends whenever we want to."

The New Thinking on Aging

THE LATEST SCIENCE BRINGS PLENTY OF GOOD NEWS, AND people are living better, longer. These days, getting older is a time for growth and change, and for new opportunities you can embrace with the benefit of a lifetime of wisdom.

That's why you may want to rethink what aging means.

Bringing outdated perceptions into this part of your life can affect your health and happiness in big and small ways, according to Becca Levy, Ph.D., a professor of psychology at Yale University and author of *Breaking the Age Code: How Your Beliefs About Aging Determine How Long & Well You Live.* "Most people don't realize they hold preconceptions about aging, yet everyone, everywhere, does," she says, and these beliefs are often negative. By examining these perceptions and considering their origin, she notes, "we'll have a basis for changing not only the narrative of aging, but the very manner in which we age."

What's Your Aging Mindset?

Take this quiz to reveal if you hold any common (and false) preconceptions about aging—and get insight into your own thoughts about it. After reading each statement, consider whether it is true or false and then circle your answer.

1. As people get older, their intelligence and their ability to learn new things decline dramatically.
  True **False**

2. People's personalities change with age.
  True **False**

3. Clinical depression occurs more often in older people than younger people.
  True **False**

4. Memory loss is a normal part of getting older.
  True **False**

5. Physical strength declines as you age.
  True **False**

6. After middle age, most older adults lose interest in sex.
  True **False**

7. Senses (hearing, vision, smell, touch, and taste) don't work as well for older people.
  True **False**

8. Retirement is often harmful to people's health.
  True **False**

9. Older workers are poor employees compared to younger ones.
  True **False**

10. Older adults don't adapt as well as younger people do when they move to a new place.
  True **False**

11. The majority of older adults view their health as good.
  True **False**

12. Old age begins at age 65.
  True **False**

Check Your Answers

You might be surprised to discover that some common assumptions about aging in healthy people are no longer true—or may never have been true in the first place!

1. **FALSE** Research suggests that intellectual ability and performance stay steady into people's later decades, and they can continue to learn throughout their lives.

2. **FALSE** People's personalities remain consistent throughout their lives; sometimes, certain traits may become more pronounced in later life.

3. **FALSE** While depression is the most common mental-health problem among older adults, it does not occur more often in older people than in younger ones.

4. **TRUE** As people get older, there is some modest memory loss, mostly for short-term memory. Retrieval of information may also slow down, but older adults generally retain long-term memories and knowledge.

5. **TRUE** Physical strength does drop with advancing age, mostly because muscle mass declines. However, doing weight-bearing exercise and resistance training can help minimize this change.

6. **FALSE** The National Social Life, Health, and Aging Project says that approximately 73% of individuals age 57–64, 53% of those age 65–74, and 26% of adults age 75–85 report being sexually active. Most older adults consider physical intimacy to be crucial to their relationship and to their emotional well-being.

7. **TRUE** In general, sensory processes—including vision, hearing, taste, smell, and touch—begin to decline with advancing age. That said, there is considerable variation among individuals.

8. **FALSE** On the contrary: As long as retirees are engaged in fulfilling activities, retirement can improve people's health by giving them more time for physical activity and reducing their stress.

9. **FALSE** Some people have negative perceptions of older workers, but research shows low turnover, less absenteeism, and fewer injuries in older workers, along with greater loyalty and congeniality.

10. **FALSE** While some people take longer to adjust to new environments, this varies by individuals across all ages. For some older people, moving presents an exciting opportunity for exploration and new experiences.

11. **TRUE** In fact, most older adults perceive their health to be good to excellent. They don't usually compare their current condition to their younger, possibly healthier, selves but to their peers who may have worse health.

12. **FALSE** There's no such thing as "old age"—it's a social construct that varies individually and across cultures. Being identified as "old" has less to do with chronological age than health status, functional ability, and self-perception.

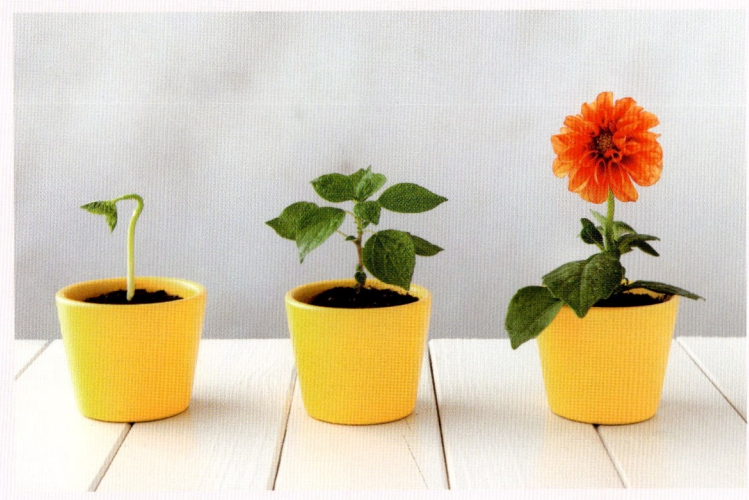

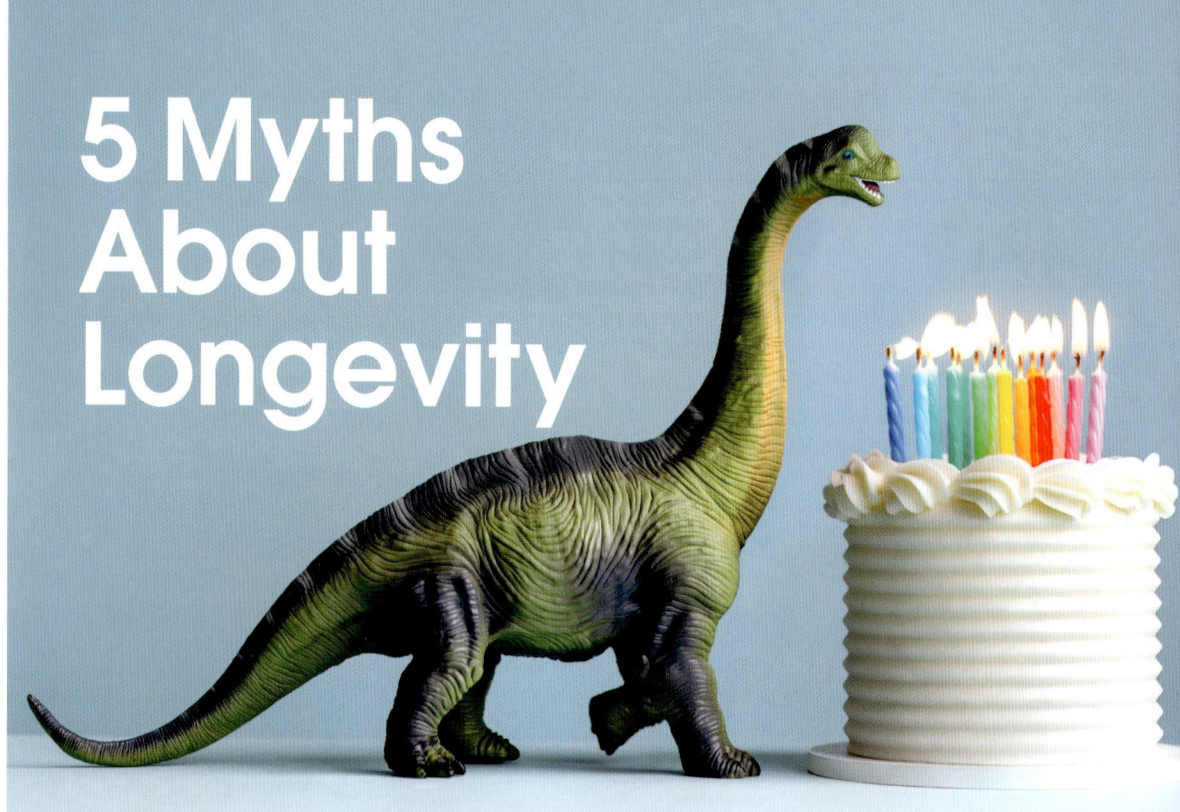

5 Myths About Longevity

1 A SUNNY DISPOSITION INCREASES YOUR LIFESPAN

An upbeat personality won't necessarily help you in the long-life sweepstakes. A Longevity Project study that followed more than 1,500 people for 80 years found that the carefree, happy-go-lucky folks actually lived shorter lives. Folks with an everything-will-turn-out-fine philosophy tended to take more risks with their health (such as skipping recommended health screenings). By contrast, those who lived longest tended to be persistent and conscientious.

That's not to say you need to be dour in order to tack on more years of life. Just try to balance life enjoyment with a conscientious approach to maintaining your health.

2 WORKING TOO HARD WILL PUT YOU IN AN EARLY GRAVE

Hard workers actually have a 20% to 30% lower risk of early death, according to the Longevity Project study. For most people, the social engagement and mental stimulation of working bring real benefits. But if your workplace causes you to take stress home, that's bad for your health.

Whether that work is paid or unpaid, it's having a sense of purpose that helps extend longevity, according to research in *Psychological Science*. Aside from paid work, you can find purpose in just about any type of activity, from volunteering to caring for a grandchild to taking up a social hobby.

3 IF PEOPLE IN YOUR FAMILY TEND TO DIE YOUNG, YOU WILL TOO

Genetics account for only a small percentage of your longevity. If you have at least one parent who lives past the age of 70, your chances of living longer go up, but lifestyle habits and your environment, both of which impact how your DNA is expressed, play a much bigger role in influencing your lifespan, says Catherine Johnson, M.D., founder and medical director of Precision Medical Care in Clarendon Hills, Illinois. When researchers studied more than 123,000 people, they found that five lifestyle habits in particular—maintaining a healthy weight, never smoking, exercising, following a healthy diet, and drinking alcohol only in moderation—greatly increased life expectancy at age 50.

Still, talk to your doc about your family medical history so you can take advantage of health screenings and find ways to lower inherited risks.

4 IT'S TOO LATE TO BENEFIT FROM GIVING UP BAD HABITS

It's never too late to improve your health and even increase your lifespan and health span. Take smoking: A study in the *New England Journal of Medicine* found that people who stopped smoking when they were between ages 45 and 54 gained about six years of life compared with others who kept puffing. And if you've been lax about slathering on sunscreen, researchers showed in a four-year study from the University of Queensland that daily sunscreen use slowed skin aging even in middle age. Giving up alcohol is another lifestyle change that yields almost immediate benefits. The World Heart Foundation asserts that no alcohol is good for you, while the American Heart Association warns that alcohol use can increase the chance of heart attack and stroke. Alcohol also increases the odds of getting cancer and Alzheimer's. On the flip side, within a month of quitting alcohol (or taking a break from it) many people report clearer skin, weight loss, better sleep, and better immune function.

5 AGING IS THE WORST!

No doubt some aspects of aging are suboptimal, but it's far from all bad—and research found that people who embrace aging live 7.5 years longer on average than those who dread it. This may be in part because people who have a bleaker outlook on getting older are less proactive about seeking health care when issues pop up; they may simply ascribe them to aging and fail to address them, another study found. So don't assume every stiff joint or energy dip is only because you're not as young as you used to be. Talk through any health changes or concerns with your doctor.

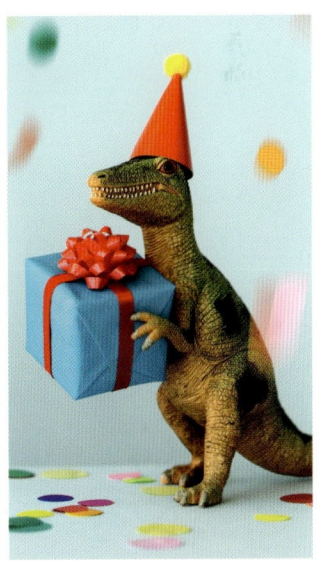

What We Know About Superagers

THERE'S A GROUP OF PEOPLE WHO SEEM TO BE WINNING against the march of time: Superagers are those 95 and older who are extra resilient against life-threatening health conditions and who maintain the cognitive and physical abilities of much younger people.

"They enjoy extended health," explains Nir Barzilai, M.D., founding director of the Albert Einstein College of Medicine's Institute for Aging Research and scientific director at the American Federation for Aging Research. And when superagers do become ill, it's in the last months or even weeks of a very long life.

While we know that healthy lifestyle choices lengthen the average person's life, in his work, Dr. Barzilai was surprised to find that superagers and individuals don't necessarily have healthier habits. Rather, several favorable genetic mutations appear to protect them against illness-causing inherited mutations.

Through his study of superagers, Dr. Barzilai says, he and others could discover ways for others to put off illness the way they do. He and others are working to help craft FDA-approved drugs that mimic genetic variants to keep bodies younger from the inside.

"To live past 100 today," Fortune. com wrote in 2024, "Barzilai says

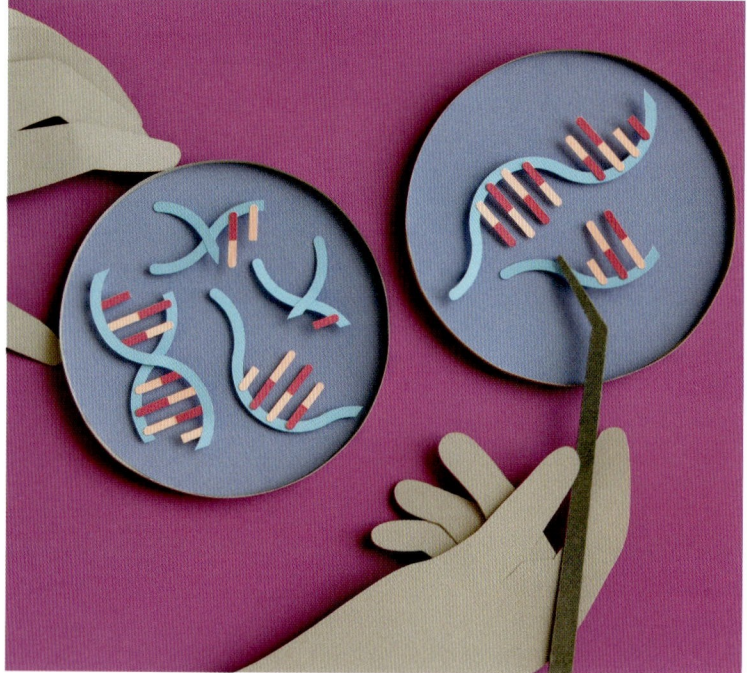

it's about following basic guidelines around exercise, nutrition, and managing stress while also keeping an eye on the next frontier of longevity science—which he believes to be a combination of precision medicine, AI interventions, and gerotherapeutics or drugs to target the underlying processes of aging."

LIFELONG VITALITY

With new scientific advances in the fields of longevity and age-related diseases, living a healthy, long life is within reach for many of us. "Longevity interventions have moved from science fiction

to science fact. We now know many processes in the body to target," says Matt Kaeberlein, Ph.D., CEO of Optispan and affiliate professor and former director of the Healthy Aging and Longevity Research Institute at the University of Washington. Here's what researchers are tinkering with in the lab, and additional studies could eventually lead to new effective drugs:

- **An anti-interleukin-11 drug** has been found to extend the lifespan in mice by up to 25%, primarily by reducing cell-damaging inflammation.

- Gene-editing snippers like **CRISPR/Cas9**, which removes mutations from genes, may one day conquer genetics-based, health span–robbing diseases.

- **Gene therapy**—i.e., inserting a healthy gene into cells to replace a defective one—is being tested to counter certain cellular aging processes, including the shortening of telomeres.

- **Metformin**, a drug commonly used to treat diabetes, has been shown to thwart various aging processes, including mitochondrial dysfunction, telomere shortening, epigenetic changes, and cellular senescence (a process where cells stop dividing and stay in an inactive state; this can weaken immune function and accelerate aging).

- The drug **rapamycin** activates natural pathways that protect and rejuvenate cells.

- **Resveratrol** is a phytochemical that may slow the aging process and increase lifespan by regulating mitochondrial function and cellular senescence, and reducing inflammation.

- A class of drugs called **senolytics** act like internal vacuum cleaners, sucking up defective, "senescent" cells that also deform other cells.

- **Taurine** is an amino acid that has been suggested in small studies to tame the inflammation behind diseases of aging.

Protecting Your Telomeres

▶ Telomeres affect how quickly your cells—and you—age. When telomeres become too short, the cells stop working and become "zombie-like" (or "senescent"). In this state, they emit molecules that promote inflammation and peptides that accelerate aging. This doesn't lead to any particular disease, but it means you may succumb more quickly to whatever your genes and environment put you at risk for, whether it's heart disease, dementia, or cancer. Research shows that you can reverse many aspects of aging if you can prevent cells from becoming zombified.

One of the best ways to fortify your cellular armor is to get moving: Exercise stimulates the production of the enzyme telomerase, which keeps them from getting worn down. In a Brigham Young University study of more than 5,800 men and women, those who jogged for 25 to 40 minutes five days a week had telomeres the length of those in people nine years younger.

Exercising your inner strength through meditation can also help protect your telomeres—researchers theorize that it may reduce damaging inflammation. Researchers at the University of California, Davis showed that people who meditated for three months had greater telomerase activity than those in a control group.

What Is Rapid Aging?

▶ While most people conceptualize aging as a steady process, a study published in a 2024 issue of the journal *Nature Aging* suggests that humans age in a much less linear fashion.

Scientists from Stanford University examined thousands of different molecules—specifically, the micro-universe of bacteria, fungi, and viruses that live within us and on our skin—in subjects between the ages of 25 and 75. The team found that the numbers of these various molecules changed drastically around age 44 and the early 60s on average.

"We're not just changing gradually over time; there are some really dramatic changes," Stanford University's Michael Snyder, a professor of genetics and the study's senior author, said in a press statement.

However, the aging process unfolded at different rates for various organs and body systems. For example, an increase in molecules related to cardiovascular disease was found in both ages, but those impacting immune function were largely seen in the early 60s.

The team hasn't discerned if these changes are the result of purely biological, behavioral, or a mixture of both influences, but evidence points to at least some being influenced by external factors.

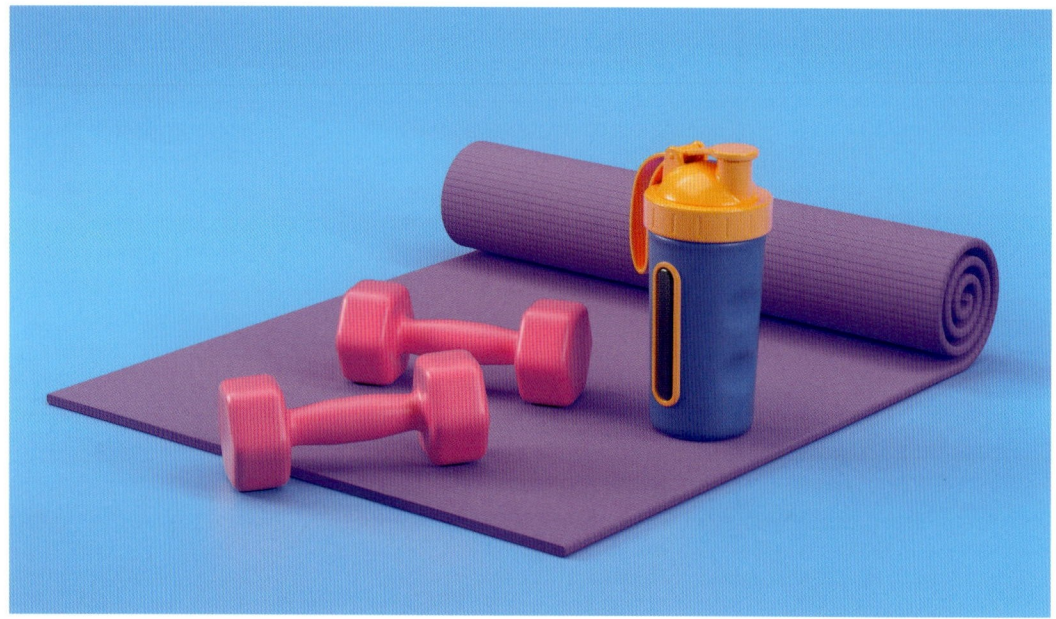

Start Today!

DO YOU THINK YOU'VE MISSED THE BOAT on making big health and wellness changes? Surprise! No matter your age, you can start turning things around right now.

EXERCISE

If your sneakers are buried under a pile of shoes, take note: Inactive folks ages 40 to 61 who upped their physical activity to about seven hours a week had a 35% lower mortality risk than those who stayed sedentary, a study by researchers from the National Cancer Institute found. Part of that longevity boost has to do with exercise's impact

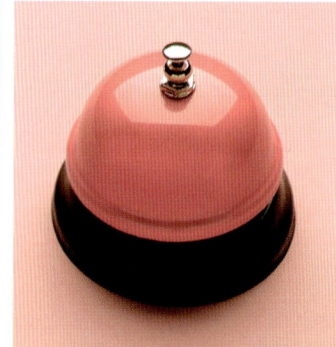

on the heart. One report found that formerly inactive 45-to-64-year-olds who increased their exercise to at least 30 minutes four to five days a week had improved oxygen uptake and reduced cardiac stiffness. Stiff cardiac tissue increases the risk

of heart failure. (See page 124 for more on exercise and fitness.)

IMPROVE YOUR SEXUAL ENJOYMENT

Yes, sex changes with age, and there are many solutions to obstacles, such as erectile dysfunction, trouble getting in the mood, or something else. Take menopause, for example: "About 60% of women who are perimenopausal or postmenopausal experience vaginal thinning, dryness, and irritation, which can bring about painful intercourse," says Lauren Streicher, M.D., medical director of the Center for Sexual Medicine and Menopause at

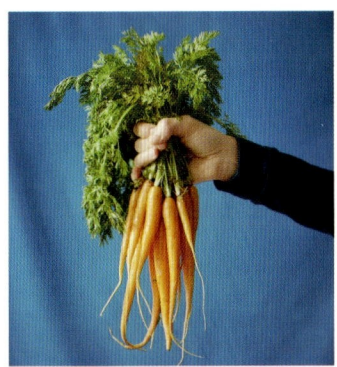

Northwestern Memorial Hospital in Chicago. But silicone-based lubricants and long-lasting vaginal moisturizers can alleviate symptoms, and prescription hormonal and nonhormonal options can restore vaginal tissue and reverse damage. "Even if it's been 20 years since you went through menopause, you can still reverse these changes," says Dr. Streicher. (See page 96.)

UP YOUR FIBER INTAKE

You probably know that consuming fiber is great for your gut. But a report in *Stroke* found that changing to a healthier lifestyle in middle age—including eating more fiber-rich nuts, whole grains, fruits, and vegetables—reduced women's long-term total risk of stroke by up to 25% and their risk of ischemic stroke by up to 36%. "And consuming 25 g to 38 g of fiber daily in midlife can help control blood pressure, cholesterol, blood sugar, and abdominal weight," says Michelle Routhenstein, R.D., a preventive cardiology dietitian and author of *The Truly Easy Heart Healthy Cookbook*. (See page 112 for more nutrition information.)

BOOST YOUR BRAINPOWER

Over the course of three months, researchers had people ages 58 to 86 take three to five different classes on subjects like Spanish, photography, and how to use an iPad. Midway through, students had already bolstered their cognitive abilities to levels similar to those of adults 30 years younger, one study found. "When you improve your cognitive abilities through learning new skills, it helps you learn more new skills, which creates a positive cycle of increased motivation for learning and social connection," says study coauthor Rachel Wu, Ph.D. Not up for a return to school? You can still acquire new knowledge and challenge your brain in other ways without setting foot in the classroom. (See page 32 for other ways to boost brainpower.)

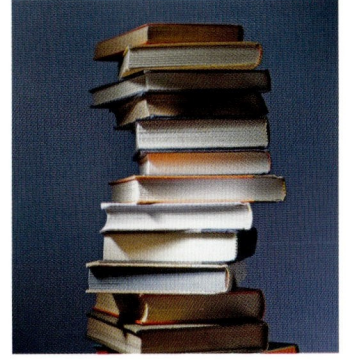

Be-Your-Best Checklist

- Question the accuracy of your assumptions about aging.

- Consider the benefits of getting older (including annoying things you won't have to do anymore).

- Reflect on your risks for age-related diseases and how you can reduce them. (See chapter 3.)

- Think about one of your less healthy habits and how you can change it.

- Add calendar entries for the coming year's preventative screenings.

- Make a wish list of what you want more of in the future (travel, relaxation, recreation, something else) and seek opportunities for those positive experiences.

- Envision the older self you want to be and think about steps you can take to become that person. (Turn the page to find out how.)

Go Ahead, Envision Your Future Self

IN GENERAL, PEOPLE ARE NOW LIVING DECADES LONGER than they were a few generations ago. And a growing number of experts say it's possible to thrive and flourish in those later years if you take the right steps now in terms of physical and emotional health, finance, and logistical planning.

First off, banish the idea that you've left your best decades behind you. That advice is straight from an expert with decades of psychological research focused on aging. Laura Carstensen, Ph.D., is the founding director of the Stanford Center on Longevity, where she studies motivational and emotional changes that occur with age and the influence these changes have on the way people process information.

Demographers estimate that by 2050 people will routinely live to celebrate their 100th birthdays. Yet while the increase in life expectancy of nearly 30 years in the 20th century is arguably one of the greatest achievements in human history, a lot of people feel more anxious than excited, says Carstensen, largely because our society is not set up to support very old people.

To address this, we need a new life map, Carstensen says. This includes a large-scale attitude shift about aging.

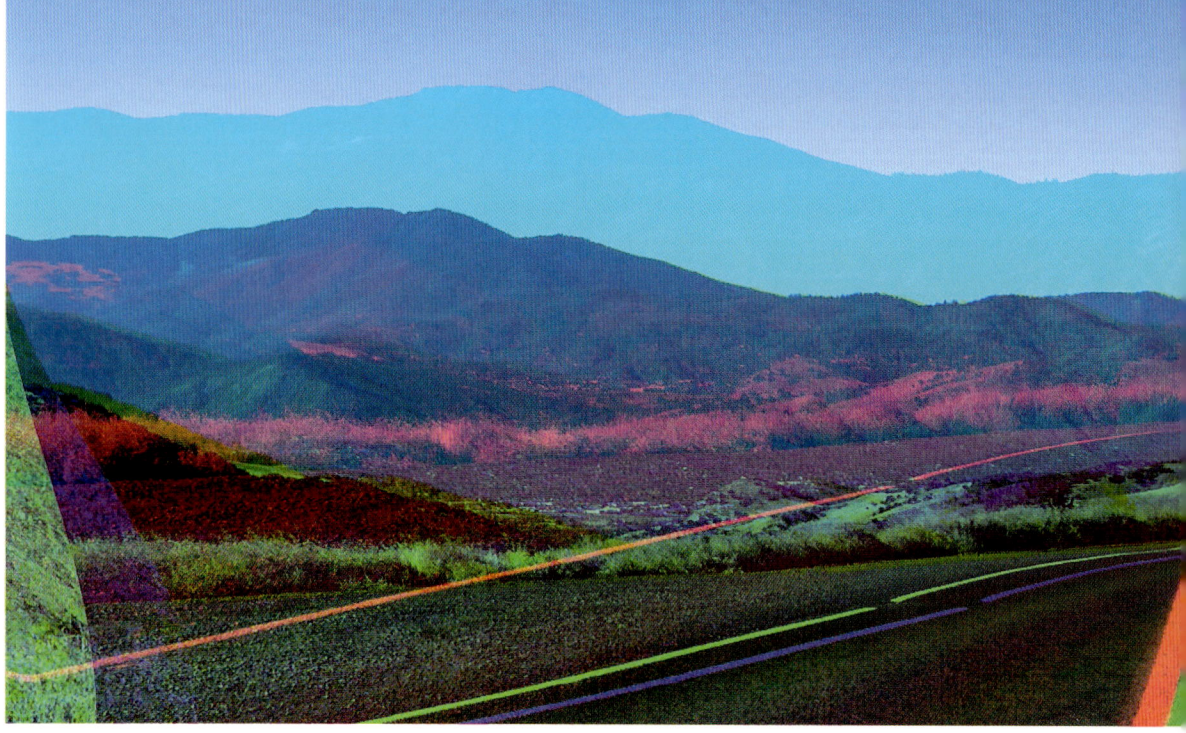

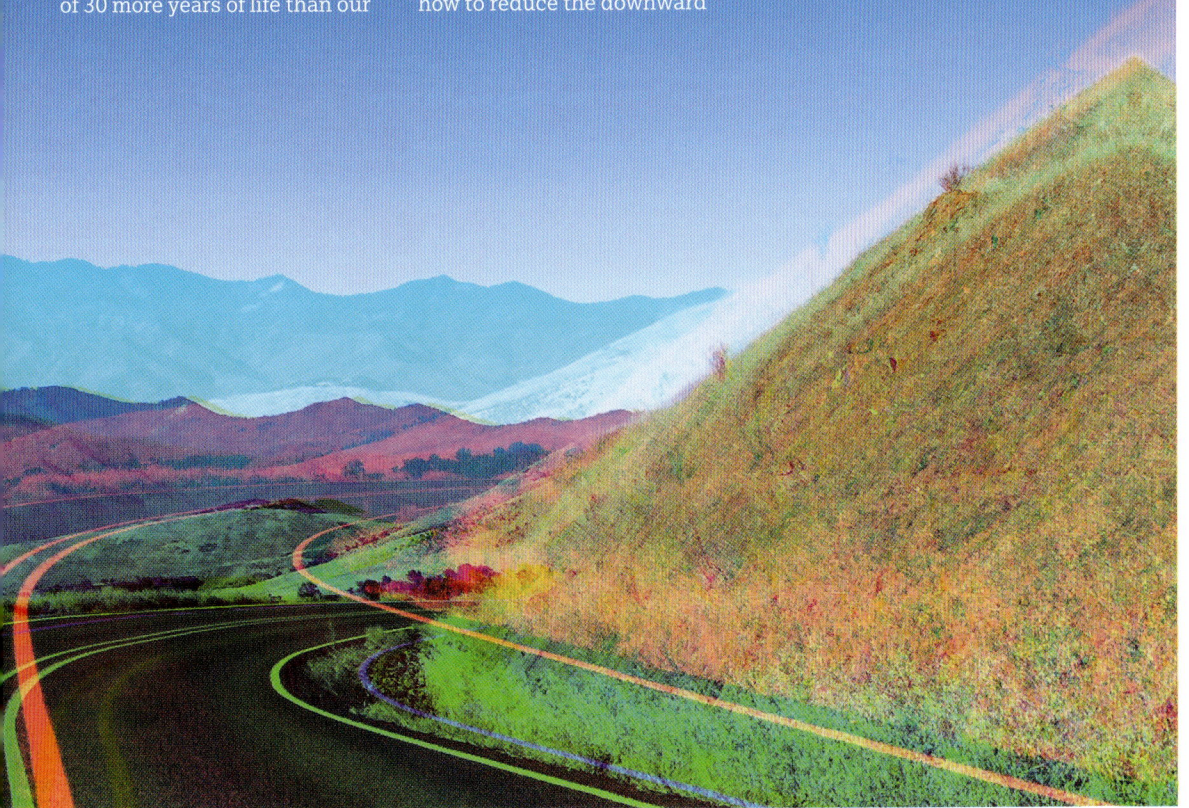

"Most of the conversations about aging and increased life expectancy focus mainly on coping with an increasingly large number of people who are declining," she says. "But this approach blocks creative thinking about how living longer could help us live better throughout our lives."

Carstensen decided to do something about this by launching an initiative called the New Map of Life. Her goal: to write a fresh narrative about longevity and the steps we'll need to take—individually, and as a society—to enhance the quality of our longer lives. After all, if we're looking at an average of 30 more years of life than our ancestors had, we want them to be fulfilling.

The New Map of Life advocates for a shift from a deficit mindset that laments the losses associated with aging—whether to health, mobility, financial security, independence, or social engagement—to a focus on the significant ways older adults can contribute to the social good, the economy, and other aspects of community. As the Stanford report notes, "many people experience good health and functional independence well into their 70s and 80s."

"At some point I realized that if we're thinking only about how to reduce the downward slide as we get older...we won't ask the right questions," says Carstensen. With this initiative, Carstensen is reframing the challenges and opportunities of a longer lifespan.

To make the most of the decades to come in your life, you can embrace Carstensen's vision of a new life map and think about what you want your later years to look like—and start planning for them wherever you're at. As Carstensen says, "You can't achieve what you can't envision."

Why Change Is Good

WHEN YOU LIVE FOR SEVERAL DECADES VIEWING yourself a certain way—as a colleague, as a parent, as a certain type of person—it's understandable that self-perceptions become solidified. Consciously or not, we all have beliefs about who we are that are based on our behaviors, abilities, feelings, and personality characteristics as well as how others see us and how they respond to us. This is what psychologists call "self-concept"—a reflection of how you see yourself as a person—and it has a powerful effect on the way you act, the choices you make, the attitudes you have, and how you move through life. If you've always been known as a go-getter or, conversely, a low-key person, you probably assume you'll always be that way.

And then you hit middle age, and maybe you start to feel not quite like yourself. One reason may be that your reactions, preferences, needs, values, and expectations have shifted over time, but your self-concept hasn't kept up. "We tend to think of ourselves as static, but we do change," says Mark Leary, Ph.D., professor emeritus in the department of psychology and neuroscience at Duke University and author of *The Curse of the Self.*

UPDATE YOUR SELF-CONCEPT

Thinking of ourselves as being one way when we have in fact changed can leave us feeling confused, out of sorts, stuck, or full of self-doubt, says Leary. Research has found that this is a common phenomenon at a certain point in life: Self-concept clarity—the extent to which someone has a clear understanding of their self and identity—increases each decade until the 60s, then begins to decline; after that, "people become less sure of their identity," the study authors noted, perhaps partly because of shifts in their work, family, and community roles at this life stage. Rediscovering a sense of self has been rated as one of the most challenging aspects of midlife for women, according to a study involving 81 women over 23 years.

Unfortunately, harboring outdated ideas about yourself can end up holding you back from taking smart risks and embracing new challenges when doing so might lead you to feel more fulfilled. "If we're looking at ourselves through an old lens of who we are, we take those outdated views into our future and make decisions based on that," says Michele Patterson Ford, Ph.D., a psychologist in private practice and a senior lecturer at Dickinson College in Pennsylvania. On the other hand, updating your self-

concept to reflect who and how you are now can help you pursue experiences and activities that feel satisfying and meaningful and skip or minimize those that may not suit you anymore. After doing some self-reflection, you might realize that you've outgrown the intense fear of public speaking you used to have and might actually enjoy giving the professional talks you've been invited to present. Or maybe you'll realize that you've had enough of the corporate grind and what you really want to do is pursue your artistic talent. And when you have a stronger, clearer sense of who you are *now*, you're likely to feel more comfortable in your own skin, maybe even happier, which is valuable in its own right. Ultimately, the goal is to make choices and changes that are in your current best interest, rather than in the best interest of you 10 or 20 years ago. So how can

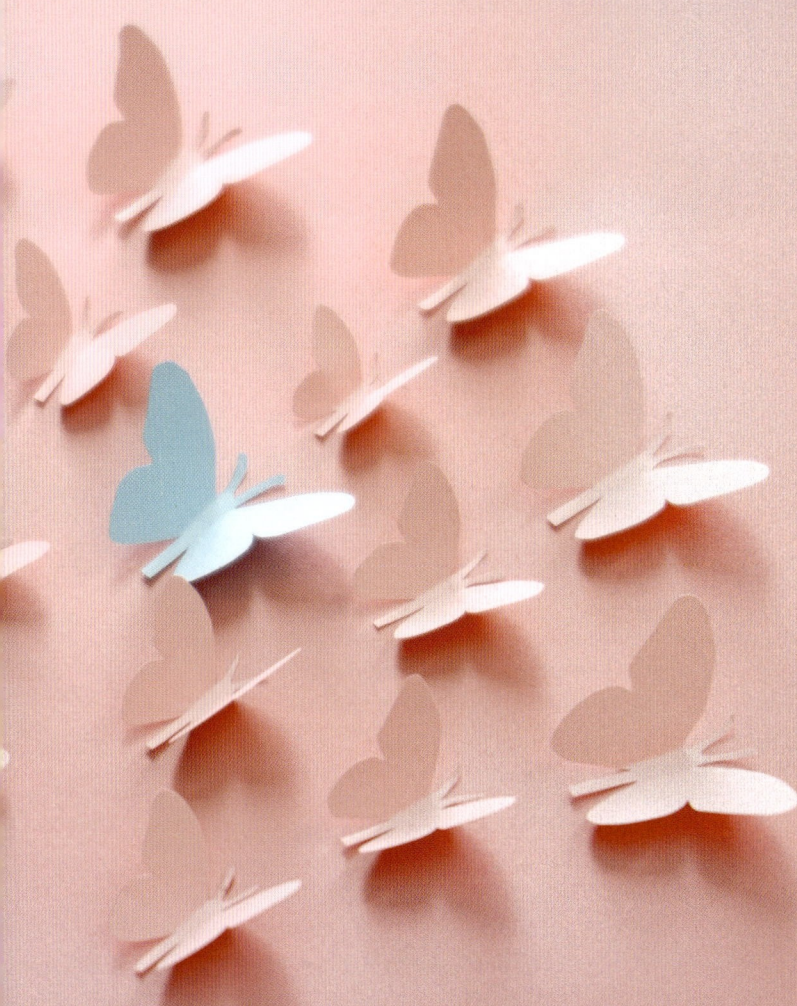

talents, values, and passions (and struggles) as much as you believe you do?

Step 3 Reflect on their answers. If everything is aligned, move on to step 4. If the answer is no, take a look at how you spend your time so you can make a concerted effort to engage in more activities that reflect the qualities and things you value. Living in a way that aligns with what you value about yourself can help solidify your self-concept, says Ford.

Step 4 Think about what was important to you 10, 20, or 30 years ago and write a letter to your younger self sharing what you've learned about yourself over time, how you've changed, and what really matters to you now.

Step 5 Stay open-minded. You might have lost some qualities you care about over time. Updating your self-concept is as much about consciously letting go of notions that no longer suit you as it is reclaiming aspects of yourself that you value.

Step 6 Rethink the terms you use for yourself. Tune in to the ways you label or describe yourself— like calling yourself an introvert or an extrovert or seeing yourself as uncreative—and assess whether these terms accurately describe your current behaviors.

Once you've completed steps 1 through 6, consider how the conclusions you reach can help you plan for the life you want to achieve. Turn the page to start charting your own course.

you figure out if you're working with a self-concept that reflects who you are now? You dig in and do an inventory.

6-STEP SELF REVIEW

Step 1 Sit down and, in writing, take stock of your current strengths, weaknesses, values, and preferences, suggests Susan Krauss Whitbourne, Ph.D., professor emerita of psychological and brain sciences at the University of Massachusetts, Amherst.

Ask yourself questions like these:
- **What are 5–10 things I am good at?** These could be anything from talents to work skills to hobbies to interpersonal qualities, etc.
- **What are 5–10 things I struggle with?** These could be daily challenges you have, things you avoid, or where you have trouble with motivation, etc.
- **What are 5–10 values I closely hold?** These might be hard work or kindness.
- **What are 5–10 things I love?** These can be as wide-ranging as hanging out with your dog to working in your business.

Step 2 Ask people who know you well if you've got the right idea. Do they think you embody these

Charting Your Own Course

NOW THAT YOU HAVE A BETTER UNDERSTANDING of who you are today, ask yourself the following questions to create a path to the future:

- **What kinds of activities make you feel fulfilled? What do you truly enjoy doing?**

- **What have you always wanted to do or try but haven't? Can you do it now?**

- **Is your social circle supportive and gratifying? If not, how can you expand it?**

- **When you imagine the future, what do you want your life to look like in five years? Ten years? Fifteen years?**

- **What do you value most in life, and are you living in a way that's true to those values? If not, what can you do to change that?**

- **What nonmaterial things would you like to have more of in your life?**

- **How would you like people to remember you when you're gone?**

- **If today were your last day on earth, how would you spend it?**

Now think about how you can set yourself up to bring more of these valuable experiences into your life. Assess this on a practical level, as well as on financial, psychological, and emotional levels. Also, think of older people you know who have these elements in their lives. Consider seeking their advice for steps you could take to cultivate them in yours.

MAKE A WELLNESS PLAN

One reason people believe that retirement is bad for your health is because research has shown that under certain circumstances, it can be. But it does not have to be. "Work, especially paid work, gives many people a sense of purpose. Losing that may lead to declines in health," says Gabriel H. Sahlgren, the study's lead author and director of research at the Centre for Market Reform of Education.

The best way for you to retain that sense of purpose after you retire is to make a wellness plan. Angela Curl, Ph.D., M.S.W., associate professor and director of the M.S.W. program at Miami University, advocates that you make that plan as concrete as possible. "If you want to volunteer when you are retired, ask yourself where and how often. Having specific plans and steps to follow will help you enter retirement more easily."

One particular point of emphasis for partnered folks is to make sure your significant other is on board with your plans. "Individuals can envision retirement one way, but if their spouse doesn't envision it the same way, it can be problematic," says Curl. "Talking to your spouse about retirement before you leave the workforce is important in reducing conflict."

GET A GRIP ON YOUR FINANCIAL RESOURCES

How much money you have (or don't have) as you get older has the potential to lead to happy-making freedom or misery-inducing stress. And a longer lifespan means it's more crucial than ever before to plan financially for the future. This means the number one thing you can do is save—and then save some more, says Michael F. Roizen, M.D., emeritus chief wellness officer at the Cleveland Clinic and author of *The Great Age Reboot: Cracking the Longevity Code for a Younger Tomorrow.*

If you're at retirement age and haven't started saving, or haven't saved enough, there are still actions you can take, from increasing your contributions to your retirement account and delaying Social Security to delaying retirement partially or altogether—which could contribute both to your health and the health of your nest egg.

Consider working with a financial advisor to evaluate your current savings plan and goals.

GET YOUR HEALTH-CARE TEAM IN PLACE

Health issues will almost certainly pop up as you get older. If you have a posse of health-care pros you trust before you need them, you'll be able to handle whatever diagnosis you're facing with more confidence and less stress, says Dr. Roizen. "And it's important to actually listen to the advice you're given," he adds, pointing to research showing that less than a quarter of people who are prescribed rehab after a cardiovascular incident or procedure actually do it. Having a team of docs you trust and respect can help you have open and honest conversations. That doesn't mean you shouldn't get a second opinion, adds Dr. Roizen: "Health and medicine are complicated—especially as you get into serious stuff—

so it's always a good idea to get multiple opinions."

FIGURE OUT HEALTH INSURANCE

According to the AARP, people in midlife (50 to 64 years old) pay a particularly high cost for private health insurance, with premiums and deductibles (not to mention covering dependents until they are 26) becoming so high that many are forced to make difficult choices about medical care and often go into medical debt. When Medicare

kicks in at 65, that doesn't mean the end of health-care costs, as individuals still pay premiums and co-pays depending on their income. In fact, AARP estimates that retired people on Medicare spend about 16% of their income on health care each year. And long-term care, such as in-home or nursing care, is a whole other question. While these are financial questions that are best addressed with a financial advisor, you can find health insurance pricing through Healthcare.gov.

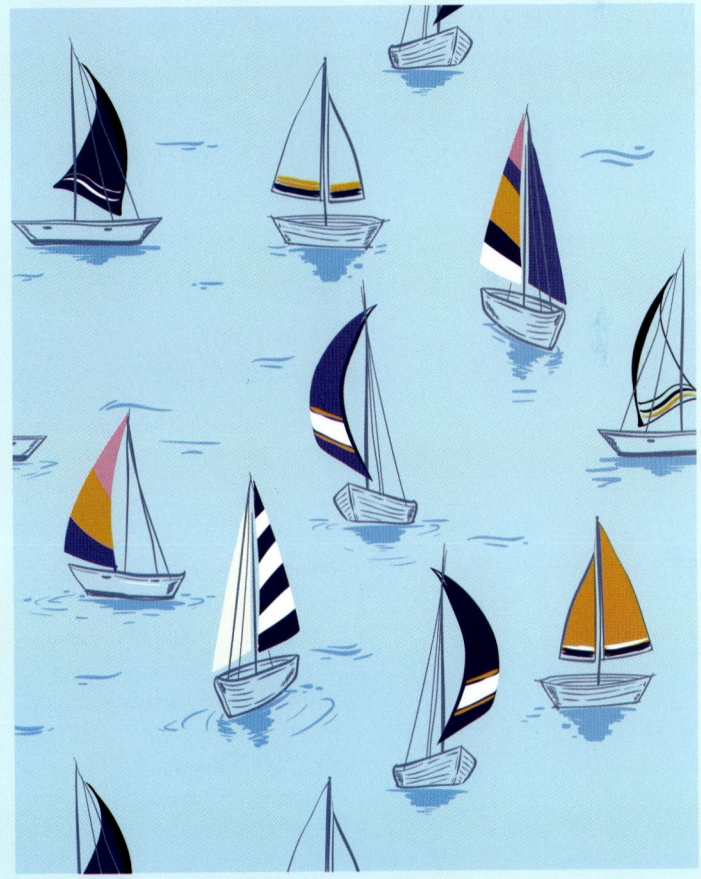

Rethinking Retirement

WITH PEOPLE LIVING LONGER THAN EVER, Stanford Center of Longevity director Laura Carstensen, Ph.D., says there are "obvious opportunities to redesign... institutions, practices, and norms and bring them into sync with the health, social, and financial needs of 100-year lives."

One problem, as she sees it, is our concept of working and retirement: "When we are working, we are working too hard, and then when we're retired, we're retired too hard. Working for 60–80 hours a week isn't good for anybody, and retiring for 30 years isn't good for anybody."

In her research, Carstensen found that across the board, people were not as cognitively sharp after they retired as they were when they were working, except for one group of people: Those who were in high-complexity jobs who retired for one year and then went back to work in some capacity. These people were in better cognitive shape than those who had continued to work steadily. In other words,

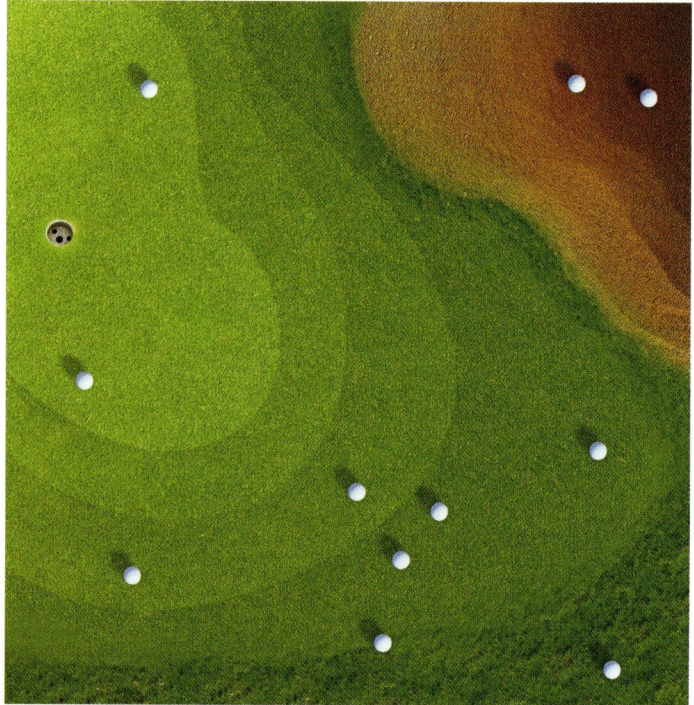

the model of working for 30 years straight and then retiring to full-time leisure isn't necessarily the standard to work toward. Instead of working full-time for 40 years and then retiring completely, Carstensen proposes that "we need breaks...we could take these 30 years [of 'retirement'] and put them anywhere we want."

Carstensen adds that people

should strive to do different things throughout their lives. "The model of work that we have in most jobs is that you train to do something, you get really good at it, and then you just do that thing. But it isn't very stimulating after a certain point."

What if instead of working 40 to 50 hours a week for 40-plus years and then retiring to play golf or tennis, you worked a little less throughout your life and were able to keep working into your 70s and 80s? What if your career allowed for more ebb and flow, enabling you to work fewer hours when your kids were young, hit it hard again as they got older, and then slow down (but not completely quit working) as you age—say, working 10 to 20 hours a week during the later decades?

"Our longer lifespans mean we have more time to separate raising our children and reaching the peak of our careers—those don't have to happen at the same time," says Carstensen. "We have an opportunity to have really creative, imaginative discussions about what our work life might look like over the course of a 100-year life."

Of course, some careers lend themselves better than others to part-time work as people get older. For example, if your job involves physical labor, you can still stay engaged by finding something to do that keeps you feeling productive and valued, says Carstensen. "If we gave up the old model of retirement and worked less through our lives but worked throughout our lives, I think all of us—both young and old—would be happier."

I Became a Pilates Teacher at Age 58
By Julie T. Chan, as told to Tula Karras

▶ When I was in my mid-50s and about 5 years from retiring, I began to think about how I wanted to live my 60s, 70s, 80s, and (hopefully) 90s. The top goals on my list: to stay connected to my Chinese roots and family, and to have fun. I'd spent a rewarding career in corporate advertising, but I didn't want to see another PowerPoint presentation or Excel spreadsheet, ever.

One day at the local Pilates studio where I'd been taking classes, I saw a sign about teacher training. I was enjoying learning to move my body in new ways, feeling the exhilaration of mastering a move through incremental progress. And I love being with people. I thought, *Why not help others discover the benefits and thrills, too?* I figured I could start teaching on the weekends to get a taste for it, and if I sucked at it, I'd move on to something else.

Pilates teacher training was the hardest thing I've ever done, and I wasn't sure I'd get through it. I was the oldest person in the teacher-training group, and it was intimidating to be surrounded by all these young people. But the group was supportive, and my director worked with me one-on-one when I was having trouble getting something. I stuck with it, and at age 58, after 9 intense months of training, I got my certification.

I'm now 64 and I've found my niche working with people who have gone through knee, shoulder, or hip replacements, because I've gone through that too! Being older and handling the changes that come along with that has really helped me relate to anyone else who is going through physical challenges.

The willingness to try new things has led me to take a writing class to sharpen my skills for a memoir. The class is aptly called "Where Do I Begin?" I want my granddaughter to know her history and be proud of being Chinese American. When I was in my 30s and 40s I was too busy raising kids and doing laundry to think about things like this. I'm freer now, not only because I have the time, but because I've learned that not everything works out, but so what? My grandmother lived to 96 and my father lived to 93. If I am going to live that long too, I might as well do something that I love every day.

We found Julie through ROAR Forward, which helps folks in the second half of their lives maximize their potential in every respect. To read other inspiring stories of Re-Imagineers, visit RoarForward.com.

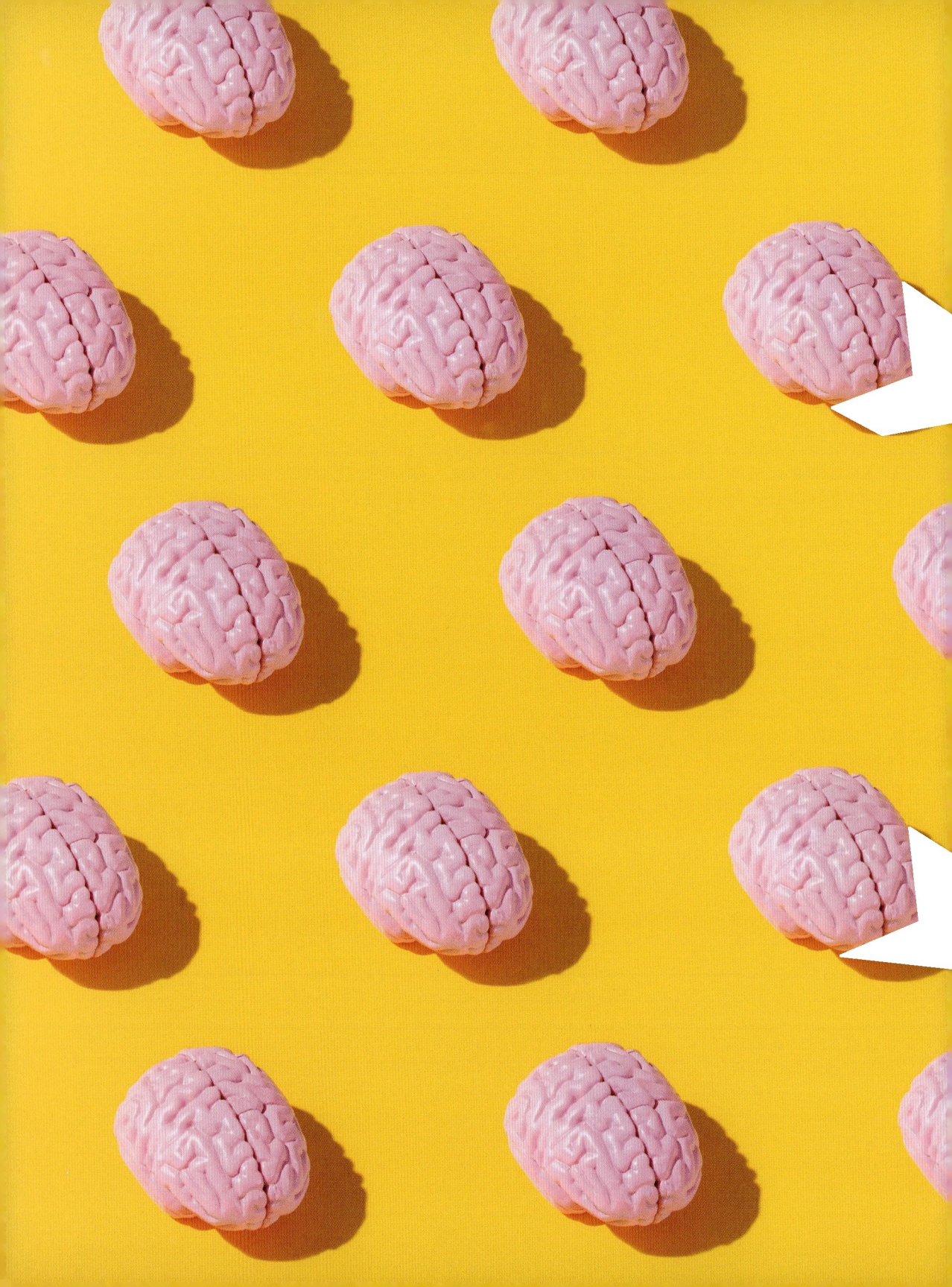

chapter two
FOCUS ON YOUR MIND

Memory, mental health, and social fulfillment are all inextricably linked to each other and to your physical health. Fortunately, you can develop these muscles at any age.

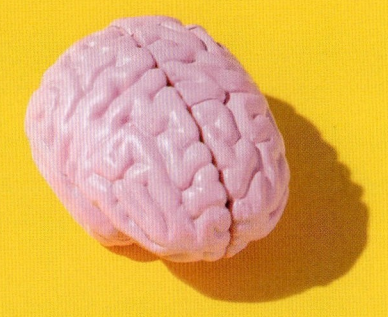
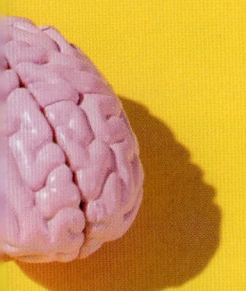
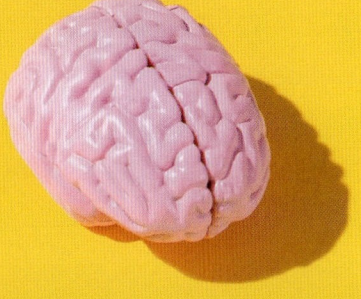

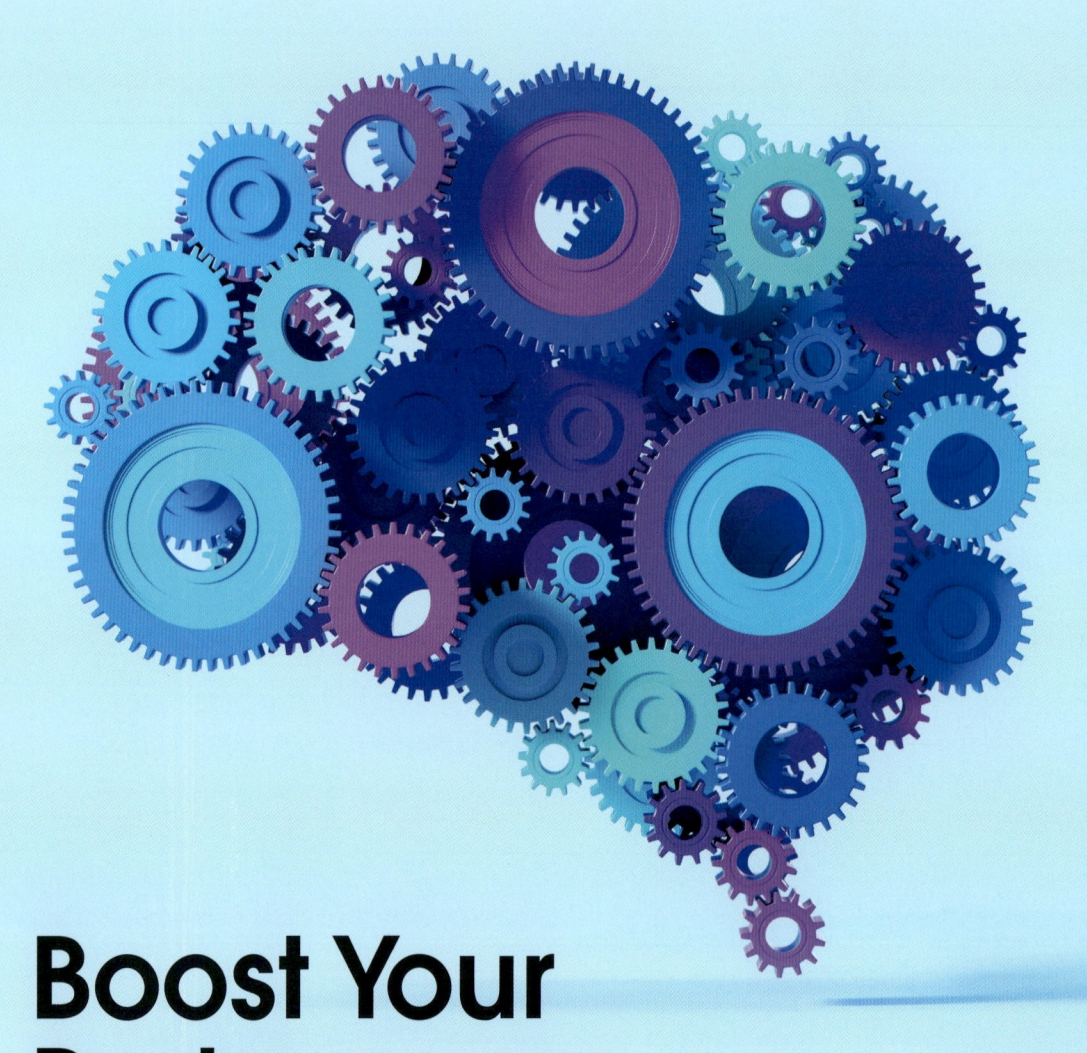

Boost Your Brainpower

THE GOOD NEWS: A REASSURING SCIENTIFIC concept called *neuroplasticity* means your brain has the ability to modify its structure and function throughout your life. New cells can be produced in your brain even when you're older. Greater neuroplasticity means denser concentrations of some brain cells and stronger, faster connections between those cells, explains Henriette van Praag, Ph.D., of Florida Atlantic University.

The upshot is that if you wish to make your brain stronger, you absolutely can. "We can't boost your IQ, but with brain training you can improve your concentration, expand your working memory, and more," explains Sherrie D. All, Ph.D., owner and director of the Centers for Cognitive Wellness and author of the book *The*

Neuroscience of Memory.

What should you expect when you're trying to make brain gains? "What's realistic depends on what people are willing to do," says Gary Small, M.D., physician in chief for behavioral health at Hackensack Meridian Health in New Jersey and coauthor of the book *The Alzheimer's Prevention Program*. Brain training isn't all fun and games (although, admittedly, some of it is). To some degree, you get out of it what you put into it.

The following strategies not only are worth your time and energy, but also have been shown to improve the way people process, focus on, store, and recall information.

EAT MEDITERRANEAN

Many brain-boosting foods are staples of the Mediterranean diet: fruits, vegetables, legumes, nuts and seeds, whole grains, fresh fish, olive oil, and red wine. And people who follow this diet (or come close to it) have significantly less heart disease and Alzheimer's disease and fewer strokes. In addition, adhering to the Mediterranean diet is associated with a lower risk of developing diabetes (and better blood sugar control in people who have it), as well as a reduced risk of hypertension, cholesterol abnormalities, and metabolic syndrome—all conditions that can affect brain health. (See more beginning on page 62.)

MOVE YOUR BODY

There's no debate: Physical activity does a body and a brain a world of good. "We have really strong evidence that exercise can help you grow more brain cells, increase the number of connections and pathways in your brain, and create more nerve growth factors—which are like Miracle-Gro for your brain cells," says All.

While there's no single type of workout that all experts recommend, studies have looked at the brain-building benefits of everything from hopping on a bike to practicing yoga. One small study in *Applied Physiology, Nutrition, and Metabolism* showed that high-intensity interval training in adults 60 and older, for example, resulted in an increase of up to 30% in memory performance. By contrast, a scientific review from the University of Illinois used MRI images to demonstrate that regular yoga practice brought about increased volume in the brain's hippocampus (which is involved in memory) and a

larger prefrontal cortex (which is essential to planning). Bottom line: Pick a fitness path you enjoy—and stay on it.

LEARN NEW THINGS AND INCREASE YOUR SKILLS

You may have heard this and thought it meant you had to learn how to play the guitar or take up Mandarin. Those things are great, but deepening your skills can also be beneficial.

"The idea is to train your brain, not strain your brain," says Dr. Small. "Each of us needs to find that entry point so the new activities we choose are engaging and we're motivated to do better at them." That might mean bringing novelty and variety into your favorite activity by, say, switching out your daily crossword for a sudoku puzzle a few days a week, or playing card games or computer games occasionally. If you enjoy painting, you might try a freehand drawing class. The idea is to ease yourself into something new by building on something you enjoy or deepening your skills on

The Perks of Wisdom

▶ The flip side of the slower processing and weaker short-term memory that comes with aging is that as the years pass, you develop a larger reserve of knowledge, says Brenna Renn, Ph.D., an assistant professor of psychology at the University of Nevada, Las Vegas. "The longer you live, the more facts you've built up, and that sort of intelligence tends to stay pretty well preserved and actually improves with age."

something you already do. You can also try something totally new but low-stakes, like a viral dance or experimenting with a language app in the privacy of your own home. Introducing a novel challenge helps your brain create new pathways instead of repeatedly activating the old ones, experts say. Think of it as cross-training for your brain.

BE MEDITATIVE AND MINDFUL

You'll never remember the name of the person you just met or the five things your partner asked you to buy from the store if you can't focus. Enter mindfulness meditation, a 7,000-year-old practice that can help sharpen your attention in less time than you probably spend looking for something you've misplaced. Research has shown that even brief bouts of mindfulness meditation can yield immediate benefits. In one small study, mindfulness novices spent 10 minutes listening to an audio-guided mindfulness meditation and saw an increase in their attention, accuracy, and reaction times in a task performed afterward, compared with a control group.

Daily deep breathing and/or meditation lets the brain and the heart relax, which is restorative for the entire body. Count down from 10, breathing in on 10, out on 9, in on 8, and so on, saying the numbers out loud as you go. If you're new to meditation, try an app like Headspace or Calm.

EXERT SNOOZE CONTROL

Aim to get an uninterrupted seven to eight hours of sleep per night. Research has shown that the effects of a lost night of sleep are similar to being drunk when it comes to performing tasks.

During sleep, your body goes through a brain-care cycle. "Deep sleep happens early in the night and allows your brain to flush out toxins, including Alzheimer's-causing beta-amyloid plaques," says All. "REM sleep happens between hours four and eight and consolidates long-term memories into really long-term memories."

"There is an established line between individuals with dysfunctional or inadequate sleep and dementia," says W. Chris Winter, M.D., a neurologist and sleep medicine physician with Charlottesville Neurology and Sleep Medicine and host of the *Sleep Unplugged* podcast. "The mechanisms that rid waste from the brain are far more active when we sleep."

When you have healthy sleep, the glymphatic system in your brain—which pumps

out waste products—is more active and efficient, Dr. Winter says. On the flip side, when you have poor sleep, your brain can't restore itself overnight.

So what are you to do if you can't get that full night's sleep? If you're having trouble getting a solid night's sleep, All recommends talking to a doctor about lifestyle modifications to help you get the zzz's your brain needs. Regular naps may also help. "Any sleep counts, although sleep that is regular in its scheduling is far more effective," Winter says. "So trying to nap 'on a schedule' can elevate the power of your naps tremendously."

PLAY GAMES

Brain-training games are a multibillion-dollar industry that has skyrocketed in the past few years. If you've ever wondered whether the apps you see advertised on your Facebook feed are worth it, know that the answer is a solid...maybe. "There are good games and bad games," says Adam Gazzaley, M.D., Ph.D., the founder and executive director of Neuroscape, a neuroscience center at the University of

The risk of developing dementia over nine years was **27% higher** among socially isolated older adults compared with older adults who were not socially isolated.

California San Francisco that's focused on the intersection of technology and brain health, whose lab has been developing and testing video game technology to enhance brain health for over a decade. And different games have different brain-gain goals. Some are slow and strategic, with the aim of enhancing your thinking skills, while others are action-packed, with the aim of speeding up your processing.

As it stands, there isn't definitive research on the benefits of commercially available brain games. It's possible that they will help, so if you enjoy the games, give them a go.

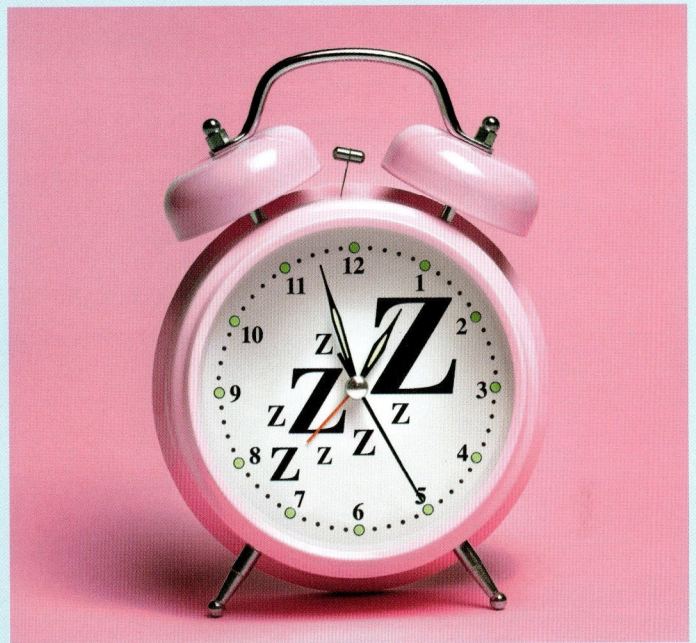

BE SOCIAL

It's not just that social isolation brings a greater risk of cognitive decline—socializing is very good for your brain because it's another way to learn new things and challenge your mind. "When you're having conversations with other people, you're working your brain," says Dr. Small. Just 10 minutes of conversation can increase executive-functioning skills like working memory and the ability to suppress distractions, says a study in *Social Psychological and Personality Science*.

But quality counts. In a study from Rush University, researchers examined the quality of social interactions and cognitive functions of 529 adults, age 50 and older, over nearly five years. Those with a higher frequency of negative interactions had a 53% higher risk of developing mild cognitive impairment. The take-home message: Surround yourself with positive and supportive people and steer clear of toxic people.

You're in Good Company

While going through a contentious divorce, Sarah's stress level was through the roof, and she found herself struggling with memory and attention issues. "I had trouble staying focused during meetings at work, and I couldn't pay attention while reading for pleasure—that was a huge bummer because reading novels was my primary way to relax," says Sarah, 49, a mother of two and a communications consultant. To stay on top of what was happening at work, she began taking detailed notes during meetings. To decompress, she started using a mindfulness meditation app. After the dust settled post-divorce, her attention and mental acuity gradually returned.

Memory Matters

OH, THERE'S WHAT'S-HER-NAME. MY NEIGHBOR, THE one whose kids were good friends with my kids. Is it Julia, Jenna, Jennifer...?

You may be familiar with this kind of tip-of-the-tongue moment—when you can't quite remember a name or word that used to be easy to retrieve. Maybe it's because you're seeing the person out of context or because you're simply blanking out on their name. As you get older, these brain blips can happen more frequently. The same is true of things like misplacing your phone, keys, or glasses multiple times in a day or opening the pantry door only to completely forget what you wanted.

People jokingly call these mental glitches "senior moments," but behind the self-deprecating humor there may be a slight shiver of dread: Is this due to normal aging, or is it an early sign of dementia? With more than 6 million people in the U.S. currently living with Alzheimer's (a number that's expected to nearly double in the next few decades as the population ages), this is not an unreasonable fear. A large national poll by researchers at the University of Michigan found that 44% of people between ages 50 and 64 admitted they were worried about developing dementia.

But—deep breath—most of these slips are perfectly harmless, and in fact there are many things other than dementia that could be putting a damper on your memory.

First, let's make it clear: If your neighbor is one of your best friends but now her name doesn't even ring a bell, that is cause for concern. But if she's a friendly acquaintance and you remembered her name as soon as someone else said it, or

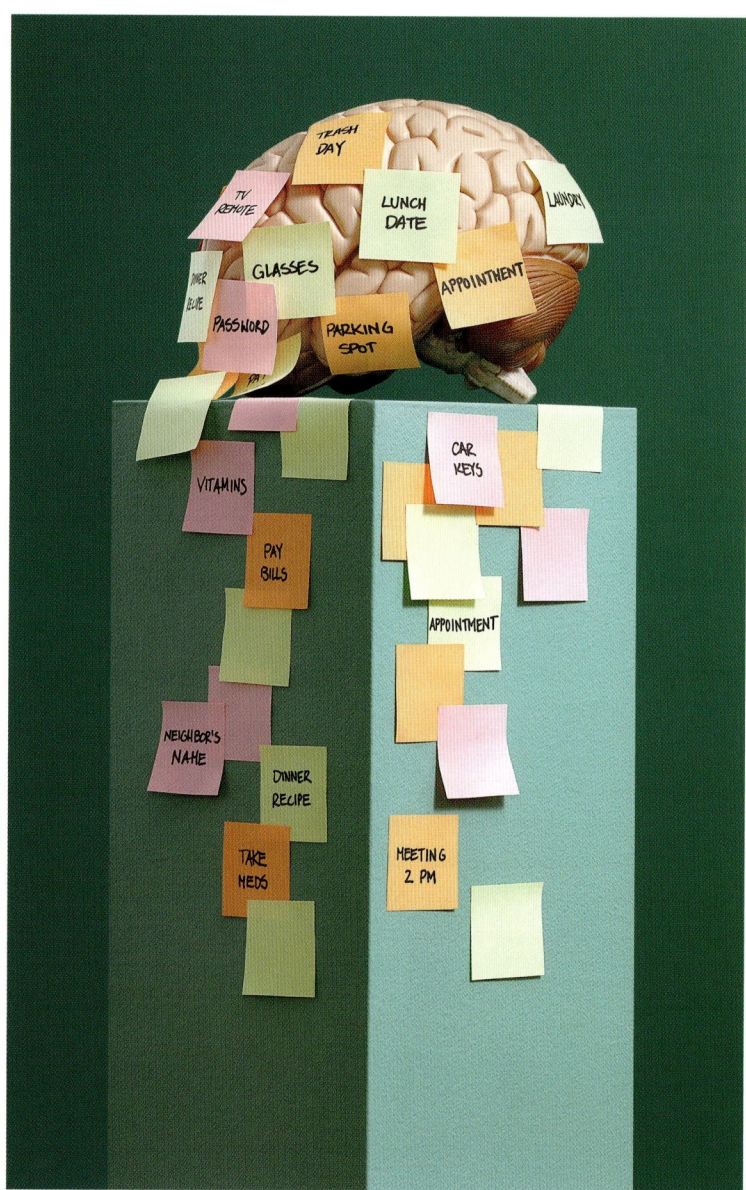

if her name suddenly pops into your head as you're brushing your teeth that night, that's not a sign that something is seriously wrong.

THE WHYS OF MEMORY LOSS

Here's why this can happen: After growing at a furious pace for the first couple of decades of your life, your brain starts to shrink when you hit your 30s and 40s, says Elise Caccappolo, Ph.D., a professor and the director of neuropsychology service at Columbia University Irving Medical Center in New York City. "When you're a child, your brain is constantly creating new neural connections, and by age 25, it should be fully developed," she explains. About a decade after that, the brain slowly starts to lose volume, and brain cells start dying off.

The first part of the brain to start shrinking is the frontal lobe. "This is where we house our short-term or working memory, sort of a scratch pad for the brain," says Murali Doraiswamy, M.D., a brain-health researcher at Duke University. Newly learned names, dates you haven't yet put on the calendar, and the location of your keys all get temporarily deposited here before being transferred to long-term memory.

This natural loss of brain

Heart Health = Brain Health

▶ Many of the lifestyle factors that keep your heart in good shape are the same ones that may lower your risk of brain-health issues as you age. That's because the brain requires fuel to function, and it gets its fill when the heart pumps lots of oxygen- and glucose-containing blood upward, says Constantino Iadecola, M.D., director of the Feil Family Brain and Mind Research Institute at Weill Cornell Medicine. Consider your heart and blood vessels as supply lines to a remote city with no grain silo, Dr. Iadecola says. "If the tracks don't work, the city doesn't [have food] and the people starve."

In fact, your cardiovascular fitness may be the most important factor in keeping your mind sharp for the long haul. The evidence overwhelmingly supports this notion: In a study from Finland, people with the best cardiovascular scores at midlife cut their risk of developing dementia later in life by up to 40% compared with those who had the worst scores. In another study, Swedish researchers found that the more quickly people developed cardiovascular risk factors, the more likely they were to experience Alzheimer's and dementia.

At any age, you can double up on actions that are terrific for your heart and your brain. A study found that 65-year-old women with four or five healthy lifestyle practices—such as consuming a healthy diet, engaging in regular physical activity, doing cognitive tasks, not smoking, and limiting alcohol—had an additional life expectancy of 24.2 years—3.1 years longer than those with none or only one of these healthy practices.

volume also affects processing speed, Caccappolo notes.

"This is why it may take a minute longer to come up with a name or a word, or it may take longer to solve a problem," she says, stressing that you still can do these things; you just do them at a slower pace.

Another reason your brain may not be quite as quick when you're in your 50s or 60s: You have a

Researchers found an improvement of **around 13%** in working memory following a strength training program in older adults.

lot going on as you balance the demands of young-adult children, aging parents, work, and home life, says Thomas Holland, M.D., a physician scientist at the Rush Institute for Healthy Aging in Chicago.

While it's important to know which kinds of memory changes are in fact worrisome signs, the key thing to recognize about the normal shifts that come with getting older is that "you can live your life as you always have, you can function independently, and [these changes won't] affect what you do on a daily basis," Caccappolo says.

6 Reasons You May Have Brain Blips

THE BRAIN IS A PART OF A VAST INTERCONNECTED system of organs, and the way you treat your body affects how well your brain works. If you're concerned about your memory, your first step should be a head-to-toe wellness check with your doctor.

If a health issue isn't to blame, it's time to look at your lifestyle. In general, whatever is good for the heart is good for the brain: Keeping blood vessels clear and blood flowing freely helps maximize the flow of oxygen and nutrients to the brain. Exercising, quitting smoking, maintaining a stable weight, consuming a healthy diet, and getting plenty of good-quality sleep will keep your brain healthier too.

These factors could be contributing to foggy moments.

1. MEDICATIONS

Many common drugs can affect cognition and memory, and if you take several, they may be interacting with one another. Talk to your doctor about any prescribed or over-the-counter drugs or supplements you're taking.

2. MOOD

Depression and anxiety are major culprits in forgetfulness for people in their 40s, 50s, and 60s, says neuropsychologist Elise Caccappolo, Ph.D. "When you're depressed [your brain is] not paying attention to things as well as it usually does." If you think mental health or mood issues may be responsible for your brain blips, speak with a professional about talk therapy and/or medication.

3. DIET QUALITY

What you eat can influence your brain function. Eating foods that provide the appropriate nutrients and bioactive compounds for brain health can help protect the neurons, Dr. Thomas Holland of the Rush Institute for Healthy Aging says. In a study he and his colleagues published in *Neurology*, they found that a diet filled with foods rich in flavonoids

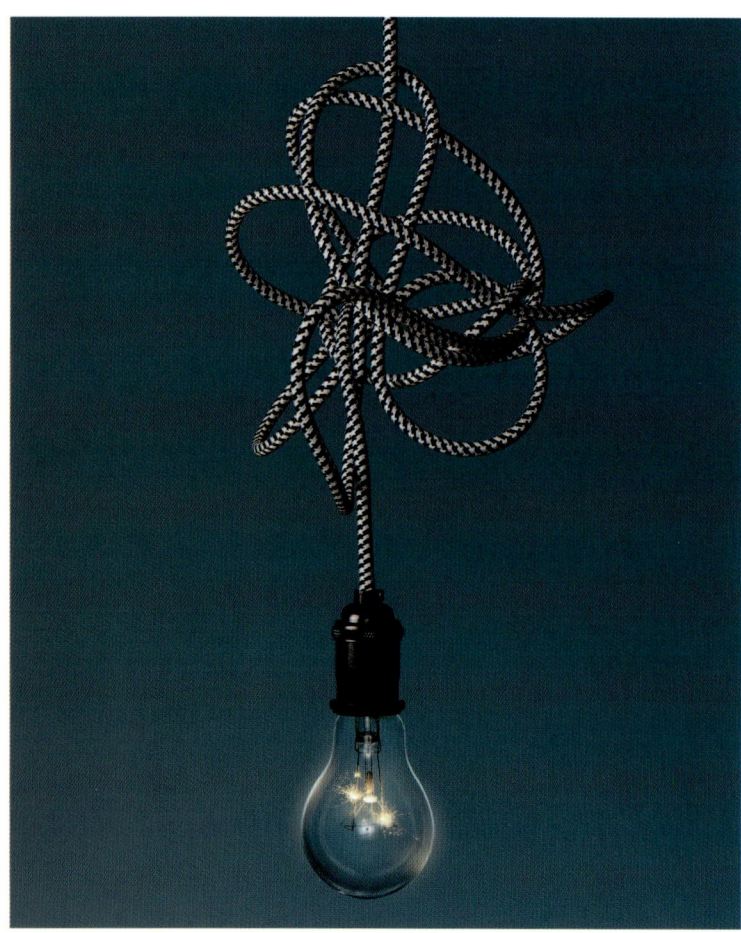

(such as dark leafy greens, tea, and tomatoes) was associated with slower rates of cognitive decline. Learn more about nutrition and how it affects your brain health on page 115.

4. SLEEP CHANGES

You could be missing out on restorative sleep for a number of reasons including menopause symptoms, stress, and other untreated causes like obstructive sleep apnea. Exhaustion can affect your ability to remember or learn new things. See ideas for getting better sleep on page 160 .

5. HEARING LOSS

Hearing loss may interfere with cognition because it means the brain is working hard just to understand speech. Fortunately, hearing aids can help by making the information clearer as it enters the brain—and new tech combining earbuds and clinical hearing devices promises to make them more discreet and less

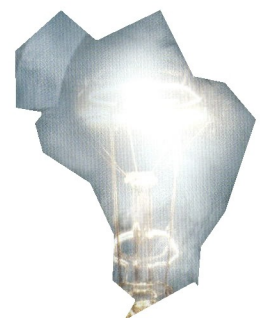

expensive. If you notice that your hearing is not what it used to be, consult with an audiologist.

6. MULTITASKING

Doing multiple things at once could be detrimental to memory. A study of young adults published in *Nature* found that media multitasking—using several devices simultaneously—in

particular was associated with attention lapses and decreased the ability to encode new memories. For older people, multitasking may be even more problematic, says Caccappolo. "As our processing speed gets slower, we're slower overall...If you're trying to do two or three things at the same time, you're going to be a little bit slower at each one."

Feeling Foggy?

▶ Brain fog isn't a medical diagnosis exactly, but a term many people use when they feel absent-minded, or fuzzy, or have difficulty focusing. Other symptoms include being more forgetful than usual or not as sharp as they usually are—almost as if you can feel your brain chugging but not firing on all cylinders, says Jessica Caldwell, Ph.D., a neuropsychologist and the director of the Women's Alzheimer's Movement Prevention and Research Center at Cleveland Clinic.

Brain fog is related to stress, lack of sleep, certain medical conditions and medications, menopause, and even COVID—anything that disrupts the healthy function of our brain. There's actually a physiological reason why it's so common, adds Gayatri Devi, M.D.,

a clinical professor of neurology and psychiatry at Zucker School of Medicine at Hofstra/Northwell, director at Park Avenue Neurology, and an attending physician at Lenox Hill Hospital in New York City. Of the trillions of neurons in your brain, just 10,000 to 20,000 secrete a neuropeptide called orexin, which is one of several circuits that keep us awake and alert. "It's astounding that our wakefulness and arousal is controlled by such a small number of nerve cells—and easy to see how this part of the brain system might be easily impacted," says Devi.

Our brains are hardwired to be alert; that's what helps us react so quickly to our environment. The fact that such clarity is our brain's go-to mode helps explain why brain fog can feel so disorienting—and stressful.

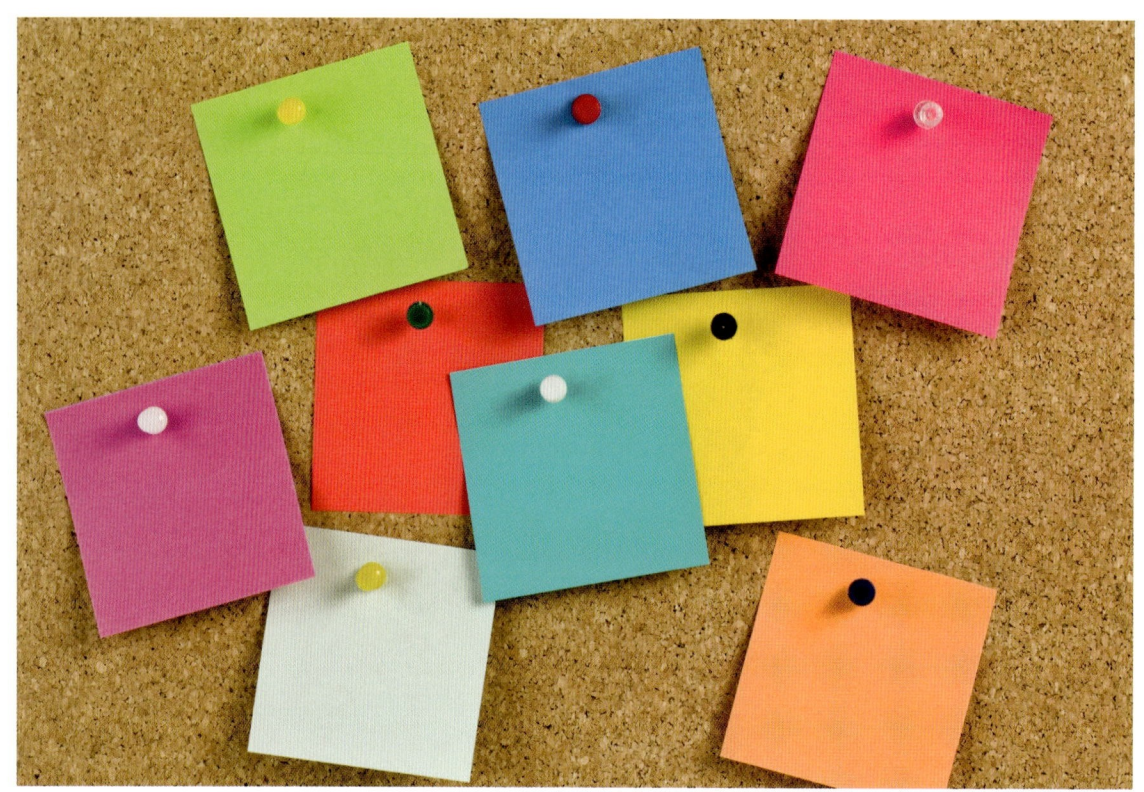

When to Worry About Your Memory

THE BRAIN CHANGES THAT ACCOMPANY THE NORMAL AGING process can lead to *age-related cognitive decline*, which may be marked by slower thinking, trouble with word finding, and subtle attention problems. These changes can be frustrating, but they're common and not cause for concern.

When doctors start to worry is when cognitive changes and memory glitches are more pronounced. These may occur on a spectrum:

<u>Mild cognitive impairment (MCI)</u> is when someone has more cognitive challenges than typical for their age but the changes in memory or judgment aren't severe enough to impact their daily activities. MCI is often a precursor to dementia, but "not everybody with MCI will go on to have dementia," says Brenna Renn.

<u>**Dementia**</u> is an umbrella term for loss of memory, language, and other thinking abilities that become severe enough to interfere with a person's daily life. Many people think Alzheimer's disease and dementia are synonymous, but they're not. While Alzheimer's disease is the most common type of dementia, affecting an estimated 60% to 80% of all people with dementia, it's far from the only one. Vascular dementia, Lewy body dementia (LBD), and frontotemporal dementia (FTD) are other forms of the disease, and people can suffer from multiple forms at one time. If you are concerned about your risk for any of these, consult with your doctor.

How Good Is Your Recall?

Occasional forgetfulness is normal, especially as you get older or during times of stress. This memory quiz from the Alzheimer's Research & Prevention Foundation can help you figure out whether your experience is within the normal range or whether you should consider lifestyle changes or check in with your doctor. Mark yes or no to each statement.

		YES	NO
1.	From time to time I forget what day it is.		
2.	Sometimes when I'm looking for something, I forget what it is that I'm looking for.		
3.	I'm more sensitive to minor challenges than I used to be.		
4.	My friends and family think I'm more forgetful than I used to be.		
5.	I find it hard to concentrate for even an hour at a time.		
6.	I use caffeine to stay focused and sharp.		
7.	I frequently misplace my keys and can't recall putting them where I find them.		
8.	I forget my friends' names at times.		
9.	Sometimes I get lost, even when driving somewhere familiar.		
10.	I often miss appointments because I've forgotten about them.		
11.	I feel less energetic than I once did.		
12.	It's hard to add two-digit numbers in my head.		
13.	People tell me I often repeat myself.		
14.	I find it harder to learn new things.		
15.	Sometimes I forget the point I'm trying to make.		

If you answer yes to more than seven questions, consider lifestyle changes, like a brain-healthy diet, better sleep, and more exercise, or give your doc a call.

TOTAL:

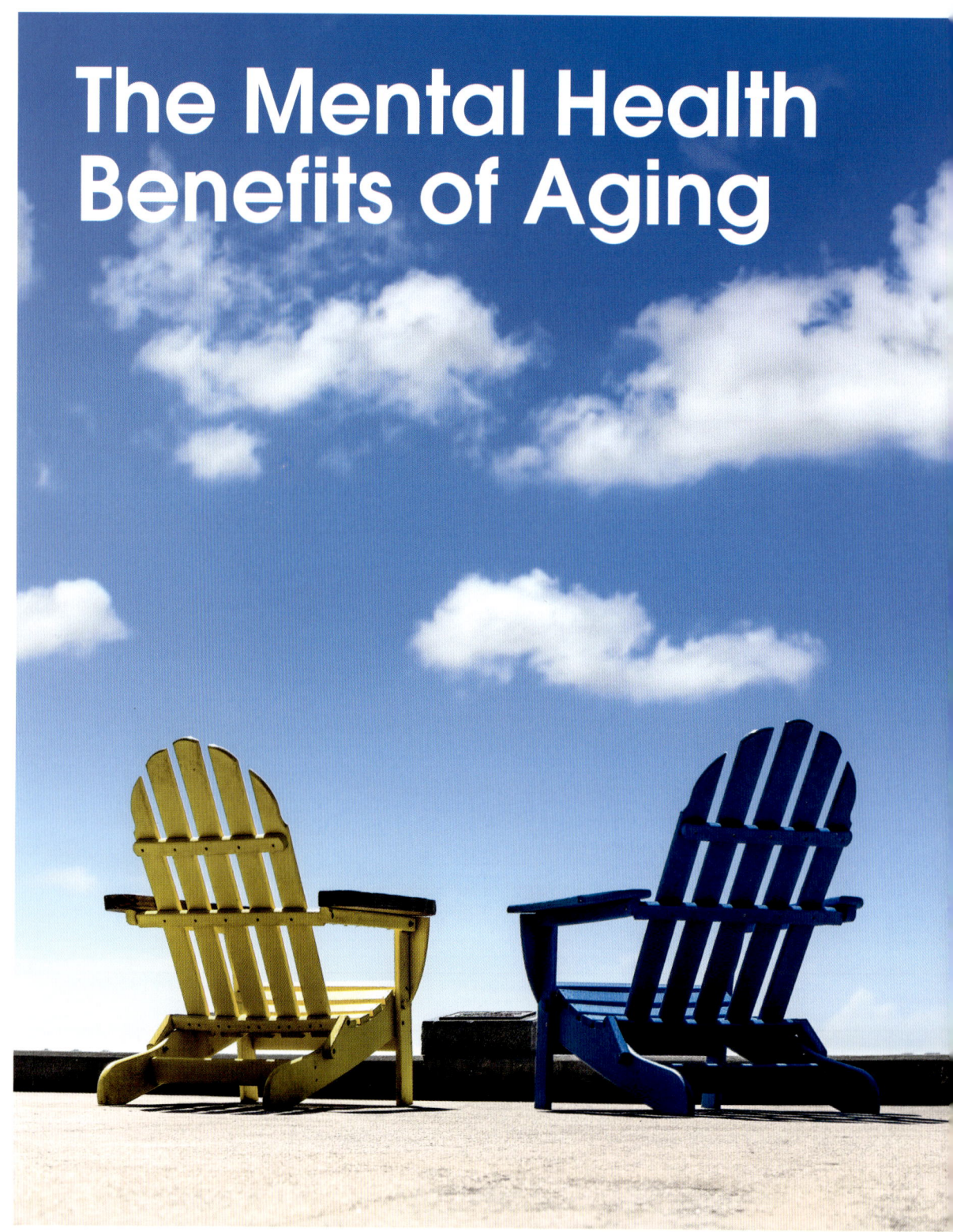

The Mental Health Benefits of Aging

IS IT TRUE THAT THE OLDER YOU GET, THE HAPPIER YOU GET?

The research seems to say yes. The U-shaped happiness curve is the research-backed theory that emotional well-being highest for ...

World Health Organization approximately 14% of adults age 60 and older have a mental-health condition, more than 23% of the general population ... ental-health disorder, ... and anxiety ... ones

some researchers (although ... not a slam-dunk—newer studies have found considerable variations around the globe and by gender).

Research has shown that the majority of older adults are not depressed or anxious, and for those that do experience mental health issues, many can address them effectively. While according to the

of purpose after ... or other big changes. Fortunately, the same strategies for healthy aging—such as staying physically active, sticking with a healthy diet, staying socially connected, getting plenty of sleep, and maintaining a sense of purpose—are also effective for preventing or alleviating mental-health disorders.

Movement Is Medicine

▶ Besides being good for your body, exercise can have positive effects on your mood and state of mind. In a review of 218 studies in a 2024 issue of *BMJ*, researchers concluded that exercise can be an effective treatment for depression, with walking, jogging, yoga, and strength training leading the way. Other research has shown that mind-body practices such as tai chi and yoga can improve anxiety symptoms. If you're experiencing depression or anxiety, talk with your doctor about incorporating exercise along with medication, therapy, or other treatments as part of your mental health plan.

Is It Anxiety or Depression?

While everyone feels blue or on edge from time to time, it's important to identify those times when you may need a little more help. Answer these seven questions to see if you have symptoms of either depression or anxiety, or possibly both.

Note: *This quiz is not an official diagnostic tool. If you think you're struggling with anxiety or depression, seek the professional opinion of a therapist. If you experience thoughts of harming yourself, dial 988 to reach the Suicide & Crisis Lifeline.*

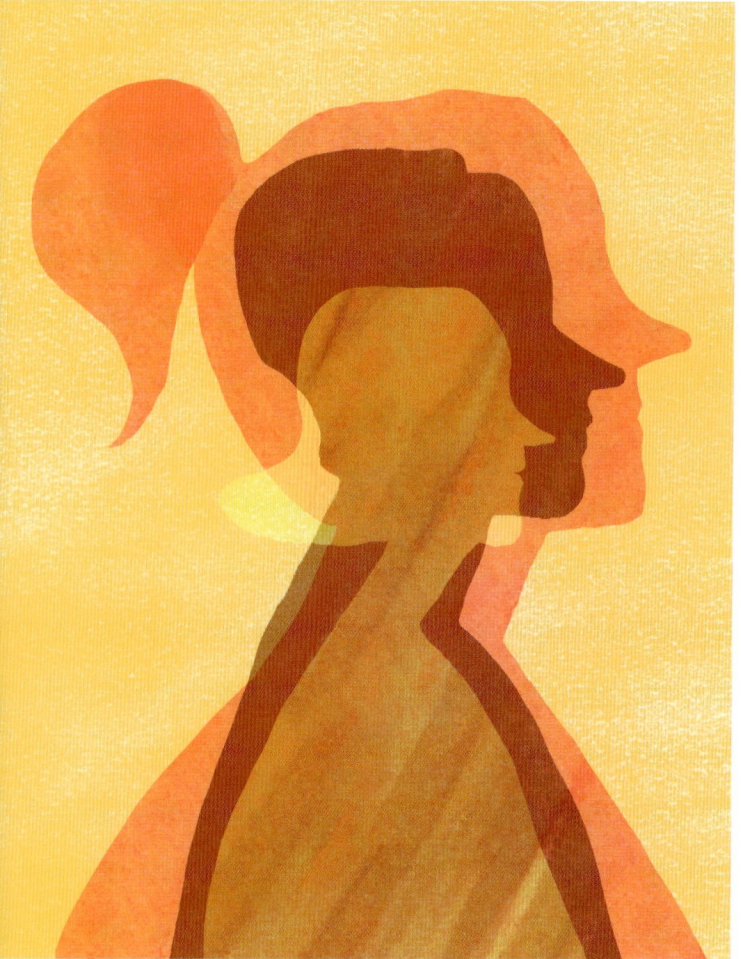

1. You feel gloomy most of the time and/or suddenly burst into tears.

   Yes (A)   **No** (C)

2. You feel tense and stressed, and you constantly dread the future.

   Yes (B)   **No** (C)

3. You often feel like there's no point in trying.

   Yes (A)   **No** (C)

4. It's hard for you to concentrate and/or relax.

   Yes (B)   **No** (C)

5. Your appetite is way bigger (or smaller), and you may have gained or lost several pounds over the last month.

   Yes (A)   **No** (C)

6. You replay the same scenario (your boss firing you, your partner leaving you, your friends ignoring you) over and over in your head.

   Yes (B)   **No** (C)

7. You're just not interested in things you used to love, like cooking or spending time with friends.

   Yes (A)   **No** (C)

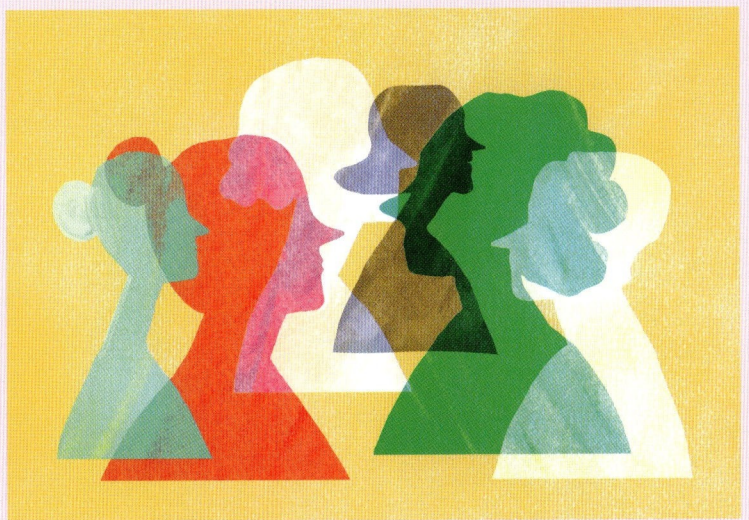

You may be suffering from both depression and anxiety

"It's very common for people to experience both anxiety and depression," says Ross. To be diagnosed with either disorder, your feelings must affect one or more areas of your life (e.g., they keep you from working, attending school, caring for your children, or otherwise living your life) and occur almost every day for at least two weeks.

MOSTLY C'S

You don't appear to be suffering from either depression or anxiety

Check Your Answers

MOSTLY A'S AND C'S

You may be suffering from depression

Sadness: If you are depressed, the most common symptom is feeling down—really down. "Of all symptoms, sadness is the most prominent," says Alison Ross, Ph.D., a New York City psychologist.

Hopelessness: People who are suffering from depression may feel like things are horrible and will always stay that way.

Changes in appetite: Some people respond to depression with a huge increase or decrease in appetite. "You may stop eating because you have no interest in food, or you may want to fill yourself up and start eating a lot," says Ross.

Loss of interest in things you used to love: Activities that used to be joyful may not feel that way anymore.

MOSTLY B'S AND C'S

You may be suffering from anxiety

Feeling stressed, tense, and worried all the time: Constantly mulling over the future and feeling on edge is anxiety symptom number one. You likely feel wound up, doubtful about your abilities, and insecure about how life is going.

Inability to concentrate or relax: "Relaxing means emptying your mind and just being," says Ross. "If you're constantly worrying whether you're going to lose your job, or if a friend is mad at you, or if you're healthy, you can't enjoy whatever it is you do to relax."

Racing or ruminative thoughts: Anxiety can mean constantly churning over the same issues until it gets in the way of getting things done.

Signs It Is Time to Seek Help

- Your feelings of anxiety or depression are disrupting your life or worsening

- You avoid the things you love

- Your work is suffering

- You feel isolated

- You're concerned about your mental wellness

- Your symptoms are physical as well as mental

- Your relationships are affected

- Your fears keep you from functioning

- The depression or anxiety has been lingering for weeks

Myths About Anxiety and Depression

DESPITE THE FACT THAT TENS OF MILLIONS OF Americans deal with depression and anxiety, the conditions are still often misunderstood. And although the percentage of older folks with one of these mental-health disorders is lower than in the general public, many contend with one or both on a daily basis. Many people assume that the signs of anxiety or depression will be easy to detect, but the symptoms aren't always consistent among individuals, and anxiety and depression may even mimic each other.

1 ANXIETY IS ALL IN YOUR HEAD

Anxiety causes real physical responses that may include trembling, chest pain, heart palpitations, nausea, and light-headedness, says Karen Surowiec, Psy.D., a psychologist with the Manhattan Psychology Group. That's because fears and worries trigger the body's fight-or-flight response, releasing hormones that make your muscles tense and your heartbeat and breathing quicken. The brain and the gut share a connection too, which is why feeling nervous can lead to an upset stomach and an upset stomach can make you feel nervous. All of which means that your worries could be associated with a very real physical reaction.

2 ANXIETY IS SIMPLY WORRYING TOO MUCH

Worry is a part of anxiety, but it's not the whole story. Regular worries tend to be tied to specific, realistic issues—losing a job, your child being bullied, missing a flight. Anxiety, meanwhile, may not be based on rational concerns, and it creates emotional distress that can be felt in your body. Some anxiety is good, but when it gets in the way of everyday functioning, it may be diagnosed as a disorder, says Aaron Telnes, a psychologist with the College of Alberta Psychologists. Sometimes the fear is not specific, or it continues even after what you were worried about is over. For example, it's common to be

nervous before a performance review with your boss, but fixating afterward on something you said or did can be debilitating and may involve ruminating, hyperventilating, sweating, and trouble concentrating or sleeping.

3 YOU SHOULD AVOID SITUATIONS THAT MAKE YOU ANXIOUS

Though it's a natural reaction, avoidance may make your anxiety worse, says anxiety expert Haley Neidich, L.C.S.W., a licensed psychotherapist who provides telehealth. "Anxiety will insist on being felt," she says. Staying silent about what's upsetting you in a relationship, procrastinating on your work, or avoiding social interactions or paying bills can have harmful ripple effects in your life. In fact, a common treatment for anxiety is the opposite of avoidance: exposure therapy. This practice involves helping people approach their fears in a safe environment, says Telnes—and, by doing so, they learn that they can handle them.

4 YOU CAN JUST SNAP OUT OF ANXIETY

Just as someone can't "snap out of" cancer or diabetes, the same is true for anxiety. "That mentality is rooted in

Nostalgia Can Boost Your Mood

▶ Believe it or not, taking a walk down memory lane can bring mental-health benefits. Research has found that reminiscing about an event from the past can help people stay in touch with who they think they truly are and what they value and improve their mood and sense of well-being.

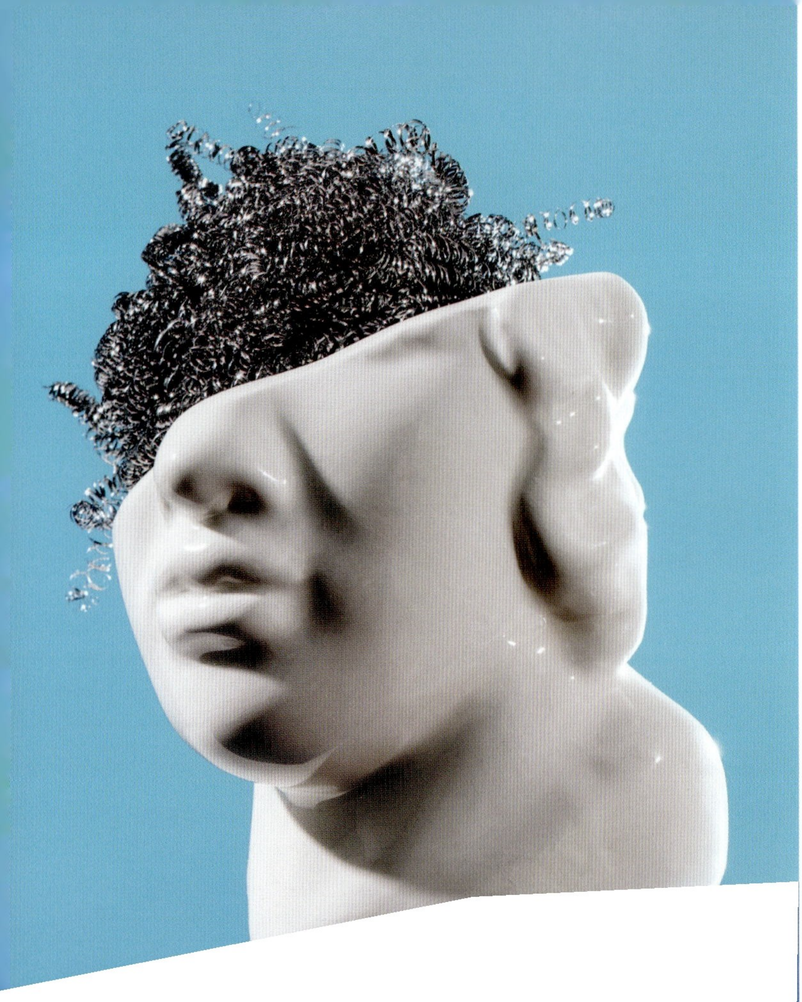

the Center for Cognitive Therapy at the University of Pennsylvania. It's also possible they might have trouble concentrating and/or speak or move slowly, says Jocelyn Smith Carter, Ph.D., director of clinical training in DePaul University's Department of Psychology, because depression's effect on the brain also affects some motor functions.

The key is to look for significant changes—the person may become more argumentative or hopeless or markedly less social, Newman says. They might start drinking more or stress eating, or stop wanting to eat. If you notice such changes, "be a good listener and recommend that they see a professional," he says.

6 EVERYONE GETS DEPRESSED SOMETIMES

At some point, most people have said, "Ugh, I'm so depressed!", but sadness or feeling down are emotions that tend to come and go, whereas clinical depression is more constant and lasts for at least two weeks and often much longer, says Newman.

Other signs: feelings of extreme guilt or worthlessness, loss of interest in activities you once liked, and/or suicidal thoughts. There's also dysthymia, a treatable and less severe form of persistent depression that can ebb and flow; symptoms can include hopelessness, low self-esteem, and fatigue. If you feel unusually down for two weeks or more and/ or have suicidal thoughts, talk to a mental health professional.

mental- health stigma and denialism of mental-health disorders as real medical issues," says Neidich. You can't just flick a switch and eliminate anxiety. And it's a mistake to deny or suppress anxiety because doing so can backfire in various ways, such as setting you up for substance abuse, chronic health conditions, dysfunctional relationships, or insomnia, she says. "If you want to feel better, you're going to have to acknowledge your anxiety, feel your feelings, and learn coping mechanisms." If you're experiencing anxiety, a professional can help you develop coping mechanisms.

5 YOU'D KNOW IF SOMEONE WAS DEPRESSED

Many people with depression go about their normal business and may seem more irritable or anxious than sad, says Cory Newman, Ph.D., director of

7 DEPRESSION ONLY AFFECTS MOOD

Yes, a downturn in mood is part of the picture, but depression can also sap people's energy and appetite and disrupt sleep. It's also connected to a host of physical symptoms, from hives and migraines to respiratory, cardiac, and gastrointestinal issues. "Your mental and emotional state can trigger specific physical reactions, and vice versa," Newman says.

There seems to be a strong connection between inflammation, autoimmune disease, and depression: A large Danish study found that patients with an autoimmune disease such as multiple sclerosis or type 1 diabetes were 45% more likely to have a mood disorder than those without one. If you have a chronic health condition, take care of your mental health too, advises Newman.

8 YOU JUST HAVE TO POWER THROUGH DEPRESSION

It's not about willing it away. The condition is partly caused by, and also causes, physical changes in the body and the brain, says Carter. That includes disruption of mood-regulating chemicals such as serotonin, and you cannot just "snap out of it."

With the help of a therapist, someone with depression can learn skills to ease symptoms or cope better, says Newman. For example, people can learn to reframe how they see things, resist defeatist all-or-nothing thinking, and celebrate small accomplishments, which makes them feel better, he adds. Therapy can also teach people to "complete tasks in small bursts and build their way back up to doing things they enjoy," Carter says, which further lifts their mood.

Keep in mind: Some people may need medication, as well as therapy, to help improve their mood and assist with sleep.

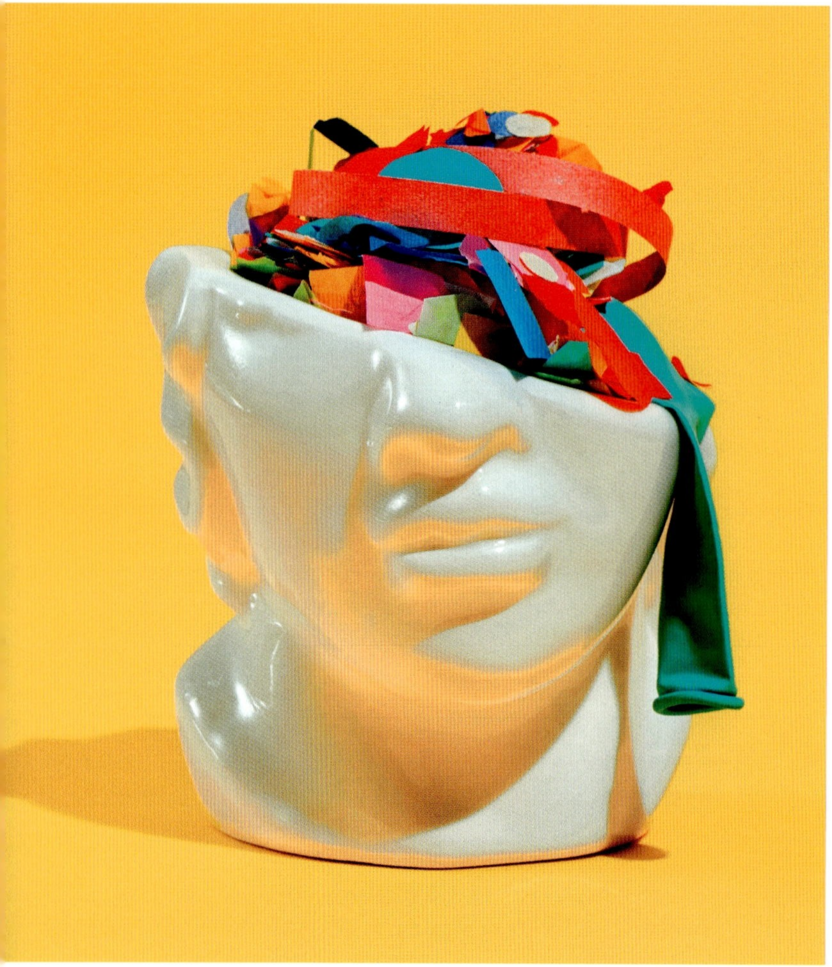

9 DEPRESSION IS REALLY HARD TO TREAT

On the contrary, "it's one of our most well-researched disorders in terms of how people respond [to treatment]," Carter says. The tricky part is landing on the right treatment, Newman says, as well as addressing conditions such as anxiety, PTSD, and substance abuse that often accompany depression. With therapy and medication (which research shows is most effective for those with moderate or severe depression), up to 70% of people with major depression show improvement.

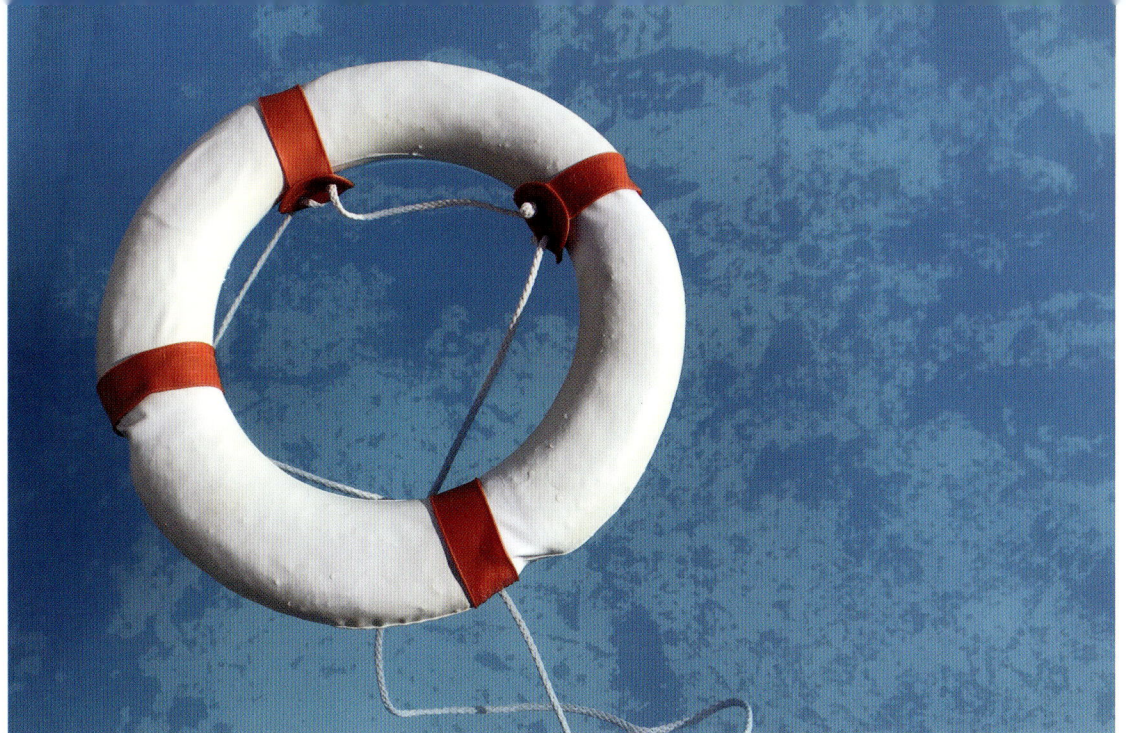

How to Find a Therapist

SOMETIMES THE **RIGHT THING TO DO FOR YOURSELF** is find a professional therapist to talk to. It will help you get an outside perspective on your life and your feelings—and strategies for coping with challenges you're facing. Finding a therapist may seem daunting, but with some time and effort, you can find the right match.

ASK A FRIEND

If you know someone who's in therapy, their therapist may be a good source for recommendations.

TRY TELETHERAPY

Some well-known companies offering telehealth for therapy include LiveHealth Online, Talkspace, BetterHelp, and MDLive.

USE YOUR HEALTH NETWORK

Contact your primary-care physician for recommendations, and if you have insurance, reach out to your insurance company to identify therapists who are covered by your policy.

SEARCH ONLINE

Try using *Psychology Today's* Find a Therapist tool.

Calling for Help

▶ **If you or someone you know is at risk for suicide, there are places that can help:**

Call or text 988
The Suicide & Crisis Lifeline is the mental-health equivalent of 911 in the U.S.

Call 1-800-273-TALK (8255)
The National Suicide Prevention Lifeline

Text HOME to 741741
The Crisis Text Line provides trained crisis counselors for free.

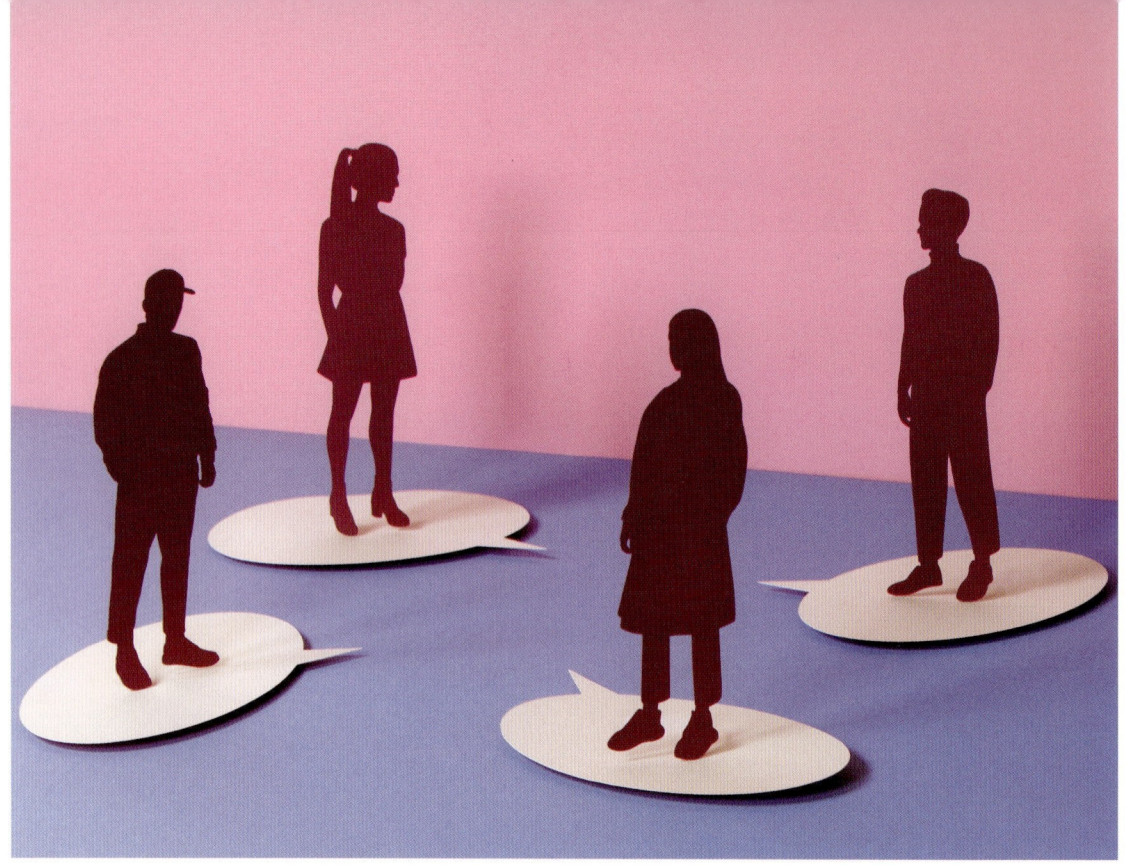

Picking Your Path

DIFFERENT FORMS OF THERAPY MAY APPEAL TO DIFFERENT PEOPLE so it's wise to know what the options are. Studies have found that older adults tend to respond well to solution-oriented therapies. These are some of the most widely available options:

▶ **Cognitive behavioral therapy** tends to be short-term, collaborative, and solutions-based, equipping you with strategies to cope with difficult thoughts or emotions.

▶ **Acceptance and commitment therapy** focuses on using acceptance and mindfulness, along with a clarification of your personal values and a commitment to making behavior changes that are in line with these elements.

▶ **Dialectical behavioral therapy** builds on cognitive behavioral therapies but tends to be ongoing and addresses four key areas: mindfulness, distress intolerance, emotional regulation, and interpersonal effectiveness.

▶ **Interpersonal therapy** is a short-term, supportive form of psychotherapy that addresses relationship issues and emotion identification and expression, in order to ease emotional distress.

▶ **Psychodynamic therapy** (including psychoanalysis) is more open-ended and less targeted; it can involve exploring themes in your life and mind or be aimed at processing past trauma.

▶ **Age-specific therapy** In addition to the usual forms of therapy—cognitive behavioral therapy, acceptance and commitment therapy, and interpersonal therapy—older adults may benefit from music therapy, art therapy, and reminiscence therapy. And some mental-health professionals—such as geriatric psychiatrists—focus on various aspects of the aging process and the issues that come with it.

Why Self-Care Isn't Selfish

▶ Although many people may still think of "self-care" as indulgence—bubble baths, goblets of wine—it's more about the ways in which you take care of yourself, says Christine Carter, Ph.D., a sociologist and senior fellow of Greater Good Science Center at the University of California, Berkeley. "Self-care is about creating a foundation that supports you so you can support others," Carter says. "Look at what truly makes you feel nourished and healthy and build on that."

Many of the lifestyle habits that can help relieve stress can also help with depression and anxiety. These include exercising regularly, getting enough sleep, consuming a healthy diet, and staying socially connected. On the stress-management front, meditation and other mind-body techniques such as progressive muscle relaxation can do a world of good.

How to Talk About Your Mental Health

▶ When you're grappling with depression or anxiety, it can be helpful to let loved ones know that you're struggling. But not everyone in your life will know how to respond or is able to be supportive around mental-health issues. Here are some ways to begin a conversation:

- **Consider who you tell:** If you suspect a friend or loved one might be insensitive or unsupportive, it's fine to not confide in them.

- **Rehearse the conversation:** Plan exactly what you want to share and what you hope the conversation provides. It might be receiving support, or it might be just letting them know why you've been more removed.

- **Set some boundaries:** Let them know why you're sharing this with them and how you want future conversations to go.

- **Tell people how they can support you:** Loved ones want to help you, but they may not know how. Ask for what you need.

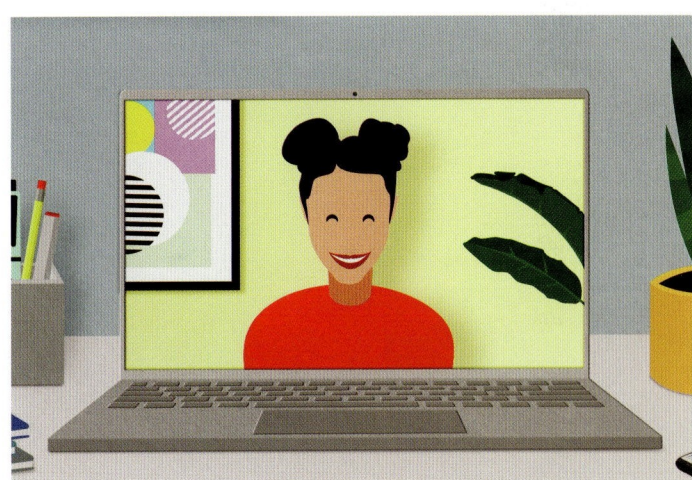

You're in Good Company

After being diagnosed with anxiety and depression, Shaundra added meditation to her treatment plan. When she first started her practice, she noticed that she felt less down about doing everyday things.

After a while, she began to notice helpful shifts in her thought processes and mindset. Problems at work became an opportunity to learn; would-be confrontations with a friend, a chance to develop her communication skills.

With mindfulness, she says, "it feels like you can observe things from another vantage point rather than immediately responding or reacting." Freed from her anxiety spiral, she felt like she was finally able to be her "full self" again.

"It's all thanks to meditation," she says. "It helped me understand that feeling anxiety is normal, but being trapped by it is a choice."

The Social Prescription

HUMANS ARE SOCIAL CREATURES, which means we don't just enjoy being social, we *need* to be social. It's how we survive—together, in groups, finding strength in numbers. Being socially isolated, by contrast, hurts us emotionally and psychologically, and its stresses take a physical toll. Persistent loneliness (lasting longer than two weeks) is linked to high blood pressure, depression, heart disease, and stroke, among other conditions, including Alzheimer's disease.

"People think of their relationships as related to emotional well-being—they don't recognize the profound effect they have on physical health," says Brigham Young psychology professor Julianne Holt-Lunstad, Ph.D. According to Holt-Lunstad's research, lonely people have a 26% increased likelihood of dying prematurely. "We need to take our social relationships as seriously as we take our diet, exercise, nutrition, and everything else that we know impacts our health," she says.

FEELING LONELY? JOIN THE CLUB

A growing number of adults in the U.S. now live by themselves, which is one reason people are experiencing greater loneliness than ever before.

According to the Pew Research Center, 27% of U.S. adults over 60 live alone (a number far higher than in most other countries). Another factor is the lightning-fast evolution of technology, particularly social media. "We have had more change in the last 24 years than we did in the previous 2,500," says Dilip Jeste, M.D., the former director of University of California San Diego's Department of Healthy Aging. "Social changes have been dramatic, and loneliness is definitely a part of that."

In a 2023 national poll, 37% of U.S. adults between 50 and 80 reported experiencing loneliness, and 34% reported

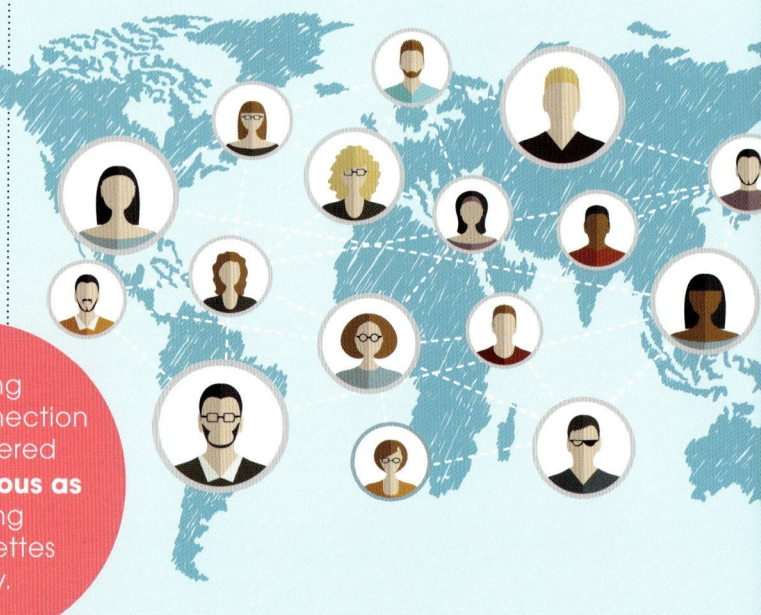

Lacking social connection is considered **as dangerous as** smoking 15 cigarettes a day.

that they felt socially isolated. Older adults may experience social isolation because of the death of a partner or other loved one or because of decreased mobility or chronic illness.

Loneliness is not simply about being alone. What it really hinges on is the quality of your relationships: The more satisfied you are with them, the less lonely you are. Middle age is when that dissatisfaction often runs highest, when you may be surrounded by family (perhaps caring for both children and older parents), coworkers, and friends but you are too busy to have meaningful connections. This is also when illness begins to brew. "The loneliness-related diseases old people get diagnosed with can take decades to develop, but often start to emerge on a cellular level in early middle age and even before then," says Steve Cole, Ph.D., professor of psychiatry, medicine, and biobehavioral science at UCLA's David Geffen School of Medicine.

MIDLIFE FRIENDSHIPS MATTER

The reasons people are lonely are different in early middle age as opposed to late middle age. The earlier years are a time when long friendships can fade as people crank it up at work and spend happy hours with colleagues who can help them get ahead. Childhood friends may be replaced with new "parent friends," people with whom we have no history

Deepen Your Relationships (and Form New Ones Too)

▶ Feeling connected to others is especially important as we get older. Research shows that social isolation increases the effects of stress as well as the risk of serious disease and death. One review found that feeling valued helped older people stave off mental-health problems.

Founding director of the Stanford Center on Longevity Laura Carstensen, says research illustrates the value of intergenerational connection, in particular. Joanne, an 85-year-old in Wellesley, Massachusetts, says having friends of all ages is one of the reasons she feels she's thriving. "My friends are mostly younger than me, and they're from all different backgrounds and nationalities," she says. "These multigenerational friendships teach me so much— I'm constantly learning."

and little in common except parenthood. Having random people around—especially those who serve more of a functional purpose than an emotional one—is often not enough to stave off loneliness.

Then once people push through their 40s, the social scaffolding starts to collapse: Parents die, couples divorce, children move away, people lose their jobs, and they may still be too busy to properly attend to the emotional fallout.

"For the first time, you become aware of mortality," Cole says, noting that it's when women enter menopause, and men go into andropause (a decline of male hormones). It's also when many illnesses—arthritis, diabetes, high blood pressure— make their debut. "It's a time when we can no longer count on

perfect health as we could when [we were] younger," he says. "Put that all together and you have a sort of situational invitation to be lonely and socially dissatisfied."

Fortunately, if you're a member of the lonely-hearts club, you can take steps to relinquish your membership. The first step is to acknowledge your feelings and try to understand *why* you feel lonely. Is it because you don't have enough meaningful contact with other people? Is it because you don't feel in tune with people around you? Is there another reason? Once you identify the underpinnings of your loneliness, you can address them and cultivate more satisfying social connections. The good news is that research suggests that from middle age, loneliness reaches a low point in the 60s and doesn't become high again until the 80s.

How to Combat Loneliness

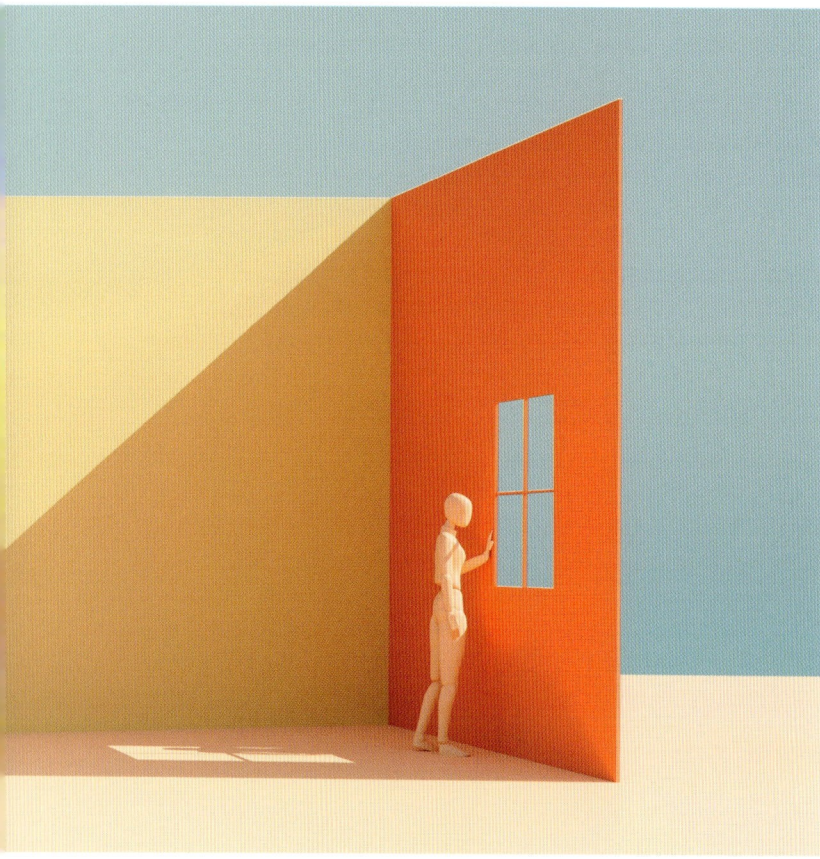

WE'RE MORE CONNECTED THAN EVER, WITH ZOOM calls, live stream events, and social media. But despite having the ability to reach out to people halfway across the world in a matter of seconds, we may feel socially isolated.

A Harvard report revealed that 36% of people in the U.S. feel "serious loneliness." But what is loneliness? Being alone isn't the same as being lonely; we may feel lonely even when we're in a roomful of people. Loneliness is "a perceived discrepancy between what we want and what we have in our relationships," says Louise Hawkley, Ph.D., principal research scientist at NORC at the University of Chicago. "It's not about the quantity of connections, but rather the quality of our bonds." In a nutshell, we feel lonely when we're not getting the level of emotional support we crave.

But feelings of loneliness can have a silver lining when they motivate us to take action. "Loneliness is adaptive and evolutionary," says Hawkley. "It's a nudge to get out there because you need something. In that way, it's like hunger or thirst." No one likes to feel socially isolated, but it's your brain's way of pushing you to foster social connections in order to survive and thrive.

While many studies have looked at techniques for combating loneliness, there's no consensus on what's most effective. But if you're feeling isolated, here are some strategies you can try.

ADMIT YOU'RE LONELY

There's always been stigma associated with loneliness, says Hawkley. But ignoring feelings of isolation continues to feed them. Giving a name to what you feel is one step toward actually doing something about your loneliness. Labeling your feelings also may reduce their intensity.

REALIZE IT'S SOMETHING MOST OF US EXPERIENCE

Ironically, loneliness is a universal feeling. "It's common for most of us at one point or another in life," says James Ellor, Ph.D., D. Min, professor emeritus of family studies at the Diana R. Garland School of Social Work at Baylor University. Acknowledging your loneliness doesn't remove it, but it can be helpful to know it's temporary.

REFRAME YOUR RESPONSES TO SITUATIONS

"Loneliness changes the brain and how you see things," says Hawkley. But you can learn to do a little introspection to re-examine your perception of social situations. For example, when you were chatty with the cashier and she didn't respond, was it really you? Or was she just having a bad day?

TAKE A CHANCE

People who are lonely often anticipate being rejected. "They may withdraw from others, so their behavior becomes a self-fulfilling prophecy which perpetuates their loneliness," says Ellor. "You've got to do something differently and put yourself out there to meet people and make new connections." Try a new activity or join a group that has similar interests such as a book club, yoga class, or dog park meetup. And don't give up. Sooner or later, something will click.

DO SOMETHING FOR OTHERS

Volunteering for a group or cause that focuses on something that matters to you—literacy, homelessness, the local food pantry—is one way to feel connected to your community at large. It also takes the focus off you, because you'll be engaging with people who have the same desires and goals to help others. Cross-generational organizations, such as those that offer tutoring or mentoring to kids, can be especially rewarding.

ADOPT A FURRY FAMILY MEMBER

Research has shown that pets offer benefits including reduced blood pressure, heart rate, and levels of anxiety, stress, and loneliness. If it's something you've always wanted to do, adopting a pet will make you feel needed (time for a walk!), may encourage you to get more active, and may help build new friendships with other pet lovers. If you can't commit to pet parenthood, consider volunteering at a local animal shelter instead.

GET OUTDOORS

Whether you're going into your own backyard to garden, hiking with a friend, or joining a birdwatching club, studies show that "being outdoors is a natural antidote to stress," says Richard Taylor, Ph.D., head of the physics department at the University of Oregon, who studies how nature's patterns affect mental health. His research shows that stress levels plummet by 60% when we view patterns like those found in nature.

EXPRESS GRATITUDE

Studies have shown that gratefulness is associated with a lower risk of depression, anxiety, and substance abuse, and may improve loneliness. Try a few basic gratitude exercises such as taking time each day to reflect on what you're grateful for, or writing a note to thank someone for something they've done for you. You can also consider participating in a religious service to connect with a higher power, as well as gain community.

KNOW WHEN TO GET SOME HELP

If you begin to feel you can't function or if loneliness begins to inhibit your capacity to be yourself, talk to your primary-care doctor or a mental-health professional.

Use Tech to Feel Better—Not Worse

▶ Social media can be good or bad, depending on how you use it, says Ellor. Constantly comparing yourself with everyone else who has an Instagram-worthy house/job/car/life is exhausting. If you catch up with faraway family members or rediscover an old friendship through social media, that's positive. If you feel worse after a scrolling session, try limiting your engagement. And ditto for news and push notifications: You don't need to consume every bit of breaking news out there. Doing so constantly ramps up emotions and may trigger feelings of anxiety, which also has been associated with loneliness.

And remember: Don't use technology to replace in-person contact. Technology can be great for connecting long-distance or when you can't be together in person. But emerging research is showing it can supplement, not replace, in-person interactions in maintaining mental health.

How to Make Friends as an Adult

HERE ARE SOME STEPS TO TAKE IF YOU WANT TO MAKE NEW friends and stay connected to the ones you already have.

THINK ABOUT YOURSELF FIRST

Start by making a list of what you're interested in, what you've always wanted to do, and things you'd try in an ideal world, says Whitney Goodman, L.M.F.T., a family relationship expert and the author of *Toxic Positivity*. Consider things you could learn, like how to play an instrument or speak a new language, that might be avenues for connecting with people who share your interests while boosting your brainpower, adds Marc Milstein, Ph.D., a professional speaker on brain health and the author of *The Age-Proof Brain*. Then come up with themes like travel or creative expression that you can begin to explore with others who have similar interests.

FIND AN "ANCHOR ACTIVITY"

Focus on pinpointing a new place to visit or class you can attend

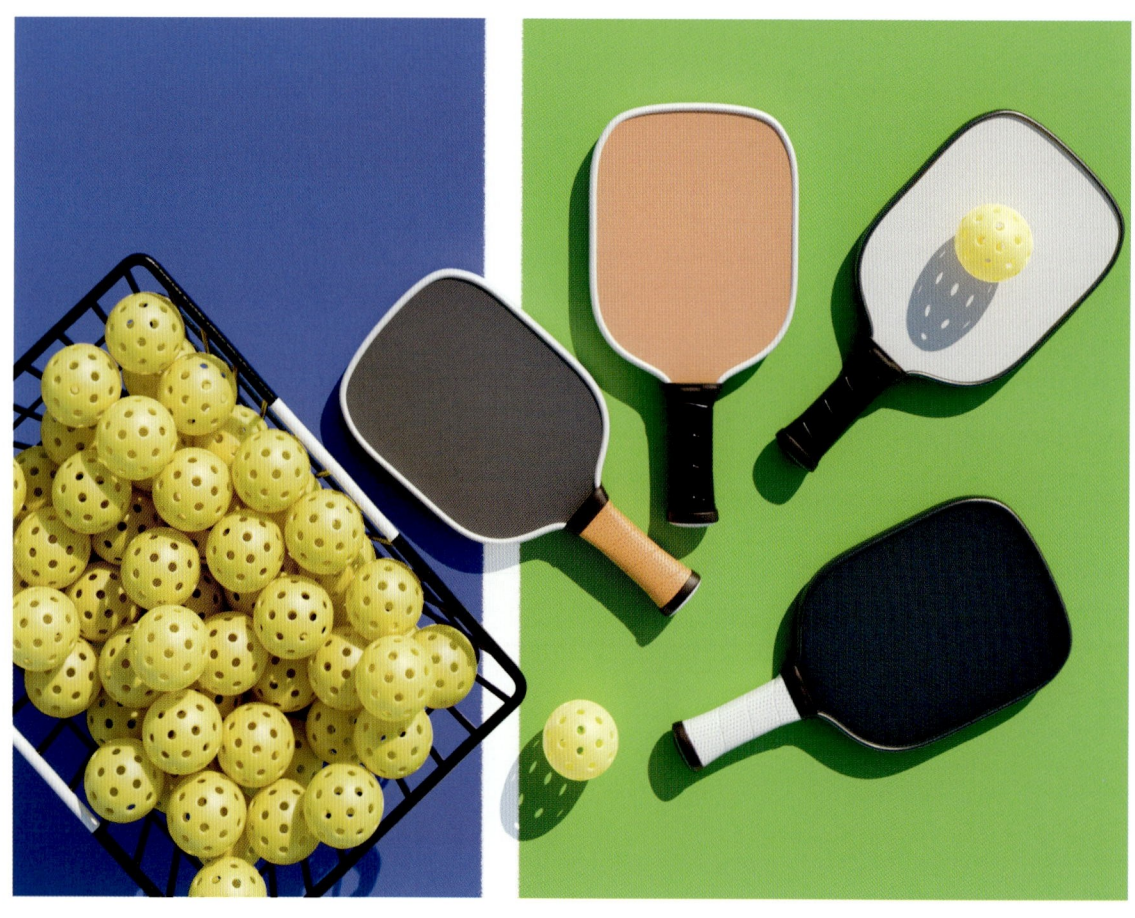

to serve as a central point as you take the next steps toward making friends. Try a religious center, gym, community center, or volunteer opportunity that will allow you to pursue the passions on your list, suggests Hope Kelaher, a licensed clinical social worker. If you live in a remote area, she recommends signing up for a group trip or joining an online community through social media or online university classes.

MARK YOUR CALENDAR

Choose three days a week for "social days." Plan something physical, like a workout class, for the first day; schedule a brain-boosting activity, like an art class, next; and plan for a more social activity, like a book club, on the third day, Milstein suggests. Once you're in a social situation, Kelaher says, allow yourself to be vulnerable and engage with other people. Introduce yourself to someone as soon as you walk in. Ask if they've been there before and what brought them to the event. And before you leave, create touchpoints to continue the conversation, like asking whether they'll be at the next meeting.

KEEP IT UP

"Friendship is like dating: It takes one person to take it to the next level and invite someone out," Kelaher says. After attending events, challenge yourself to reach out to people you felt a connection with and schedule a phone call, walk, or coffee date. Then as return invitations come in, try to say yes to as many as possible, Kelaher adds. Finally, be sure to set reminders for birthdays and

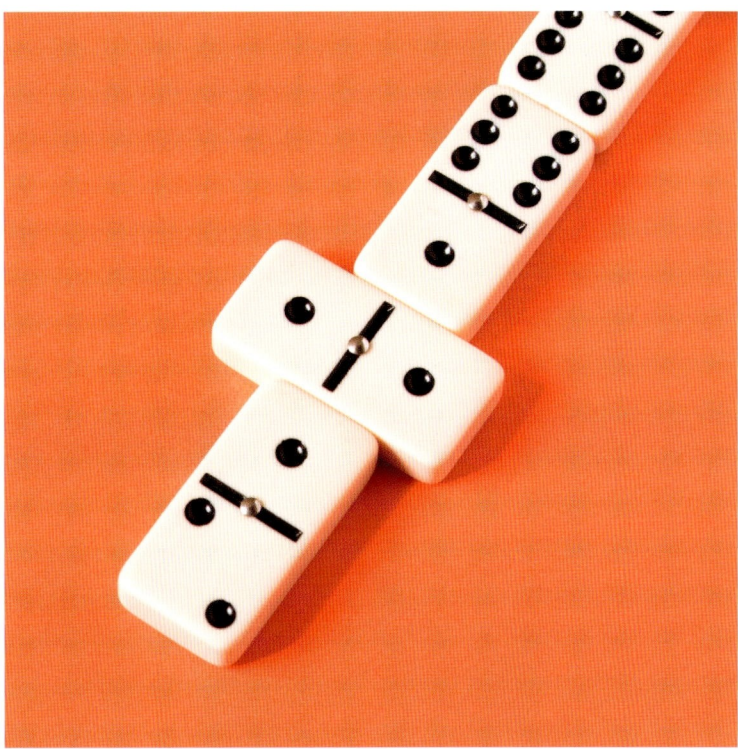

special occasions so you'll always have an excuse to reach out to friends old and new.

It takes work to maintain friendships, says Tami Zak, a licensed therapist at Grow Therapy. "You need to be intentional and make time for friends and...be committed to working through challenging periods." If you are willing to invest time and energy in friendships, the results will be positively life-changing, says Zak.

One thing Melissa Klosk, Psy.D., senior clinical psychologist at Well-Being & Psychological Services, often speaks to clients about is maintaining "friend files," which can be metaphorical or literal. "Take time to remember conversations you've had with your friends: Do they have a

new hobby? Do they have a big interview coming up? Write it down or make a mental note of it. Reach out with an email, text, direct message, or phone call when something reminds you of the conversation you had," Klosk suggests. These small gestures can go a long way in maintaining friendships and making your friend feel valued and heard.

MAKE IT MEANINGFUL

Forming deep friendships is absolutely vital to not only longevity but also to feeling a greater sense of purpose, life satisfaction, and well-being, says Zak. "One study revealed that people who have strong social connections are 50% less likely to die prematurely than people with weak social relationships," she notes.

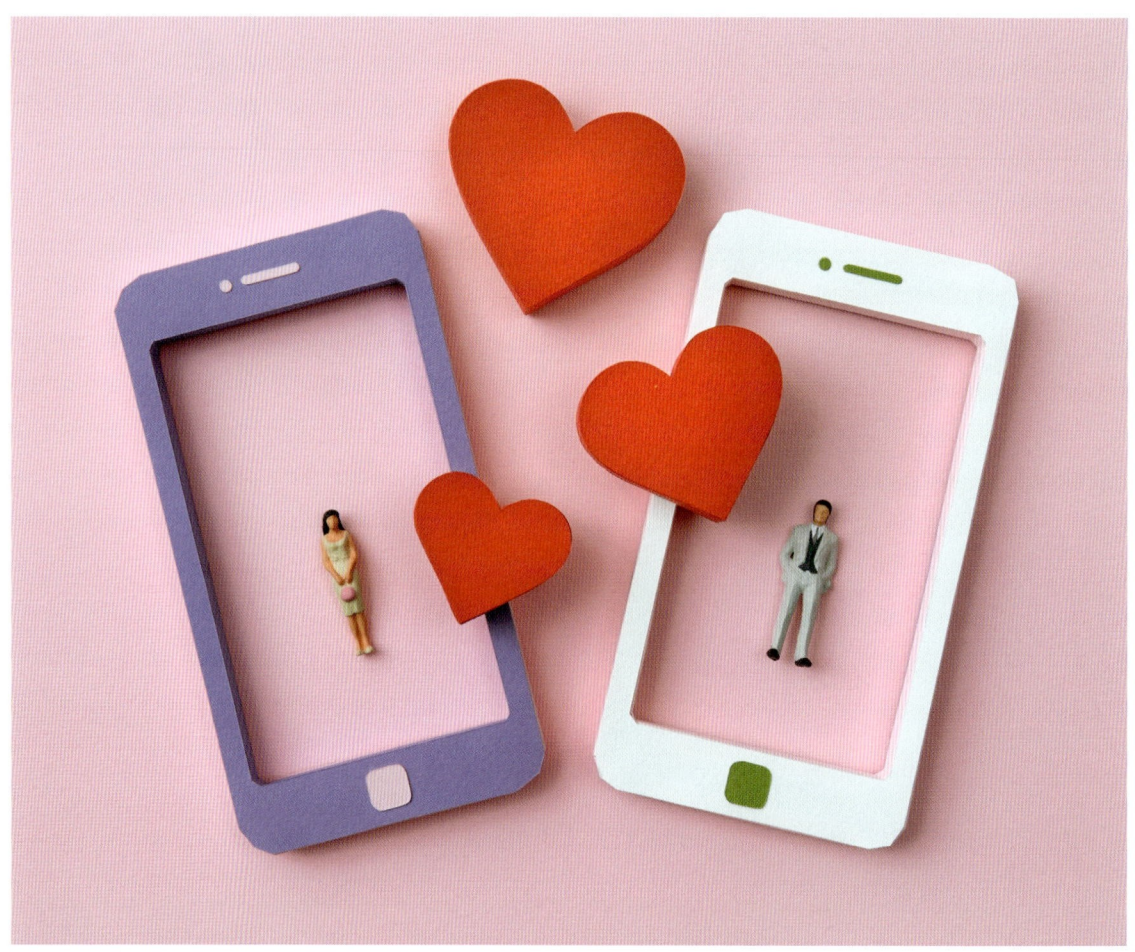

Dating After 50

WHILE THE DATING POOL FOR 50+ MAY BE A different depth and shape than in the past (newspaper classifieds, anyone?), the water's still fine if you're willing to jump in.

People are living well into their 70s on average, and many are starting over after divorce or the loss of a spouse in midlife and later. In fact, 28% of people aged 50 to 64 are single, and that number goes up to 36% for those 65 and older.

According to the late Helen Fisher, Ph.D., an esteemed biological anthropologist and senior research fellow at The Kinsey Institute at Indiana University, there are three distinct brain systems for mating and reproduction: sex drive, romantic love, and feelings of deep attachment. While sex drive can diminish to a degree with age, Fisher says, romantic love and feelings of deep attachment don't.

Meaningful dating, whether online or in person, often comes down to being in "receptive mode," explains Marissa Nelson, L.M.F.T., a certified sex therapist and sex educator who's currently the relationship and intimacy expert at BLK, a dating app for Black singles. "You have to be in a place to be able to invite love into your life," she says.

Curiosity is also key, adds Laurie

Sloane, L.C.S.W., a psychotherapist with experience helping women navigate midlife and beyond. "To be open, you have to be curious about who is the person you're looking at on an online app, who is the person sitting across from you on that first coffee or drink or evening dinner," she says. "That curiosity can take you very far."

DOWNLOADING APPS AND HIRING MATCHMAKERS

Just like younger people, those over 50 are giving digital dating a try. Paula Pardel, the CEO of Bloom Matchmaking, who typically works with heterosexual middle-aged people, says, "A lot of people come to me because they just don't know how to navigate the dating world right now." They ask, "What are the new rules and what do I do?"

Pardel helps her clients regain confidence and coaches them through how to write eye-catching bios, choose appropriate photos,

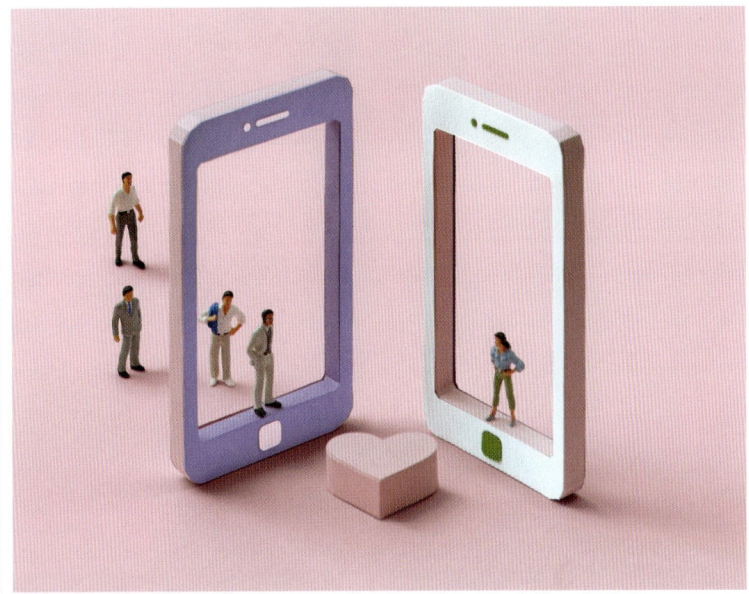

and stay safe. Thinking about safety—not disclosing too much personal information before meeting, and picking a public space for a first date, for instance— is important. About half of online daters age 50 and older say they encountered someone they thought was trying to scam them while

using a dating website or app.

"I try to warn people about texting too much before you're in a relationship because you can't get a good picture of who someone truly is through text," Pardel adds. "You can't hear the inflection in their voice. There are misunderstandings."

You're in Good Company

Ilene, 71, never turned to the Internet after her longtime husband passed away nine years ago. "But I dated a fair amount," she shares. Formerly a diabetes educator and registered dietitian, she was often set up by her patients.

Still, there's no escaping the perils of modern dating. "A friend introduced me to somebody who I really liked a lot, and he ended up ghosting me, which was pretty horrifying," she recalls. (Note: He called back two years later to apologize. "He had stuff going on, blah, blah, blah.")

Despite the challenges, "you have to put yourself out there," says Ilene, who notes she was once advised to never decline an invitation.

She also practiced manifestation in her recent search for love. "I wrote a vow...and every morning I lit a candle and [read] the vow out loud, and two months later I started dating Mark, the man I'm with," she says.

Mark was a friend of a friend whom she'd seen at many special occasions—bar mitzvahs, weddings, holidays—over the years while they were married to other people. But when they both found themselves widowed, they connected in a new way." It didn't come immediately," she explains, noting that she was guarded in the beginning. "I wasn't allowing myself to go there. I was taking it very slow. And then it just took off," she says. "It was magical, and it was really..." She pauses. "There's a lot of chemistry there."

chapter three
CARE FOR YOUR BODY

Advances in medicine and new information on how you can prevent and manage health conditions are changing the way we experience common conditions of older age.

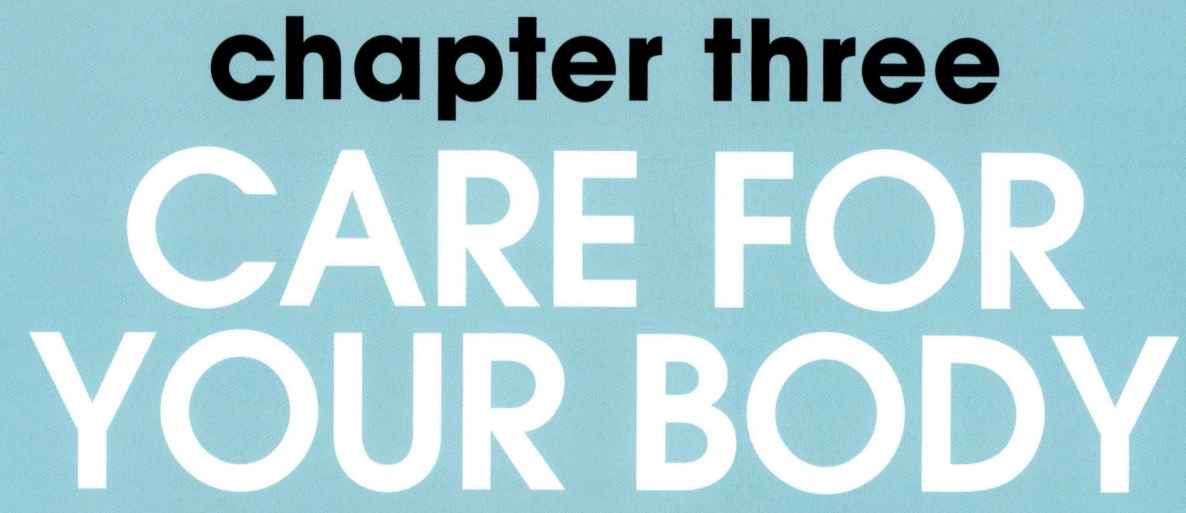

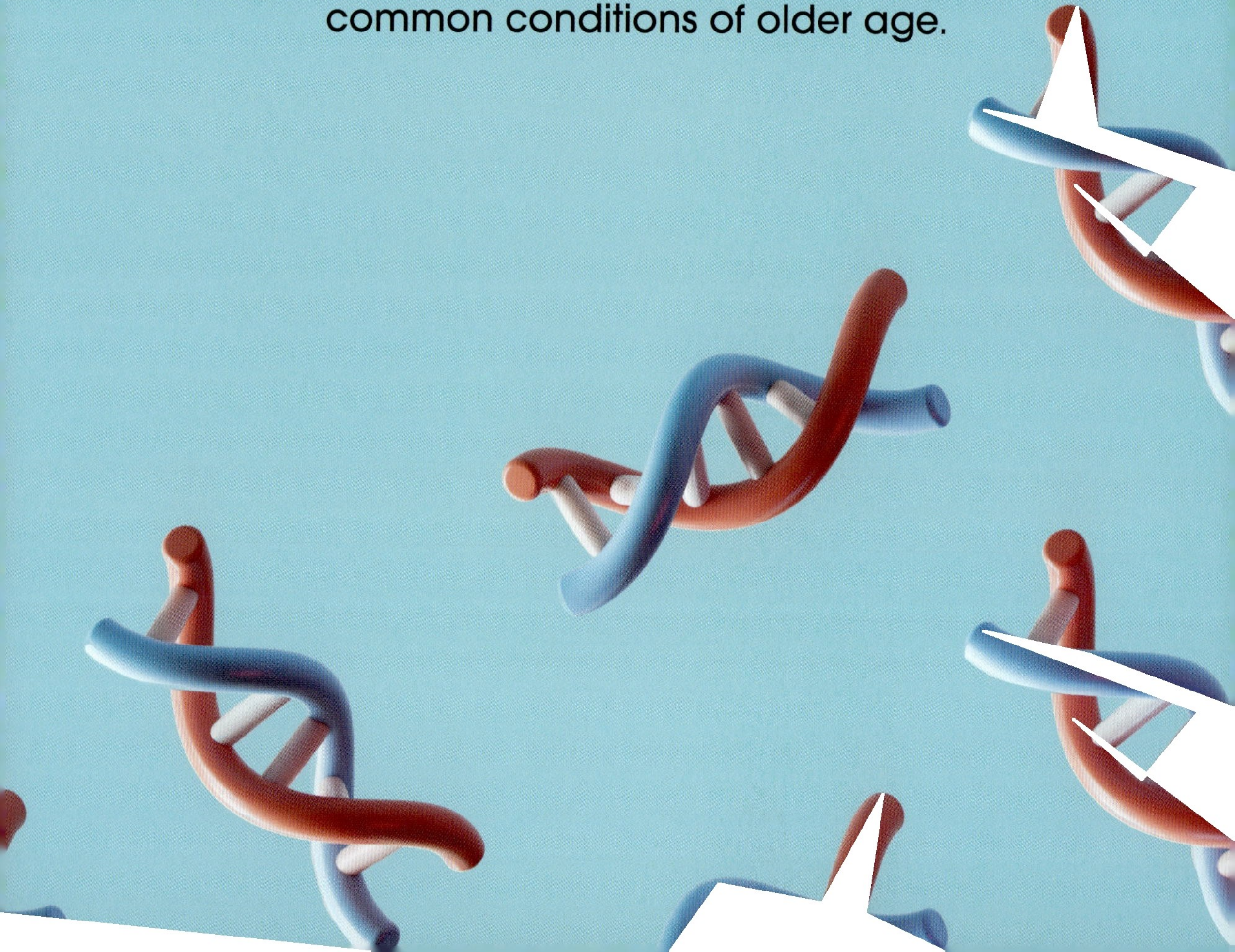

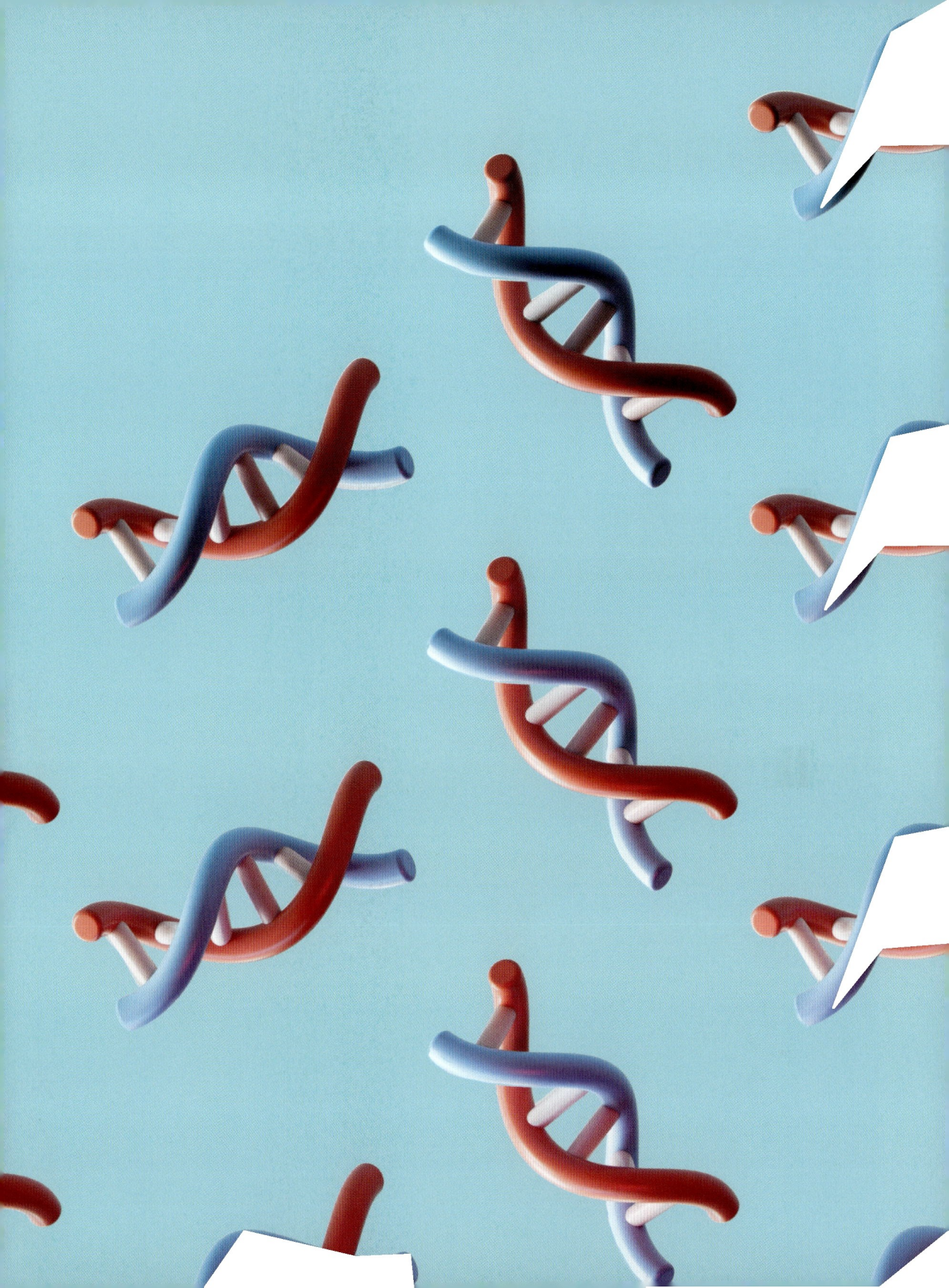

Keep Your Heart Healthy

AS THE DECADES PASS, SOME OF THE CHANGES to the human body are visible (hello, wrinkles and that unwanted spare tire!), while others are not. Among those unseen changes could be chronic conditions that affect your heart—and that could compromise the quality and length of your life.

Heart disease is the leading cause of death for both men and women of any age, and the risks increase with age: Most people who die of heart disease are 65 and older. Yet few of us have a good grasp on how to protect ourselves. Step one is to understand what, exactly, could be putting your ticker in danger. Then we'll give you some tools and lifestyle changes to help you focus on preventing cardiovascular disease.

86 million American adults live with the "silent" condition of high cholesterol.

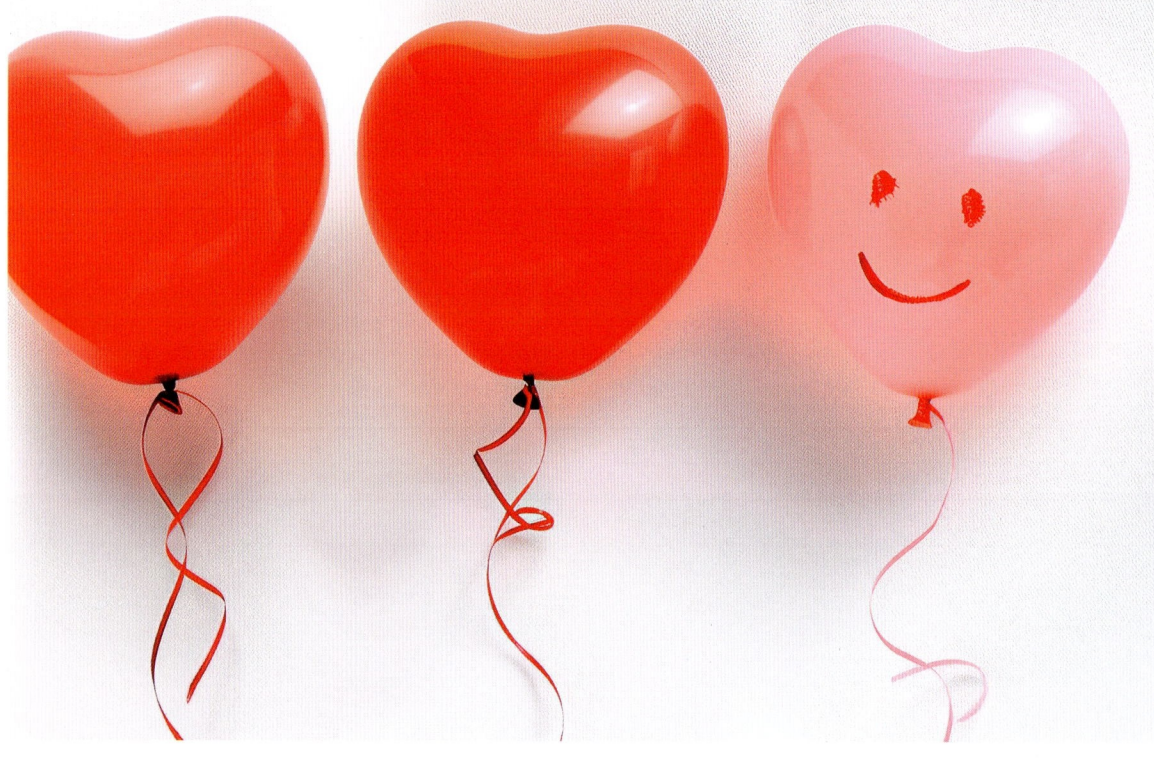

You've probably heard that having high cholesterol and/or high blood pressure, getting older, having a family history of heart disease, smoking, and being overweight or obese can raise your chances of developing heart disease. But there are lesser-known risk factors too—including some health conditions that might seem like they have little to do with the heart: Diabetes/prediabetes, preeclampsia and gestational diabetes (even in a pregnancy decades earlier), thyroid conditions, erectile dysfunction, and autoimmune disorders can all affect heart health.

Know the Symptoms

▶ While chest pain is the most common symptom of a heart attack in both men and women, women are more likely to have other, more subtle symptoms. These can include indigestion, nausea, vomiting, jaw, neck, or upper-arm pain, fainting, and extreme fatigue. What's more, women are more likely to have more than one heart attack symptom. If you have symptoms that could signal a heart attack, call 911 right away.

Other less-known contributors to heart conditions include poor dental health, depression and social isolation, poor sleep, menopause, cancer treatments, stress, and trauma.

If you have experienced or are experiencing any of these conditions or circumstances, schedule a chat with your doctor to discuss monitoring of your heart and steps you can take to prevent or mitigate the impact on your heart.

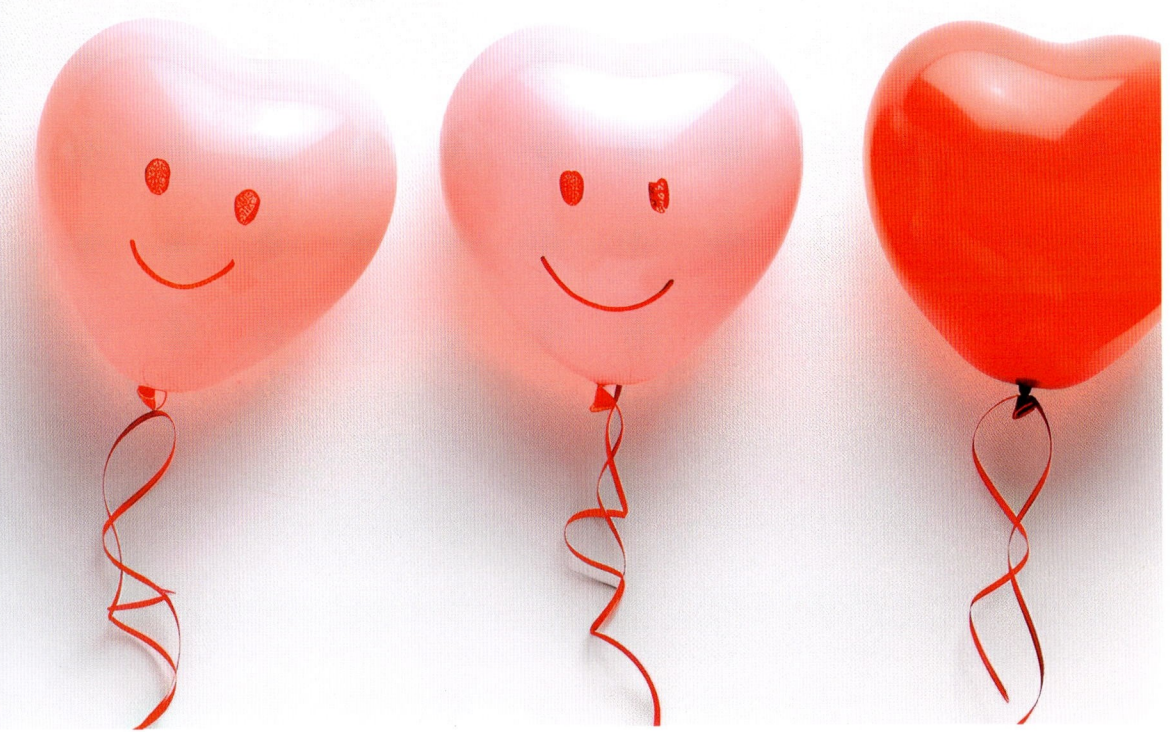

High Cholesterol and High Blood Pressure

THESE ARE AMONG THE TWO BIGGEST CULPRITS FOR heart disease, so let's break down exactly what we're talking about.

WHAT IS HIGH CHOLESTEROL?

Cholesterol gets a bad rap, but our bodies need this molecule to build cells and make hormones. "Cholesterol is a fatty substance in the blood that is produced mostly by the liver, though some of it is obtained through your diet," explains Demilade Adedinsewo, M.D., a cardiologist in Jacksonville, Florida. If certain cholesterol levels get too high, deposits can collect in the walls of the arteries, creating plaque that builds up in blood vessels. This increases the risk of heart problems.

There are three types of cholesterol: low-density lipoprotein (LDL), which is sometimes called "bad" cholesterol; high-density lipoprotein (HDL), dubbed "good" cholesterol because it helps remove cholesterol from the arteries; and total

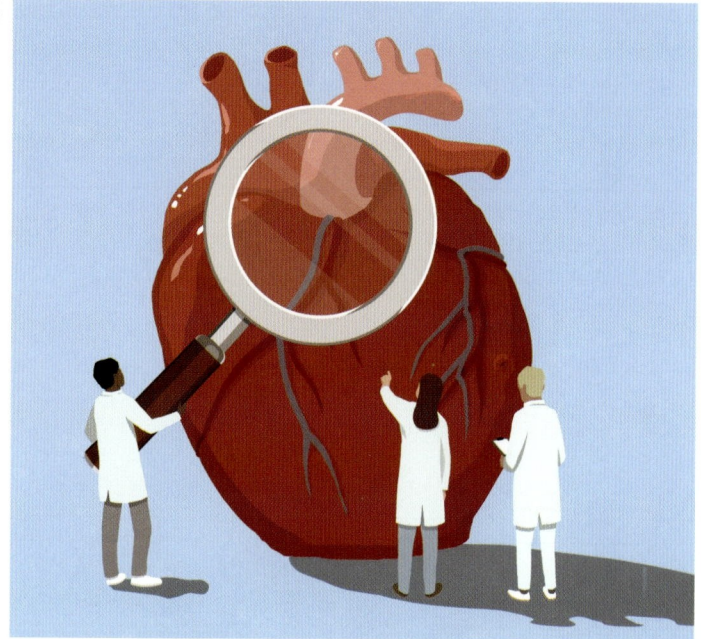

cholesterol, which is a combination of these and triglycerides, another type of fat in your blood.

As you grow older and your metabolism changes, your liver becomes less efficient at removing LDL cholesterol from your blood. This is the type of cholesterol most often associated with disease. On the other hand, with HDL, the higher, the better.

A blood test called a lipid panel measures your levels of total, LDL, and HDL cholesterol, as well as triglycerides. See the next page for optimal numbers.

WHAT IS HIGH BLOOD PRESSURE?

Blood pressure is the pressure of blood pushing against the walls of your arteries, which carry blood from your heart to other parts of your body.

It's normal for your blood pressure to rise and fall during the day. But, if it stays elevated—130/80 mm Hg and above—it's considered high blood pressure, or hypertension. Hypertension is one of the leading causes of cardiovascular disease and can lead to heart attack and stroke.

Your blood pressure is measured two ways:

- **Systolic blood pressure**, which measures the pressure in your arteries when your heart beats.
- **Diastolic blood pressure**, which measures the pressure in your arteries when your heart rests between beats.

When you get a blood pressure reading, the systolic blood pressure number is on top, and the diastolic blood pressure number is on the bottom.

The 3 Numbers to Know

Blood Sugar
What It Is: The amount of sugar (or glucose) in your blood, measured by hemoglobin A1C and/or fasting blood glucose tests

Ideal Goal: HbA1c less than 5.7%; fasting glucose less than 126 mg/dL

Why: Too-high sugar levels can damage blood vessels, making you more susceptible to heart disease.

Blood Pressure
What It Is: The force of your blood pressure against artery walls

Ideal Goal: Less than 120/80 mm Hg

Why: High blood pressure increases your risk of stroke and heart attack.

Blood Cholesterol
What It Is: A fat-like, waxy substance in the blood

Ideal Goal: *Total cholesterol:* Less than 200 mg/dL, *Triglycerides:* Less than 150 mg/dL, *"Good" HDL cholesterol:* Greater than 60 mg/dL, *"Bad" LDL cholesterol:* Less than 100 mg/dL

Why: Higher levels of cholesterol may block blood flow to the heart.

You're in Good Company

Two weeks after giving birth to her third child, Erin experienced a severe headache, swollen feet, and excessive bleeding. At the hospital, it was discovered that her blood pressure was very high, and she was told she was in danger of having a stroke.

She was diagnosed with postpartum preeclampsia and hospitalized for three days. "I knew there was preeclampsia during pregnancy, but I didn't know it could happen after birth," says Erin, co-owner of a small business. "It was shocking to me because during pregnancy my blood pressure was the best it had ever been."

That was surprise number one. The next one came when she heard that this diagnosis increased her risk of developing cardiovascular disease in the future.

To protect herself, Erin now monitors her blood pressure at home, takes hypertension medicine twice a day, and sees a cardiologist regularly. "This really drove home the importance of taking care of myself," she says. "As an older working mom, I kept putting everything else before my daily walks or not taking the time to de-stress, thinking I could put it off until I had more time. Now that I track my blood pressure regularly, I understand more how everyday stress, food, and movement affect my body."

Improve Your Heart Health Today

YOU MAY HAVE GONE A LIFETIME (SO FAR) without thinking about how lifestyle choices can affect your heart. The changes you make to improve your heart health don't have to be drastic: Little by little, you can start making tweaks to your routine. Many of these lifestyle changes can help address high blood pressure and cholesterol abnormalities, and ultimately lower your risk for heart disease. But make sure that you talk to your doctor about heart health, especially if you've been diagnosed with high blood pressure or high cholesterol, as medication may be necessary.

EAT FRUITS AND VEGETABLES

Your mom was right: Eating your fruits and veggies (especially leafy greens and berries) is good for your health! And while access to fresh produce may not be easy for all, canned and frozen vegetables are also great—just avoid those with added sugar. (See the diet and nutrition information beginning on page 112 for more heart-healthy foods.)

CUT BACK ON ADDED SUGARS

Occasionally indulging your sweet tooth is okay—but if you're concerned about your heart health, reducing your added sugar intake will benefit you in the long run. There are natural sugars that occur in many foods such as fruit (fructose and

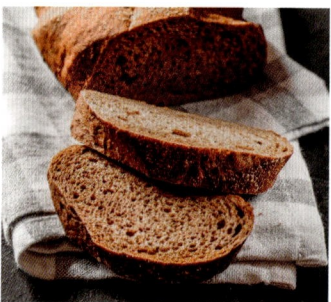

glucose) and milk (lactose). Added sugars are put in foods during preparation and are listed on a nutrition label as so. The American Heart Association recommends that no more than 6% of your daily calorie intake comes from added sugar—that's about 9 teaspoons/36 grams for men and 6 teaspoons/25 grams for women. You can start anywhere: Try one sugar instead of two in your coffee, or substitute sparkling water for soda pop. Keep in mind

that added sugars aren't just in sweets: Sugar is often added to salad dressings, tomato sauce, barbecue sauce, and more. Get in the habit of reading labels!

CUT BACK ON ULTRA-PROCESSED FOODS

Avoiding foods that have been processed in some way is nearly impossible, but if you can opt for foods that have been minimally processed and packaged, like nuts and salad mixes, you can avoid the added sugars and sodium usually connected with processed foods.

EAT MORE WHOLE GRAINS

Whole grains are a great source of dietary fiber, which can help improve your cholesterol levels and lower your risk of heart disease, stroke, and type 2 diabetes. Look for foods like whole-wheat bread, oats, barley, steel-cut oatmeal, brown or wild rice, and quinoa.

INCREASE YOUR OMEGA-3 INTAKE

Omega-3 fatty acids are a type of unsaturated fatty acid that may reduce harmful inflammation throughout the body. According to the Mayo Clinic, eating two servings of fish like salmon, trout, tuna, herring, and mackerel per week can reduce the risk of sudden cardiac death.

PICK HEALTHY PROTEINS

Fish and shellfish are great options for lean protein intake, as is chicken, but also try to include plant proteins like beans, peas, lentils, and nuts. Plant sources of protein do not contain saturated fats, which are found in meat and dairy products, and provide dietary fiber and other nutrients. Nuts, peanuts, and soybeans also contain healthy unsaturated fats. (See the diet and nutrition information beginning on page 112 for more ideas.) Other plant-based sources of protein: peas, corn, dark leafy greens, and Brussels sprouts.

ADD DIETARY FATS

It sounds counterintuitive to add fat to your diet for heart health, but monounsaturated fats can actually have a positive impact by reducing your cholesterol level. When eaten in moderation, foods like avocado, peanut butter, canola oil, olive oil, and sesame oil can be good for you.

LOWER YOUR ALCOHOL INTAKE

No amount of alcohol is good for you, so cutting back is smart. Excessive alcohol consumption is associated with an increased risk for heart disease, liver disease, and premature death. An excess is typically considered 100 grams of alcohol (or 7 drinks) per week. In 2023, the World Health Organization declared that no amount of any alcohol is good for you—not even those "heart-healthy" red wines (which studies have found are not heart healthy at all).

LOWER YOUR SALT INTAKE

The American Heart Association

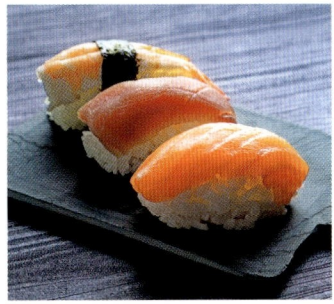

says the average adult should eat no more than 1,500 milligrams of sodium per day. But even if you are eating significantly more than that, cutting whatever your excess sodium is by 1,000 milligrams a day can improve your blood pressure. Check nutrition labels to see how much salt is in your favorite foods, and look for labels that say "low sodium" or "no salt added" when grocery shopping.

GET YOUR WORKOUTS IN

The American Heart Association recommends adults get about 2.5 hours a week of physical activity. See page 146 for heart-healthy workout options.

STOP SMOKING AND VAPING

This can be a big life change for many, but it is one that can be the most impactful. Quitting any tobacco product can lower your blood pressure, improve your circulation and lung function, and dramatically cut your risk of coronary heart disease.

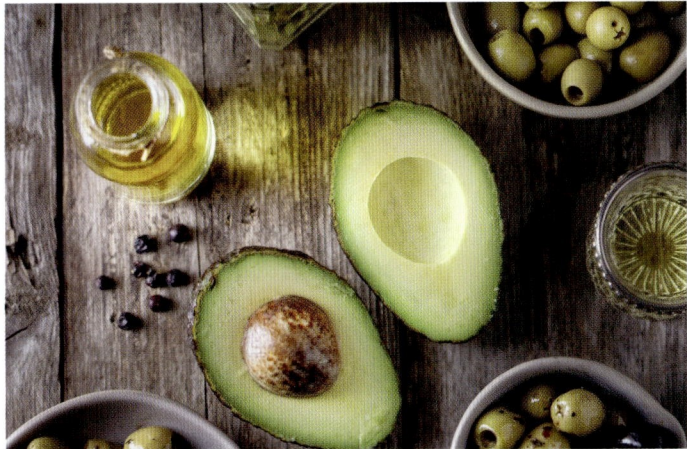

Inflammation Overload and How to Tame It

INFLAMMATION IS ESSENTIAL: IT FIGHTS infections and fixes wounds. Acute inflammation happens in response to an injury or illness, alerting your white blood cells to flood the area that's hurting and then quickly receding.

But when these defenders refuse to stand down after the problem is gone, or when they launch an offensive against something that's not a threat, that's a problem. That's called *chronic inflammation*, a long-term, low-grade condition that persists in your cells and tissues and plays a key role in many health problems. In fact, inflammation is involved in 8 of the 10 leading causes of death in the United States—heart disease, cancer, chronic lower-respiratory diseases, stroke,

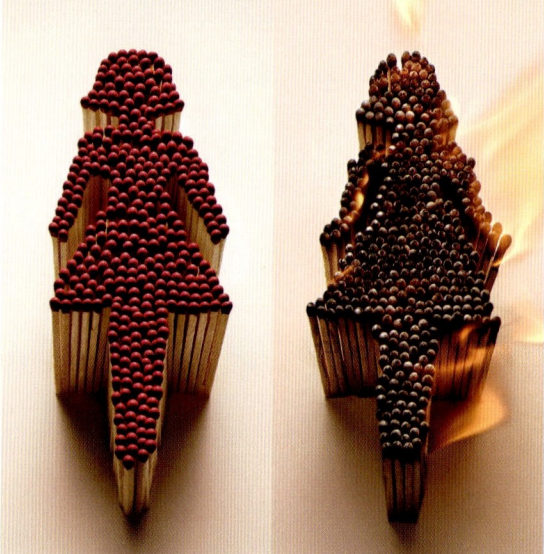

Alzheimer's disease, diabetes, pneumonia/influenza, and kidney disease. It's also associated with anxiety and depression, and autoimmune diseases.

For example, inflammatory cells in your arteries can cause plaque to develop and build up, which could lead to a stroke. How? Your body views the plaque as a foreign substance, and uses even more inflammation to "fight" it—and this causes the plaque to thicken even more. It's a vicious cycle.

THE REPERCUSSIONS OF INFLAMMATION

Harvard University Medical School data indicates a wide range of issues that can be linked to chronic inflammation:

- Acne
- Allergies and asthma
- Alzheimer's and other forms of dementia
- Anxiety and depression
- Arthritis
- Different types of cancer
- Eczema
- Heart disease
- High blood pressure
- Psoriasis
- Stroke
- Type 2 diabetes

The good news: For low levels of inflammation, easy changes in your habits can make a huge impact. "Controlling your weight, eating a healthy diet, improving your sleep—these things can

Inflammation Prescription

▶ If you are diagnosed with a condition linked to inflammation, your doctor may prescribe medications to help with the symptoms of the specific condition, which in turn can stop the inflammatory response.

nip so many health problems in the bud," says Erica L. Johnson, Ph.D., associate professor of microbiology, biochemistry, and immunology and the co-director of the Vaccine Trials Unit Laboratory at Morehouse College School of Medicine in Atlanta.

Here are some easy, science-backed steps to help reduce it.

EAT THE RIGHT STUFF

According to the Cleveland Clinic, you want a good balance of carbohydrates, protein, and fat to lower chronic inflammation. Eating a nutritious mix of healthy foods helps your tissues repair themselves and promotes healing. Following a Mediterranean diet, as detailed on page 112, can be a good start. In addition, a study from Stanford University School of Medicine finds that food and beverages that promote microbial diversity in the gut can reduce inflammation. Foods to try include yogurt, kefir, kimchi and other fermented vegetables, vegetable brine drinks, and kombucha.

LOOK AT YOUR LIFESTYLE

Turns out, lifestyle habits that reduce inflammation are also the ones that promote longevity. Prioritize these steps to maximize your health and combat inflammation.

- **Get enough sleep** The National Sleep Foundation recommends that healthy adults get seven to nine hours a night. Make it a nonnegotiable in your life. (See more on rest on page 158.)

- **Move your body** A Duke University study showed that

How Do You Know If You Have Chronic Inflammation?

▶ Most of the time, you don't. As chronic inflammation persists in your system, you could develop some symptoms, such as feeling tired, experiencing achy muscles and joints, having GI problems like constipation or diarrhea, getting headaches, or gaining weight. (Yes, these symptoms could be caused by so many things, including, well, life!) However, a regular checkup with your doctor may well reveal the problem.

"There are no specific tests to diagnose inflammation," explains Sadiya Khan, M.D., Magerstadt professor of Cardiovascular Epidemiology at Northwestern University Feinberg School of Medicine in Chicago. "You're not trying to identify inflammation as much as look at why it's there. Routine screenings, specifically your annual physical, are the way to do that." The standard blood tests you get at the doctor's office can help diagnose inflammation. Cardiovascular disease screening and blood testing are two other key aspects you need. "Basically, you want to get a complete profile of your health, and then treat any condition that the inflammation is related to," Dr. Khan says.

when muscles are exercised, damage from chronic inflammation is stopped. Aim for those key 150 minutes of exercise a week. (See exercise inspiration beginning on page 124.)

- **If you smoke, quit** Get help from your doctor if needed.

- **Limit alcohol** Keep it to no more than a drink a day, but if you think it's become a habit that you want to address, think of the health benefits you'll enjoy by quitting.

- **Stay connected** Some research indicates that loneliness causes inflammation. Cut your risk by staying in touch with people you care about. Connect with your friends and

family in person or remotely. (See more about the power of connection on page 52.)

- **Stress less** Yoga and meditation can really help. And do things that make you happy; a proactive, joyful attitude can make a huge difference in your health. (See more on stress management on page 150.)

"You can improve inflammation, and improve your health every day as well, by staying active and addressing any underlying conditions," Johnson says. "Most of the time, lifestyle remedies can really help with the conditions that cause inflammation, if you know what you're dealing with in terms of those conditions. Knowledge is power!"

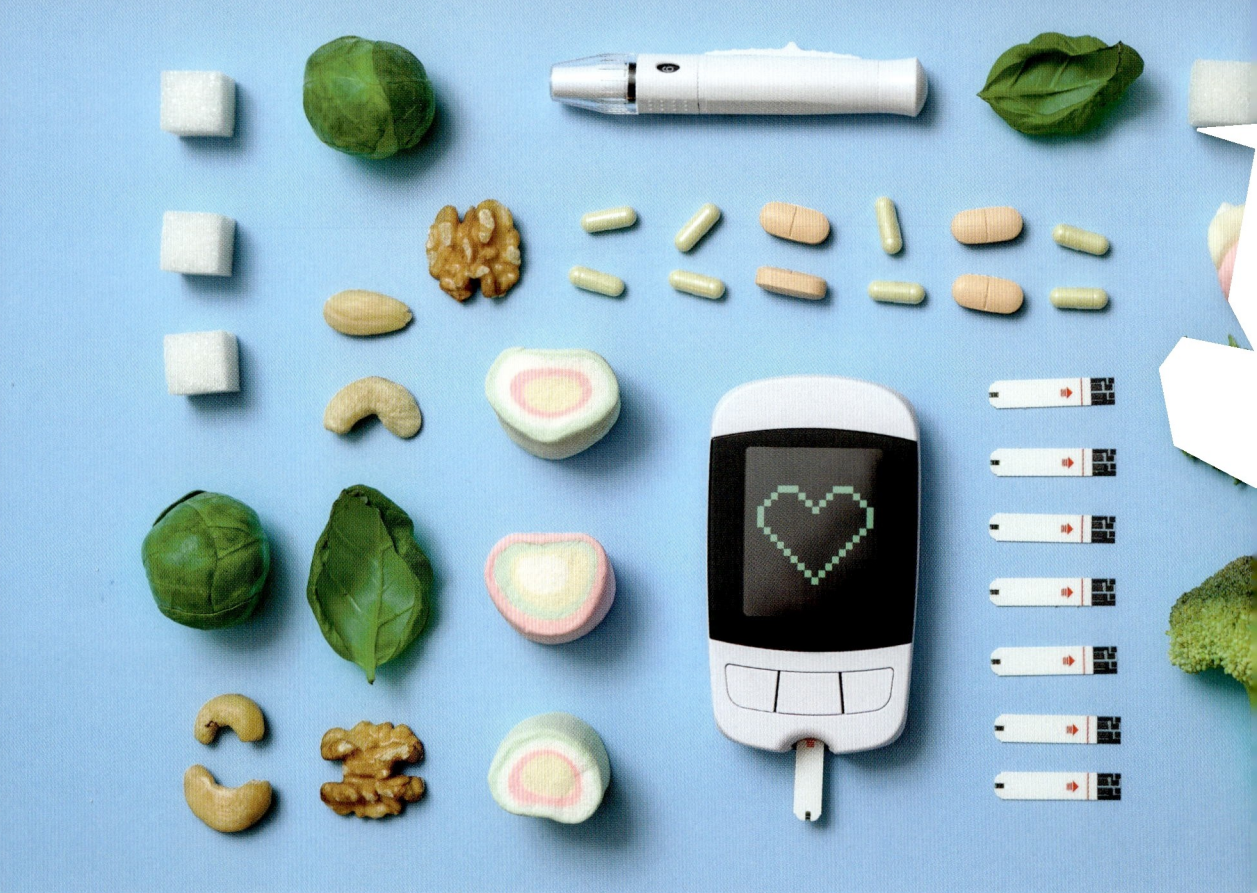

Diabetes 101

NEARLY 1.5 MILLION PEOPLE IN THE U.S. ARE DIAGNOSED with diabetes each year, and there are 38.4 million Americans living with diabetes. The Centers for Disease Control and Prevention (CDC) defines diabetes as "a chronic health condition that affects how your body turns food into energy." When we eat, the food is broken down into glucose and travels into the bloodstream, raising your blood sugar levels. That sends a message to your pancreas that it's time to release insulin, a hormone that helps that blood sugar find its way into your cells for use as energy.

If you have diabetes, one of two things happens: Either your body doesn't make enough insulin, or it can't use insulin as well as it should. So too much sugar remains in your bloodstream, which isn't good for your body long-term and brings on the possibility of serious health problems like heart and kidney disease and vision loss.

THE COMMON TYPES

Type 1 diabetes is an autoimmune disease that happens when the body mistakenly destroys the insulin-producing cells in the pancreas. Type 1 diabetes is more commonly diagnosed in children but occurs in adults as well. By contrast, type 2 diabetes—which accounts for a majority of cases in the U.S.—occurs when there is insulin resistance and insulin can no longer effectively reduce blood glucose levels. Type 2 diabetes is most common in adults over 45 due to increased insulin resistance and diminished pancreatic function.

THE SYMPTOMS

The CDC and the Mayo Clinic list the following common symptoms of diabetes:

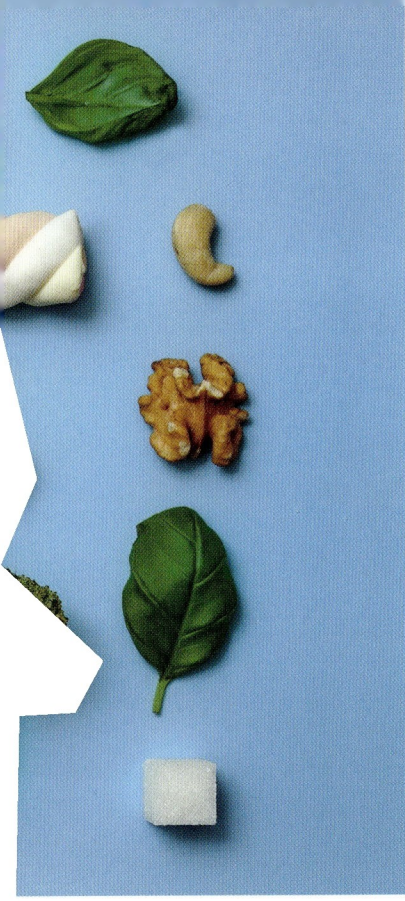

- You're very thirsty.
- You have to urinate frequently, often at night.
- You're extremely hungry.
- You're losing weight for no obvious reason.
- You're very fatigued.
- You're irritable.
- Your vision is blurry.
- You have sores that are slow to heal.
- You have frequent infections, such as in your gums, skin, or vaginal area.
- Your hands or feet feel numb or tingly.
- Your skin is very dry.

YOUR POSSIBLE RISKS

Family history Having a parent or sibling who has type 2 diabetes.

Age Being 45 or older.

Weight Being overweight or obese, particularly if you have a high waist circumference.

Inactivity In addition to helping control weight, regular exercise can help lower blood sugar by increasing insulin sensitivity and uptake of glucose from the blood.

Race According to the American Diabetes Association, some races have higher rates of type 2 diabetes, including African American (13.2%), Native Americans (ranging from 6% in Alaskan Natives to 24.1% in southern Arizona Native American groups), Asian American (9%), and Hispanic (12.8%).

Gestational diabetes A diagnosis of diabetes during pregnancy or giving birth to a baby weighing more than nine pounds.

Polycystic ovary syndrome

High blood pressure

High cholesterol

If you're experiencing any symptoms of diabetes or have risk factors for diabetes, talk to your doctor about screening. Diabetes can be diagnosed with a simple blood test—either an A1C test that measures average blood sugar over a three-month period, a fasting blood sugar test, or a glucose tolerance test, which measures blood sugar two hours after drinking a glucose solution.

What Is Prediabetes?

▶ Prediabetes refers to blood sugar (plasma glucose) levels that are higher than normal but do not meet the criteria for full-blown diabetes, explains Aleem Kanji, M.D., endocrinologist at Ethos Endocrinology. More than 86 million people in the United States—that's 1 out of every 3 adults—are prediabetic, yet 90% of them have no idea. That's because prediabetes doesn't often have symptoms.

The American Diabetes Association recommends that everyone 45 and older get their blood sugar checked, though you might need to be tested earlier if you have a family history or risk factors for diabetes.

Those diagnosed with prediabetes may have an increased risk of developing type 2 diabetes and cardiovascular disease. "Prediabetes can remain unrecognized for years," Dr. Kanji says. "Prompt diagnosis and treatment [are] necessary to prevent the progression to diabetes and reduce the risk of cardiovascular disease." If you think you're suffering from prediabetes, reach out to your primary care physician to talk about your symptoms and testing options. See "The 3 Numbers to Know" on page 65 for optimal glucose levels.

Cut Your Cancer Risk

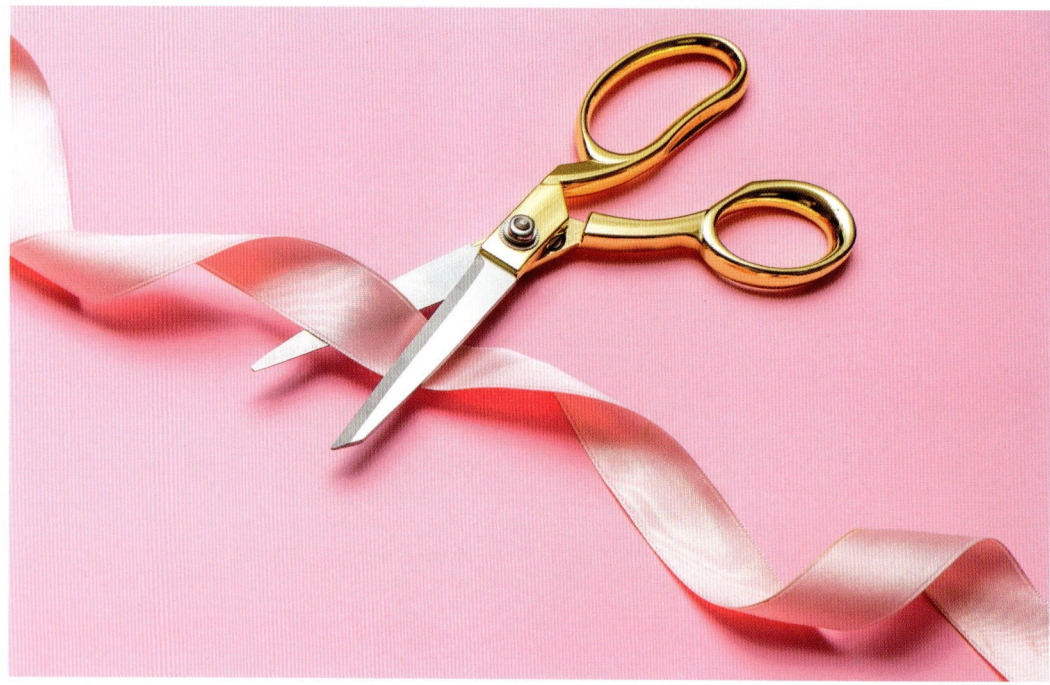

CANCER RATES ARE INCREASING IN MIDLIFE. Given this alarming information, it's natural to wonder how you can cut your risk. New research shows that nearly half of cancer deaths could be prevented with changes to lifestyle habits.

A study published in *CA: A Cancer Journal for Clinicians* by the American Cancer Society looked at 30 types of cancer and 18 risk factors that could be changed by lifestyle habits. These included smoking, body weight, alcohol use, poor diet, lack of exercise, sun exposure, and missing cancer screenings, among others. (Cigarette smoking was the leading risk factor for cancer, contributing to nearly 20% of all cancer cases and 30% of all cancer deaths.)

It is very important to understand that cancer develops when there is damage to cellular DNA, says Nelly Awkar-Lazo, M.D., hematologist and oncologist with the Oncology Institute of Hope and Innovation. The known causes of DNA damage are mainly genetic and environmental, she says.

THE BOTTOM LINE

The good news is that the effects of many of these risk

factors are reversible over time, says Neil Iyengar, M.D., breast medical oncologist at Memorial Sloan Kettering Cancer Center. The first thing to do to lower cancer risk is to eliminate or minimize exposure to risk factors such as smoking, alcohol, obesity, poor diet, and inactivity, he notes. "Smoking is still responsible for the majority of preventable cancers, so stopping smoking will have the greatest impact on lowering cancer risk. Excess body weight is the next risk factor, second to smoking," he explains. Alcohol is the third leading preventable cause, accounting for 6% of all cancers, according to the American Cancer Society.

Fortunately, many of the interventions to reach and maintain a healthy body weight will also address several other risk factors including diet, exercise, and alcohol, Dr. Iyengar points out.

"Eating a plant-forward diet in which at least 80% of food intake is comprised of minimally processed, whole plant-based foods will help to lower cancer risk by improving diet quality, improving body weight, increasing fiber intake, and increasing intake of other [cancer-protective nutrients]," he says.

The American Cancer Society study shows us that approximately 40% of cancers in the U.S. might be preventable by improving several modifiable risk factors, says Dr. Iyengar. However, these findings also tell us that the other 60% of cancers may not be preventable, he notes.

That's why it's crucial to talk to your health-care providers about when to start age-appropriate cancer screening that will help detect cancer at very early stages, says Dr. Awkar-Lazo. Early detection is essential to more effective treatment and a better chance of survival.

The American Cancer Society recommends doing the following to lower your cancer risk:

- Try to keep your body weight in a healthy range.

- Get 150 to 300 minutes of moderate-intensity or 75 to 150 minutes of vigorous-intensity activity each week.

- Limit sedentary behavior as much as possible.

- Eat a healthy diet, including a variety of fruits and vegetables.

- Limit red and processed meats, sugar-sweetened beverages, highly processed foods, and refined grain products.

- Limit alcohol to no more than one drink a day for women and no more than two drinks a day for men.

- Stop smoking.

Cancer Cases Are Also Increasing in People Under 50—Here's Why

▶ A growing number of studies have found that cancer rates are on the rise in younger people. A study published in *Nature Reviews Clinical Oncology* analyzed data from 14 different cancer types that showed an increasing number of cases in adults before the age of 50 from 2000 to 2012.

While more widespread cancer screening may account for some of the cases, it isn't the only reason. One theory is that the Western diet and lifestyle could be boosting cancer rates. That links up with recent research suggesting that eating ultra-processed foods can heighten the risk of cancer. Other possible reasons: Obesity, type 2 diabetes, a sedentary lifestyle, and alcohol consumption have gone up since the 1950s, which the researchers say could impact the gut microbiome and raise a person's risk of cancer earlier in life.

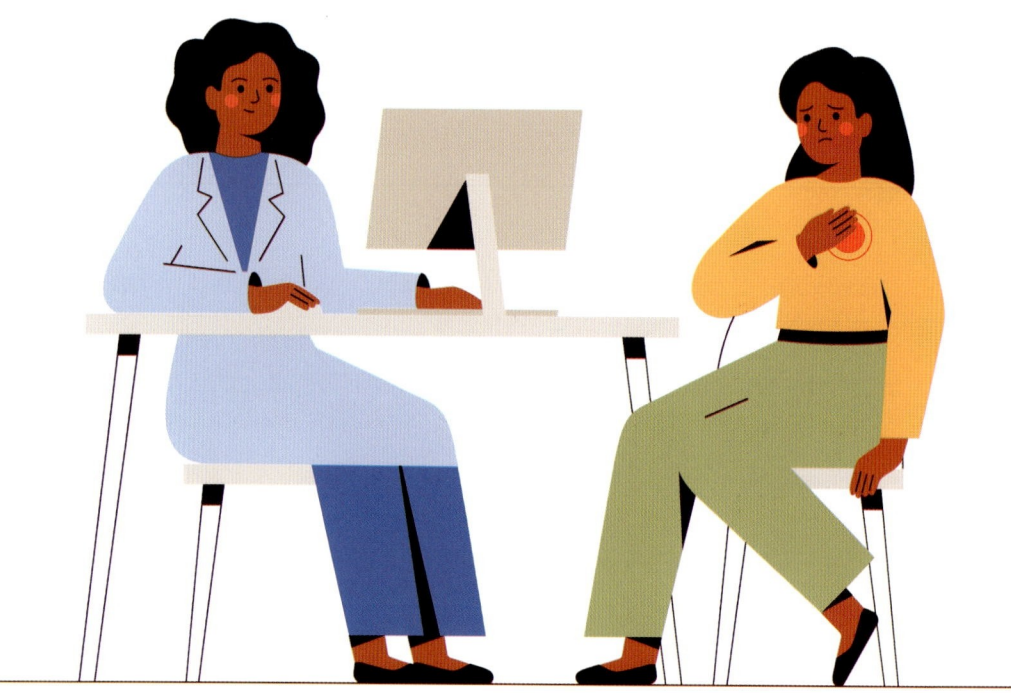

Questions to Ask Your M.D. About Your Cancer Risk

THERE'S NO QUESTION THAT KNOWLEDGE is powerful. But when the average doctor's visit lasts about 20 minutes, your questions about your cancer risk factors might take a back seat to other immediate health concerns. And you may feel confused about which questions to prioritize. Here are some of the most important questions to bring up at your next checkup, based on doctors' advice.

WHICH CANCER SCREENINGS SHOULD I HAVE AND WHEN?

First of all, you should have an annual checkup with your primary-care doctor. Based on your age and family history, your doctor may recommend certain cancer screenings. For example, mammograms to screen for breast cancer should begin at age 40. But if you have a family history of breast cancer, your doctor may recommend one sooner.

If you're between the ages of 45 and 50, the American Cancer Society recommends getting a colonoscopy. "If you have a first-degree relative with cancer, the first screening colonoscopy should be at age 40 or 10 years [before] the youngest person was affected with colon cancer in the family," says Smitha Krishnamurthi, M.D., an oncologist in the department of hematology and medical oncology at Cleveland Clinic.

IS MY FAMILY HISTORY CONCERNING FOR MY RISK OF CANCER?

Inform your doctor about your parents', siblings', children's, aunts', uncles', and grandparents' cancer diagnoses, Dr. Krishnamurthi says. A subset of many cancers, such as colorectal, breast, ovarian, pancreatic, and uterine, is caused by inherited gene mutations.

It's also important to know the age at which your family member was diagnosed, as it can help your doctor come up with individualized screening recommendations.

WOULD I BENEFIT FROM GENETIC TESTING?

Having a family history of certain cancers increases the chance of inheriting these mutations, so your doctor may recommend genetic testing to see if you carry any.

"This knowledge is powerful," Dr. Krishnamurthi says. "If a person is found to have a mutation that puts him or her at risk for

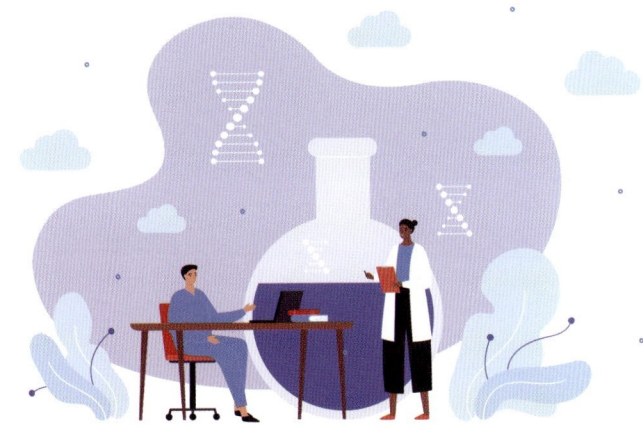

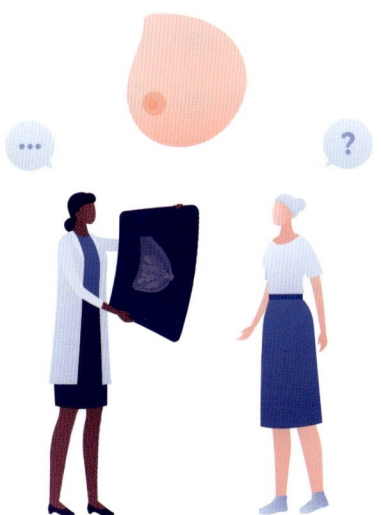

developing cancer, he or she can undergo screening tests more often and earlier to try to detect any cancers that occur at an early, curable stage," she explains.

Because various psychological and emotional issues come into play with genetic testing, it's best to talk to your doctor and a genetic counselor. "If genetic testing reveals an increased risk of disease, there may be different screening recommendations, lifestyle modifications, medical or surgical interventions, and [other recommendations]," says Adrienne Phillips, M.D., a hematology and medical oncology specialist at New York–Presbyterian/Weill Cornell Medicine.

SHOULD I BE CONCERNED ABOUT MY WEIGHT?

Being overweight has been shown to increase the risk of developing breast, uterine, and pancreatic cancers, and even blood cancers such as leukemia, says Putao Cen, M.D., an associate professor of oncology with McGovern Medical School at UTHealth in Houston

and a member of the Cancer Center at Memorial Hermann-Texas Medical Center. In fact, research from the American Cancer Society shows that excess body weight is thought to be responsible for about 8% of all cancers in the U.S., as well as about 7% of all cancer deaths.

WHAT KINDS OF EXERCISE WOULD WORK WITH MY BODY AND HEALTH STATUS?

Research suggests that exercise and regular physical activity can help reduce the risk of cancer, including breast cancer recurrence and colon cancer. And because exercise already plays an essential role in preventing heart disease, diabetes, and other conditions, it could improve your overall health.

CAN I TALK TO YOU ABOUT SOME UNUSUAL SYMPTOMS I'M HAVING?

Dr. Cen recommends talking to your doctor if you notice a change in bowel movements and bladder habits, such as constipation, diarrhea, or bloody or very dark urine. They could be early signs of

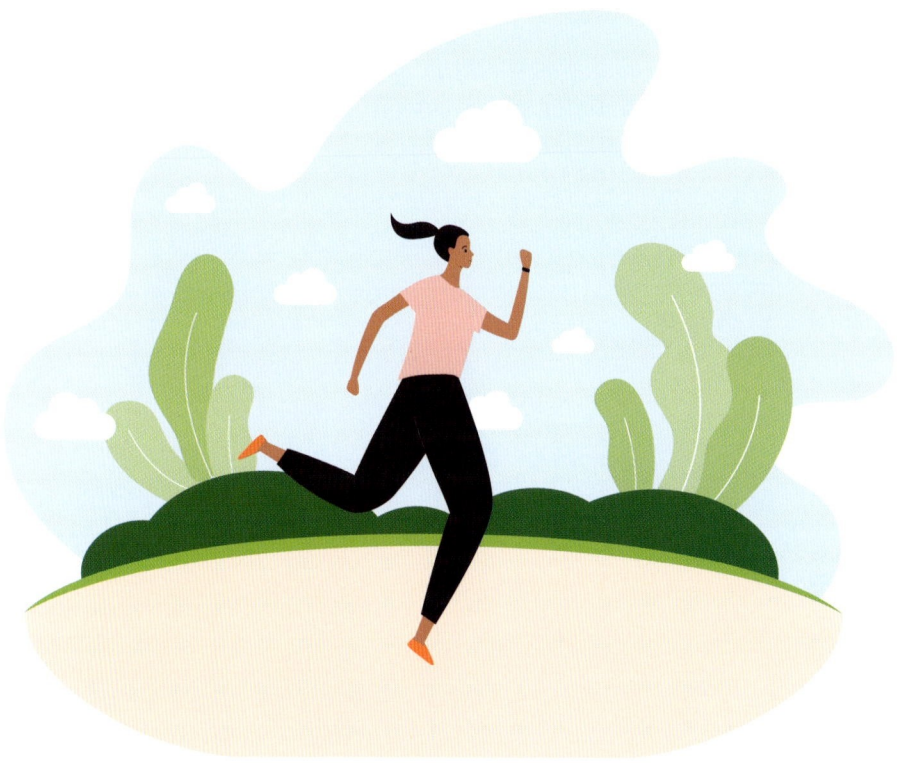

colon, bladder, or kidney cancer, respectively. Unusual bleeding from the genital area could also be a sign of uterine cancer.

A new lump anywhere on the body could be a tumor, or a sign of lymphoma or head and neck cancer, Dr. Cen says. Additionally, difficulty swallowing might be a sign of esophageal cancer. Changes in the voice might signal throat cancer, and a nagging cough or shortness of breath could be signs of lung cancer.

ANY TIPS TO MINIMIZE MY ENVIRONMENTAL CANCER RISKS?

Sun exposure and air quality can affect cancer risk, Dr. Cen says. While you should take preventive measures, such as wearing sunscreen every day, you should also talk to your doctor about the possibility of a vitamin D deficiency, which has been linked to certain cancers. Moreover, if you live an area with poor air quality, you should take steps to minimize spending extended periods of time outdoors as well.

WHAT CAN I DO TO PREVENT ILLNESSES THAT MAY CAUSE CANCER?

According to Dr. Cen, hepatitis B and C have been linked to liver cancer, so it's important to make sure you've received the hepatitis B vaccine. You can avoid hepatitis C by avoiding intravenous drug use or sharing personal care items that can come in contact with blood.

HPV (human papilloma virus) is one of the most common causes of cervical cancer. Getting a pap test at your well-woman exam every one to three years will screen for unhealthy cells.

If you have a history of stomach ulcers or gastrointestinal pain, you should also get tested for *Helicobacter*—or *H. pylori*—an infection in the stomach lining that has been linked to stomach cancer.

DO I NEED TO CUT DOWN OR QUIT DRINKING?

Alcohol is known to raise the risk of cancers of the head and neck, esophagus, colon, and rectum, liver, and breast, Dr. Krishnamurthi says. In fact, a study from *The Lancet* shows that there is no safe level of alcohol, yet many of us are unaware of alcohol's link to diseases.

Even just one alcoholic drink a day is associated with an

increased risk of head and neck cancers and esophageal cancer as well as a small increased risk of breast cancer. The Dietary Guidelines for Americans recommend women drink no more than one alcoholic beverage per day, if at all.

WHAT ARE MY OPTIONS FOR COLORECTAL CANCER SCREENING?

"The gold standard is a colonoscopy, because it evaluates the entire colon, and polyps—noncancerous growths of the intestine that have the potential to develop into cancer—can be removed in this procedure before they can become cancer," Dr. Krishnamurthi says.

But since a colonoscopy requires cleaning out the colon the day before and taking a day off work to do the procedure, it can deter people from having one. Ask your doctor about other methods, including tests that can detect colon cancer or large polyps early. Flexible sigmoidoscopy or a stool DNA test are more convenient options.

DOES MY JOB AFFECT MY CANCER RISK?

Certain toxic exposures can predispose some people to certain types of cancer, Dr. Phillips says.

For example, if you work in a hair salon and handle hair dyes, research has shown that this might put you at an increased risk for certain cancers. Or if you've been exposed to asbestos, you will have an increased risk of developing lung cancer or mesothelioma. Your doctor might recommend additional screenings.

HOW OFTEN SHOULD I GET A FULL-BODY SKIN EXAM?

Dr. Phillips advises going through the ABCDE's of potential skin cancer often, looking for **a**symmetry, irregular **b**orders, **c**hanges or uneven color, large **d**iameter, and **e**volution of changes for existing or new moles.

"If a skin lesion is not uniform and is evolving over time in terms of size, shape, or color, you should definitely bring that to your doctor's attention," Dr. Phillips says.

Additionally, depending on your personal and individual risk and history of sun exposure, your dermatologist may recommend an annual full-body skin exam, she says.

CAN YOU HELP ME QUIT SMOKING?

Quitting smoking will lower your risk of cancer among many other diseases. Doctors have numerous tools available to help patients quit smoking, depending on the patient's interest and readiness to quit, Dr. Phillips says. Whether it's behavior counseling or medications, review your goals with your doctor to receive support and appropriate referrals or treatments.

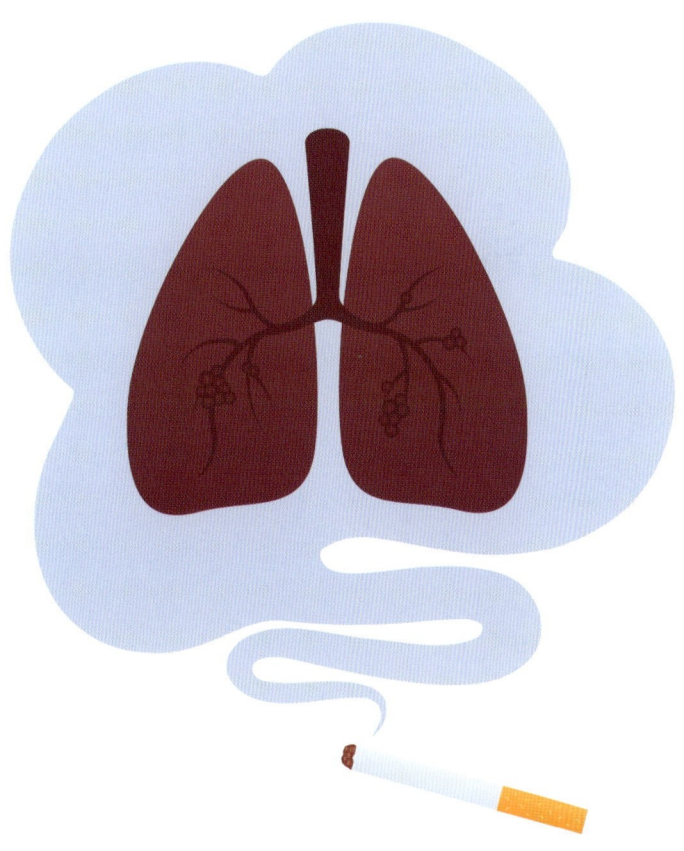

How to Prevent Osteoporosis

ADD YOUR BONES TO THE LIST OF THINGS YOU have to take care of as you age—it's time to support the bones that have been supporting you. Everybody needs to be concerned about preventing osteoporosis—a medical condition in which bones weaken and become easier to break. About 10 million Americans suffer from it, while another 44 million have low bone density, which is a precursor to the disease.

One in two women, and up to one in four men, will break a bone because of osteoporosis. And while it mostly affects women over 50, everyone loses bone density as they age.

YOUR BONES OVER A LIFETIME

From puberty until about age 30, people build more bone than they break down, a process kicked off by estrogen in girls and testosterone in boys. From the age of 30 until menopause for women, and about age 50 for men, "there is a balance between the amount of bone we break down to get rid of old bone and the amount of bone being replaced," says Ejigayehu Abate, M.D., an endocrinologist who treats osteoporosis and other conditions at the Mayo Clinic in Jacksonville, Florida.

Around age 50, because of the reduction of estrogen in women and, to a lesser extent, testosterone in men, bone breakdown overtakes bone building. This is a natural part of the aging process, so you can't reverse it. But through smart nutrition and lifestyle choices, "we can certainly slow down and reduce our chances of breaking bones," says Dr. Abate. This is a good time to speak to

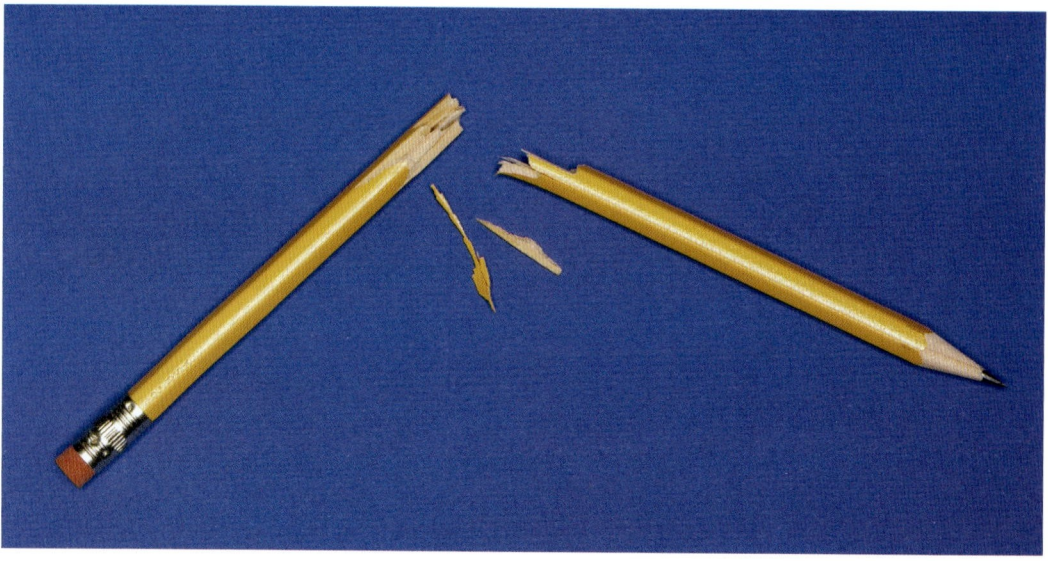

your doctor about preventive measures and screening.

WAYS TO SUPPORT HEALTHY BONES

Whatever your situation or age, there are lifestyle choices that can prevent bone loss and reduce your risk of developing osteoporosis.

Get a bone-density screening

Forty-four million people in the U.S. have low bone density (a.k.a. osteopenia), a precursor to osteoporosis that causes a decrease in the minerals in bones, potentially leading to fractures. This is just one reason to ask your doctor about having a DEXA scan, a simple test that measures bone density. Women who have experienced menopause should talk their doctors about the right time to schedule this test.

Consume calcium

When it comes to bone health, calcium is king, because it makes up most of both bone and teeth—nearly 98% of the mineral in the body is stored there. And since the human body can't produce it, it's imperative to get calcium from food, or failing that, from supplements.

The recommended amount for women is to consume is 1,000 milligrams a day prior to menopause or age 50, and 1,200 a day after menopause. Men should consume 1,000 milligrams per day until age 70

and 1,200 milligrams after that. The best way to get it is through calcium-rich foods.

To ensure that the calcium you eat is absorbed by your body, pair it with vitamin D, which can be found in eggs, fortified foods (many dairy foods are fortified with the vitamin), and fish.

Reduce inflammation

Inflammation is a condition that many people experience as they age. It can lead to various health problems, including fragile bones that in turn may contribute to osteoporosis, osteoarthritis, rheumatoid arthritis, and periodontitis. A bone scan can be helpful in diagnosing inflammation-related bone problems. See page 119 for simple lifestyle changes to reduce inflammation.

Consider supplements

If you aren't getting enough calcium through food and drink, a calcium supplement may be right for you. But these supplements can interact with many drugs, including blood-pressure medications, antibiotics, and even foods, so be sure to discuss this with your physician.

Exercise

Physical activity is key in preventing osteoporosis and promoting bone health, and specifically, regular weight-bearing exercise helps slow bone loss. Think walking,

jogging, dancing, playing tennis or pickleball, and the like for about 30 to 40 minutes per session, adding up to at least 150 minutes per week. And gentle exercises like tai chi and yoga can also help improve your balance and avoid falls.

Strength training or resistance training is especially good for your bones. According to the National Institute of Arthritis and Musculoskeletal and Skin Diseases, strength-training exercises put pressure on your bones in a good way, making them stronger.

How to Avoid Falls

▶ The Centers for Disease Control and Prevention report that older adults suffer about 36 million falls per year, and many of these result in broken bones. Fortunately, there are simple steps you can take to protect yourself:

- Wear shoes with nonslip soles indoors.
- Remove items from your floors that you could trip over, including throw rugs.
- Keep hallways and corners in your home well-lit.
- Take extra care if you take medications that can affect your balance or make you drowsy.

Your Sexual Future

REAL TALK: YOUR SEX LIFE DOESN'T HAVE an expiration date. In fact, sex is like a fine wine—it improves with age. "The presumption is that sex is for younger, fitter, and—according to what we see reflected in our media—more attractive people," says Melanie Davis, Ph.D., a nationally certified sexuality educator and creator of "Our Whole Lives: Sexuality Education for Older Adults," a series of workshops for adults over 50. But a comprehensive national study of sexuality and health among older adults shows that most people want and need sex well past 60, and continue to have it often—even well into their 80s.

"You can be sexual as long as you want to be," says Lonnie Barbach, Ph.D., a clinical psychologist, author of *The Pause: Positive Approaches to Menopause and Perimenopause*. If you have a history of enjoying sex, there's no reason to believe that you'll suddenly stop liking it when you hit a certain age. That said, some things may evolve.

YOUR DEFINITION OF "GOOD" SEX MAY CHANGE

Sexual activity when you're young is sometimes frantic, explosive, and athletic. As your body ages, sex can change into more of a slow burn, but it can still be just as hot. "It's not about how often you have sex, and it's not about how many positions you can be in. It's really about sexual pleasure, and your relationship and connection you have with your partner," says Barbach. By focusing less on your sex stats and more on good communication, you'll have just as much—or more—pleasure and passion as you did when you were young.

YOU CAN GET PAST PHYSICAL OBSTACLES

There are physical changes that are normal in aging bodies but may seem like potential barriers to sex. Menopause. Erectile dysfunction. Libido changes. Conditions and medications that affect your sex life. But there's no need to throw in the towel at the first sign of trouble. Talk to your doctor about treatments that can get you back in the business of getting busy. Taking good care of yourself will go a long way toward lifting your libido too. "Exercise and good nutrition can help a great deal, both physically and emotionally, to help older adults feel vigorous, healthy, and sexually interested," says Davis.

YOU MAY NEED MORE TIME TO REACH ORGASM

Your days of "the quickie" may be behind you, as both men and women tend to take longer to get aroused and to experience orgasm as they age. "What once literally came easily takes more time and attention, and that's not a bad thing," says Davis. In fact, it can be more satisfying to go slowly and intentionally. You can get creative and find new ways to enjoy yourself or your partner. This way, sex becomes

Snuggling Counts Too!

▶ Spend time lingering in bed, cuddling, caressing each other, and engaging in "pillow talk." Besides promoting the release of oxytocin, often called "the love hormone," research has found that time spent with your partner can enhance relationship and sexual satisfaction.

more about the journey and less about the destination.

Even couples with a fantastic sex life can benefit from taking time to tease out pleasure—especially if they're longtime partners. But good communication is crucial. "That's the major thing that makes a difference between couples who have a good sex life and keep it going, and those who don't," says Barbach. "If you don't talk about it, you can't adapt."

You're in Good Company

As couples get older, sexual timing can become a bit tricky, as Helen discovered in her 50s. To get aroused ahead of intercourse, she started needing more foreplay. "But there's a sweet spot, because if foreplay lasts too long, I'll start to get dry and sex is uncomfortable," says Helen, a realtor. Her husband Jack sometimes takes Viagra for better erections, and when he does, "he's ready to go quickly," she says, which adds an extra challenge to the timing and duration of foreplay. "I keep plenty of lube nearby and we've gotten creative with vibrators—the combination usually helps," says Helen.

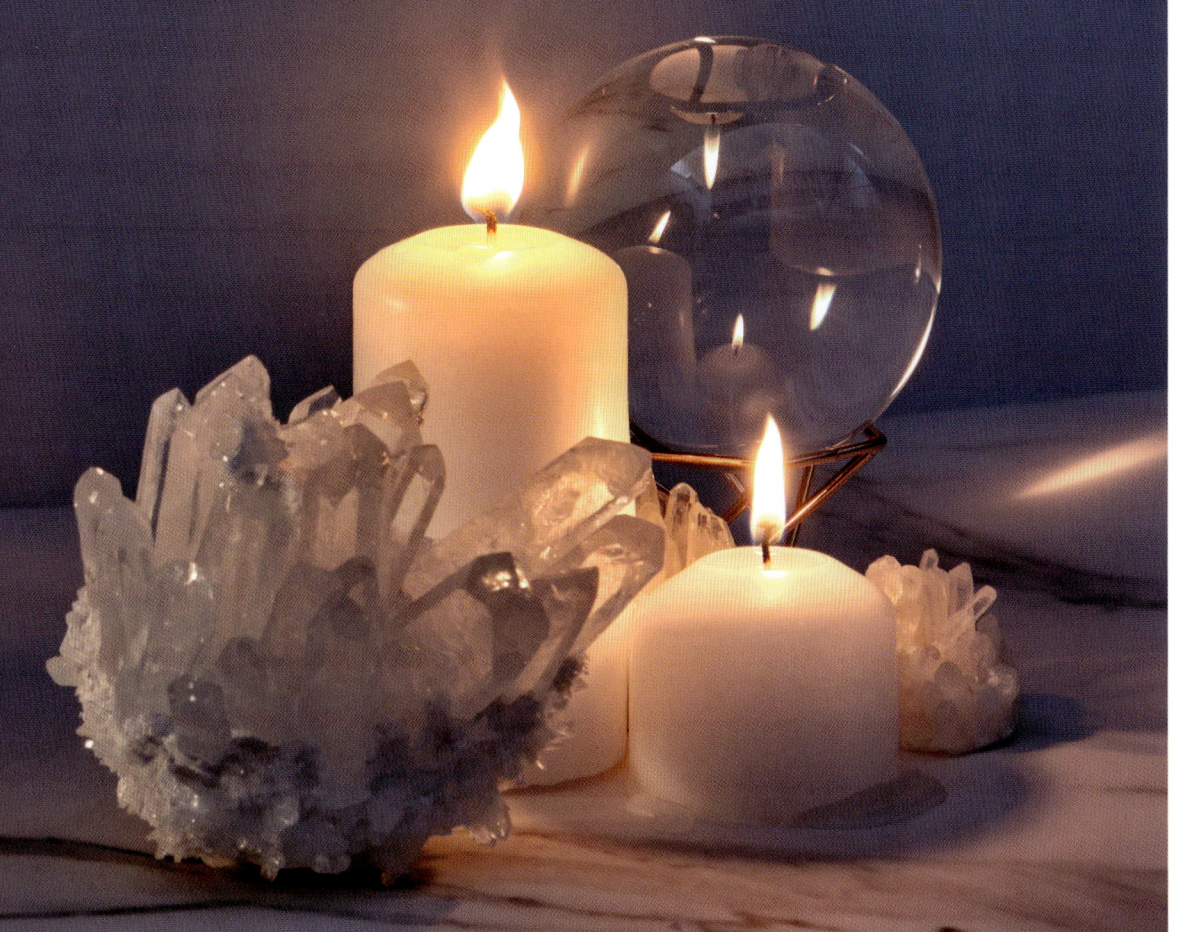

How to Have Better Sex—Now!

A **SPARKLING SEX LIFE IS SOMETHING** we'd all like to have, regardless of age. But as today's leading physicians and sex researchers are discovering, there's a profound link between the female libido and the constantly fluctuating hormones that ovaries produce. Find out how understanding your body's unique chemical balance—during every decade of life—can make the difference between a sex life that's so-so and one that soars.

IN YOUR 40S

The Advantages As women age, they become more clear about what they want, even as estrogen, progesterone, and testosterone begin to drop, says Laura Berman, Ph.D., the author of *Loving Sex: The Book of Joy and Passion*. More good

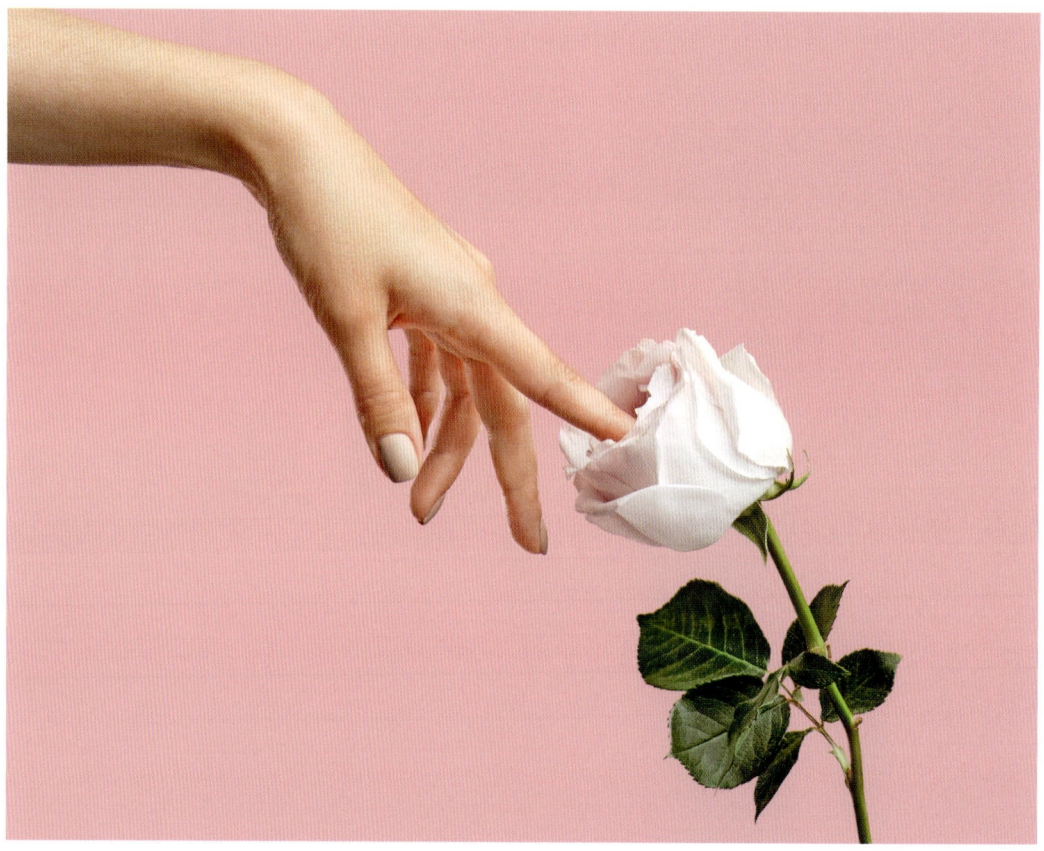

news: Studies have shown that as women age, they become less anxious about their physical "flaws," which eases anxiety in the bedroom.

Female sex drive may actually increase as a woman's sex hormones and fertility decrease in her 40s, according to a University of Texas study. "Women with declining fertility think more about sex, have more frequent and intense sexual fantasies, are more willing to engage in sexual intercourse, and report actually engaging in sexual intercourse more frequently than women of other age groups," the study authors say.

The Challenges After childbirth, testosterone falls to extremely low levels. For nursing moms, the hormone prolactin can suppress ovulation, as well as the production of estrogen and progesterone. All of that combines to make the thought of sex a big fat snore.

"By 40, a woman's testosterone levels will be about half the level they were at 25," says Glenn D. Braunstein, M.D., an endocrinologist and chair of the department of medicine at Cedars-Sinai Medical Center in Los Angeles. And yes, that drop affects libido. For the average woman who enters perimenopause in her 40s, fluctuating estrogen, progesterone, and testosterone levels may put a damper on bedroom bliss.

One suggestion? Masturbation. Regardless of age, the old adage to use it or lose it applies. Just using the equipment you were born with will improve circulation and help balance your hormones. Some doctors recommend low-dose birth control pills to even out estrogen production. Lubricants and estrogen therapies can also help.

IN YOUR 50S, 60S, AND BEYOND

The Advantages "The middle years, between 50 and 65, constitute the apex of adult life," as the late feminist author Gail Sheehy noted in *Sex and the Seasoned Woman*. "For women, the passage to be made is from pleasing to mastery." Mastery is right: The National Survey of Sexual Health and Behavior found 71% of 50-somethings said their last sexual experience resulted in an orgasm.

The Challenges Because of dramatically reduced testosterone and virtually nonexistent estrogen, sex drive drops after menopause. To boost libido, physicians sometimes prescribe very small off-label doses of testosterone along with menopausal hormonal therapy, though there can be side effects and it's not for everyone. Also, the more body fat you have, the less libido-boosting "free-floating" testosterone you have. If you're obese, losing 10% of your total weight can do wonders for your sex drive, found researchers at Duke University Medical Center. Multiple studies have also shown that after just 20 minutes of exercise, blood flow to the genitals increases, resulting in more lubrication, better arousal, and better orgasms.

Orgasms Over 60 "More Satisfying Than Ever"

▶ A survey from the Kinsey Institute in partnership with *Cosmopolitan* found that women over 60 are not only sexually active but many are enjoying the best orgasms of their lives.

The survey tapped a national demographically representative sample of 3,001 women in the U.S. Nearly three-quarters of them reported that age has had no negative impact on the quality of their orgasms, 20% said they are experiencing orgasms that are more satisfying than ever before, and 57% said they reach climax with their partners always or almost always. (Hello, wisdom and improved communication!)

The survey also found that nearly 40% of women over 60 are in the mood for love as often as they were 10 years ago.

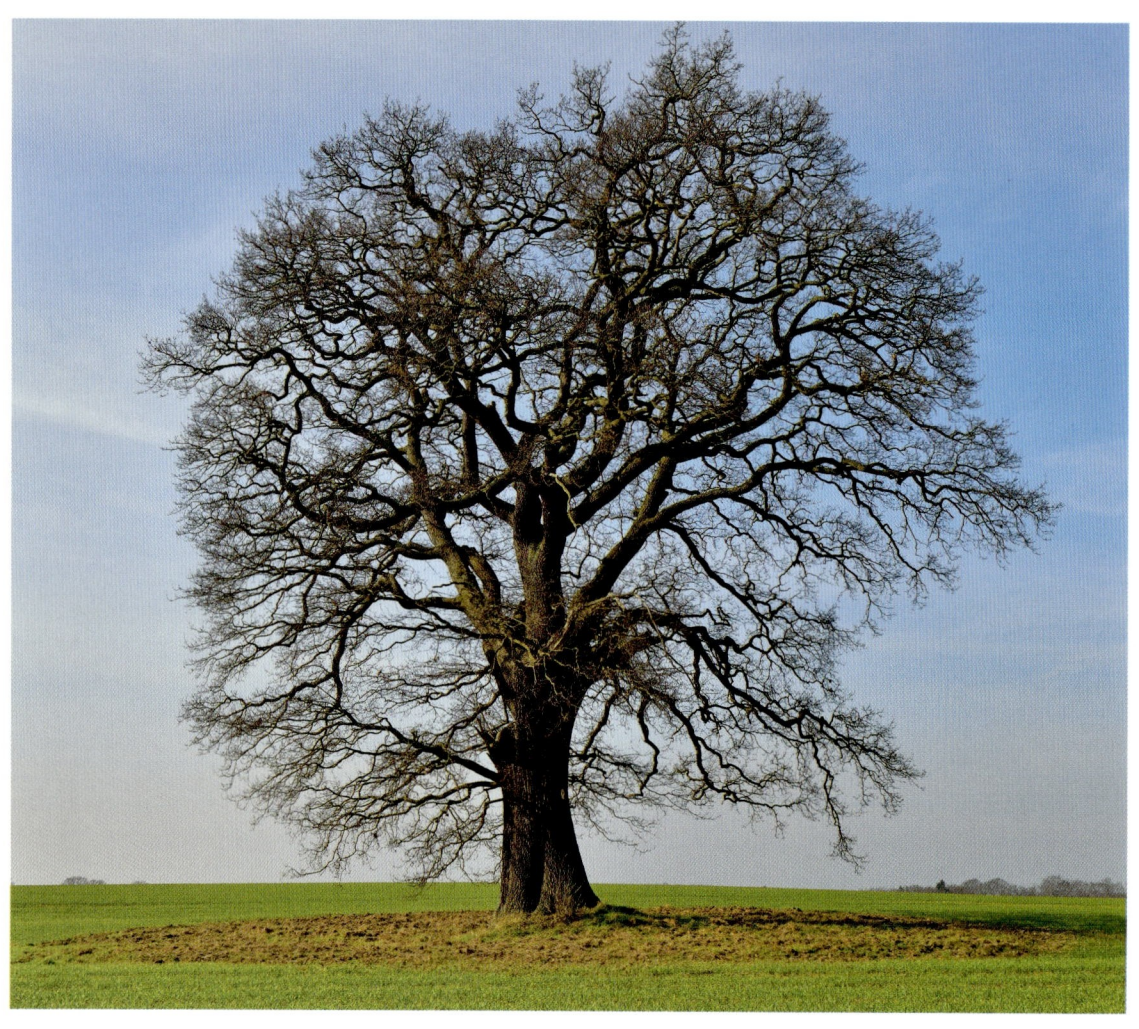

Why Your Sex Drive May Be Slowing

NUMEROUS ISSUES CAN AFFECT YOUR LIBIDO AT ANY age. As you get older, some issues may become more prevalent. Here are some of the most common culprits behind a sexual dry spell:

This is the number one factor that affects libido, experts say. Not only can the daily onslaught of work, money, and relationship worries dampen desire, but stress often starts a negative-feedback loop in which people end up sleeping less, drinking more alcohol (a depressant that impedes sexual function), and skipping self-care, which perpetuates the stress and low libido.

Yes, Older People Get STIs

▶ Older women may be especially vulnerable to sexually transmitted infections. Condoms are less often part of the sexual playbook, and postmenopausal women have vaginal and vulvar tissue that's thin and easier to infect than that of younger women. To prevent STIs, use condoms and dental dams and seriously consider regular screening for STIs.

YOU'RE ON DESIRE-DAMPENING MEDS

An estimated one in eight Americans takes antidepressants, and many don't realize that some types can quash desire. Their effects on libido are "a major reason people stop taking them," says Tami Rowen, M.D., an ob/gyn and an associate professor at the University of California San Francisco. (If you're taking Paxil or Prozac, for example, and are experiencing low libido, ask your doctor about adjusting your dosage or switching to a different antidepressant.) Meds for allergies, diabetes, and high blood pressure can affect sexual desire as well.

YOUR DIET COULD USE A RESET

If you've ever felt bloated and not in the mood after a dinner date that featured heavy food, you know that what you eat can immediately affect your desire. Your nutrition from day to day is important too, says Tameca Harris-Jackson, Ph.D., a sex therapist and director of Hope & Serenity Health Services in Altamonte Springs, Florida. "If blood flow is impeded by a high-sodium or high-sugar diet, there can be difficulty feeling sensation

and having full function of sexual organs."

YOU'RE TIRED

According to a study in the *Journal of Sexual Medicine*, for some women just one more hour of shut-eye can lead to higher levels of sexual desire and better arousal the next day.

YOU HAVE HEALTH CHALLENGES

Chronic pain from arthritis or fibromyalgia, for example, may prevent you from focusing on pleasure cues. Conditions like anxiety and incontinence can also make sex more challenging.

SEX IS UNCOMFORTABLE

Vaginal dryness can happen at any time in life as a result of illnesses like diabetes or autoimmune conditions, medications or cancer treatments, breastfeeding, hormonal contraception, or, significantly, menopause. For more information about vaginal dryness and menopause, see page 93.

Men Slow Down Too

▶ Libido in men is just as complex as it is in women. Some men want sex every day; some are perfectly happy with once every few months. Both patterns are normal. There's a normal decline in the amount of sex most couples have over time, but if you're concerned, here are some considerations.

What He's Going Through

Some think a shift in desire is due to age or low testosterone, but this doesn't match the science; however, there's a strong correlation between low desire and sexual issues like erectile dysfunction, premature ejaculation, and difficulty with orgasm. These challenges can be associated with medical issues and medication side effects, notably blood pressure meds and antidepressants. Anxiety, depression, or severe stress may also block desire. A thorough medical examination can help solve issues.

Talking It Out

Once medical issues are ruled out, the challenge is to get curious instead of defensive. Try to have a conversation while fully clothed about what has changed. Has his work stress gone up? Is he distracted by family needs? Are the two of you fighting a lot? Shifts in your relationship may help sex become a priority again. Counseling with a sex therapist can help these talks. In the end, the more you feel like an intimate team, the better you can work toward a mutual and authentic sexual relationship.

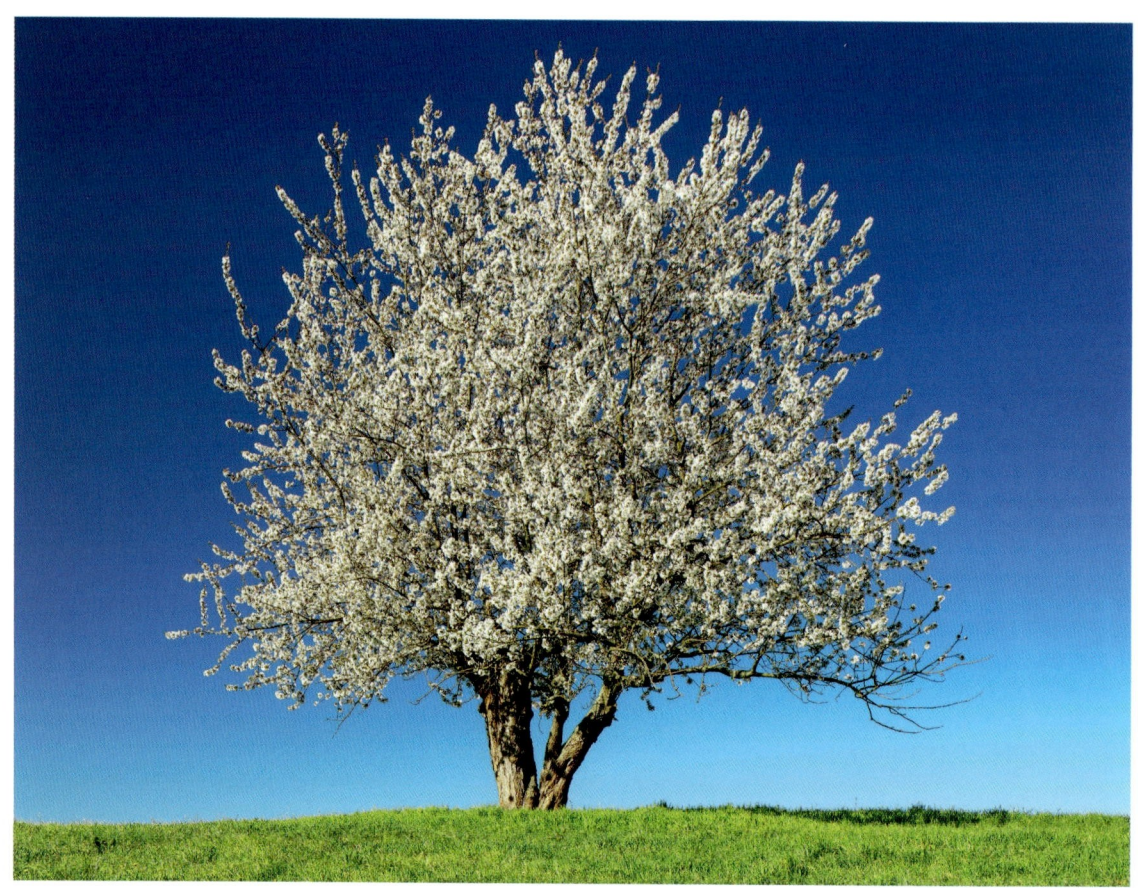

How to Get Your Desire Back

SCIENCE-BACKED STRATEGIES CAN HELP PERK UP a low sex drive. Try these techniques to relight the fire.

BE MORE MINDFUL

Experts theorize that libido could boil down to a balance (or imbalance) in brain chemicals. There are some neurochemicals that get you amped up for sex, like dopamine, oxytocin, and norepinephrine, says Stephanie S. Faubion, M.D., director of the Center for Women's Health at the Mayo Clinic. Then there are others, like opioids and serotonin, that can get in the way and inhibit your excitement.

That's where mindfulness exercises—like focused breathing or meditation—come in. "Being more mindful might alter the balance of brain chemicals in a good way," Dr. Faubion says. One review of research found that mindfulness-based therapy improved sex drive in women. The practice also aids in reducing stress hormones, which are known to cause low libido.

Try 15 to 20 minutes of meditation a day to start. In the heat of the moment, try syncing your breathing with your partner's or focusing on what they smell like, suggests Leah Millheiser, M.D., a physician at the Palo Alto Medical Foundation and cofounder of LegalizeV in California. "This brings you back to the room instead of going through the motions while your brain is somewhere else."

TAKE YOUR TIME

Most people dive right into sex, but at least 15 to 20 minutes of foreplay is crucial for building arousal, says Stephanie Buehler, Psy.D., the director at LearnSexTherapy.com and president of the Buehler Institute.

Once you spend some time kissing and touching, your desire will spike both emotionally and physically. You'll not only feel more connected to your partner, but the vagina will produce lubrication to make sex feel more pleasurable and enjoyable. There's also no shame in using a good lube! All of this boosts your chances of wanting to do it again.

SKIP THE ALCOHOL

While a few glasses of wine can loosen you up and put you in the mood, alcohol actually makes it more difficult for you and your partner to enjoy sex. One study from the University of Missouri at St. Louis found that among 3,000 people who had sex while intoxicated, 11% of them were unable to reach orgasm and 7% had inhibited sexual desire, with 33% of women experiencing some kind of sexual dysfunction after drinking.

Why does this happen? Alcohol is a depressant and slows activity in the part of your nervous system that controls arousal and orgasm, so even if you and your partner have sex, it may not be satisfying. So try skipping or limiting the alcohol on your next date night—it may help you cross the finish line.

STICK TO A WORKOUT ROUTINE

Research has shown that women who do moderate to vigorous aerobic exercise see an increase in libido and sexual performance, says Sherry Ross, M.D., women's sexual health expert and author of *She-ology* and *She-ology: The She-quel*. "During exercise, endorphins—the feel-good hormones—are released," she explains. What's more, "all of those things lend themselves to a woman wanting to engage in sexual activity because she feels good about herself," says Dr. Millheiser. Other research has shown that exercise has a similar effect on men, boosting their ability to get and maintain an erection. "Sex isn't just about desire. It's about body image, self-esteem, and confidence—and exercise boosts all of those."

USE LOTS OF LUBRICANT

Lubricants can be applied on your partner and on the opening of your vagina before intercourse to reduce friction, or you can use a

Zero Libido?

▶ If your libido has lowered and that bothers you, talk to your primary care provider, or an ob/gyn. They may diagnose you with hypoactive sexual desire disorder (HSDD), a condition that occurs for unknown reasons and produces a persistent lack of interest in sexual activity and fantasies about sexual activity that causes personal distress. It affects 12.3% of women between 45 and 65 and 7.4% of women 65 and older. Your doc will ask questions about your medical and sexual history, may perform a physical exam, recommend extra testing to rule out underlying medical issues, and refer you to a specialist before making a diagnosis.

long-acting vaginal moisturizer that alters vaginal tissues by increasing the water content of the cells. Both are available over the counter. Another option is estrogen or non-estrogen prescription treatments. Talk to your doctor about the ways to get back to pleasurable sex.

PRIORITIZE SEX

Pick a day of the week or have a cue that only you two know means sex (something like "I think we need to go out to eat"). The more this intimacy becomes part of your routine, the better. It helps physically too. If you make an active effort to schedule time for sex, you'll also boost pelvic blood flow and vaginal moisture, which leads to increased comfort and (hopefully) pleasure, notes Dr. Faubion.

The Sexual Seesaw

▶ Research found that when a woman's partner has erectile dysfunction, she may have decreased sexual desire or problems with arousal or orgasm. Coincidence or sexual ping-pong? Either way, talking about how each of you feel can help.

Welcome to Menopause

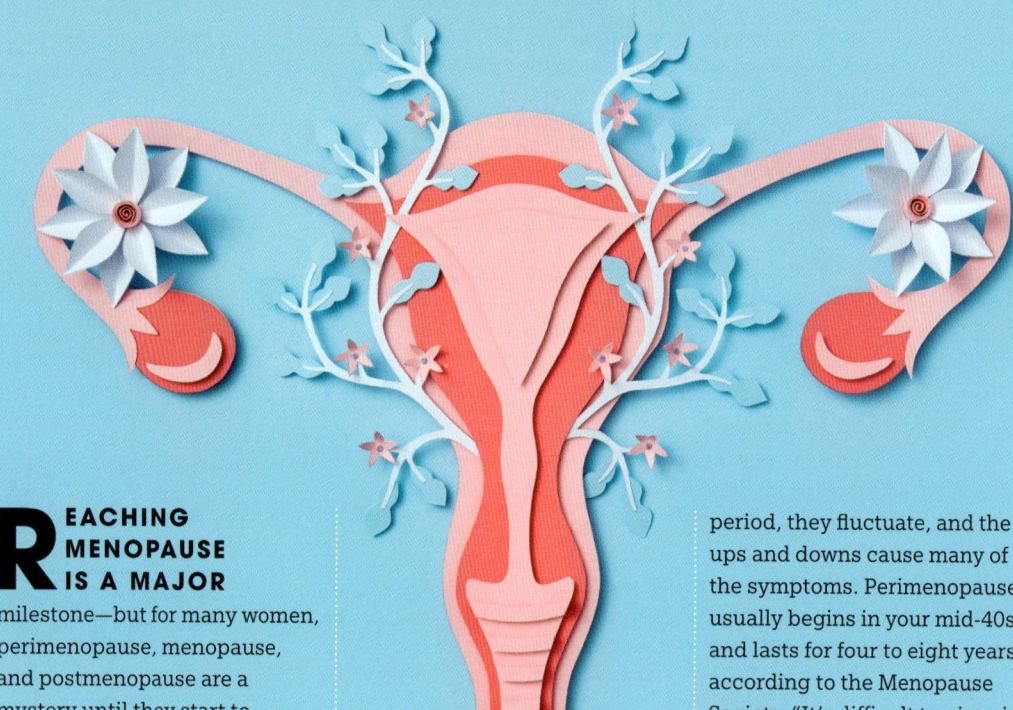

REACHING MENOPAUSE IS A MAJOR milestone—but for many women, perimenopause, menopause, and postmenopause are a mystery until they start to happen. Until recently, public discussion of menopause was virtually nonexistent. Luckily, that's changing, and so is treatment of menopausal symptoms. "Every woman will go through the stages a little differently," says Mary O'Toole, M.D., an ob/gyn at Hoag Hospital in Laguna Hills, California. That said, there are certain things you can expect throughout each phase as your estrogen levels decrease and

your period becomes a thing of the past (which, for many women, is one of the benefits!). There's a lot more to this transition than hot flashes, so let's get started.

PERIMENOPAUSE

This is the first phase when estrogen and progesterone start to decrease over time, explains Dr. O'Toole. But within that

period, they fluctuate, and the ups and downs cause many of the symptoms. Perimenopause usually begins in your mid-40s and lasts for four to eight years, according to the Menopause Society. "It's difficult to pinpoint the onset [of perimenopause], but irregular menstrual cycles may be the initial sign," says O'Toole. You can still get pregnant during this time, so it's important to use contraception if you're not looking to conceive.

What to Expect With estrogen fluctuations, your periods may become irregular (you might even skip one, two, or three months before they restart) and the periods themselves may get longer or shorter, according to the Mayo Clinic. You may also notice your period is heavier than usual, or it could be lighter. "Along with menstrual cycle changes, there may be emotional and psychological changes including anxiety, depression, brain fog, and forgetfulness," says Dr. O'Toole.

MENOPAUSE

A woman has officially reached menopause when she hasn't had her period for 12 consecutive months, notes Dr. O'Toole. This defining moment can happen in your 40s or 50s, but in the U.S., the average age is 51, according to the Mayo Clinic. At this point, estrogen production has drastically decreased and your ovaries have stopped releasing eggs. Menopause isn't so much a phase as it is a line in the sand when your periods stop.

What to Expect Hot flashes are common and they can vary in frequency and duration. Night sweats are hot flashes that happen while you're sleeping. "They may affect sleep and be a source of chronic sleep disturbances, fatigue, or brain fog," says Dr. O'Toole. But they are just one symptom. "Other symptoms that may be present are vaginal dryness, decreased libido, anxiety, and depression." (See p. 92 for relief!)

POSTMENOPAUSE

As the name implies, postmenopause is the time period after a woman has reached menopause, per the Cleveland Clinic. Once you arrive at this stage, you'll be here for the rest of your life. During this time, estrogen levels continue to decline.

What to Expect "Symptoms like hot flashes may gradually diminish," says Dr. O'Toole. "But you may experience vaginal issues like dryness or irritation; some women may also find that intercourse is more painful."

Additionally, postmenopausal women have an increased risk of osteoporosis and heart disease because the decline in estrogen speeds up bone loss. Lower estrogen also impacts the way the body uses calcium and maintains cholesterol levels in the blood.

You may also notice changes to your skin after menopause, says Cynthia Bailey, M.D., a board-certified dermatologist and founder of Dr. Bailey Skin Care. After menopause, skin tends to be more delicate, and can be drier.

How Do You Know You're Menopausal?

▶ Most often, women can tell they're going through perimenopause—the time leading up to menopause— because their periods become irregular. A woman is considered menopausal a year after she has had her final period—it's that simple. After that, she is considered postmenopausal.

While blood work isn't necessary to determine menopausal stages, sometimes your health-care provider may check for an increase in your levels of follicle-stimulating hormone, which increases in the years leading up to menopause. They may also check your levels of estrogen (estradiol), which decreases, to confirm where you are in the menopausal transition.

When you see your doctor, come prepared to discuss the symptoms you're experiencing and any treatments you've tried, from home remedies to mind-body practices to dietary changes. Also, familiarize yourself with your family's health history of various diseases so you can discuss those with your doctor as well. Some menopause treatments and herbal supplements to mitigate symptoms come with health risks and may be best to avoid if, say, breast cancer runs in your family.

4 Myths About Menopause

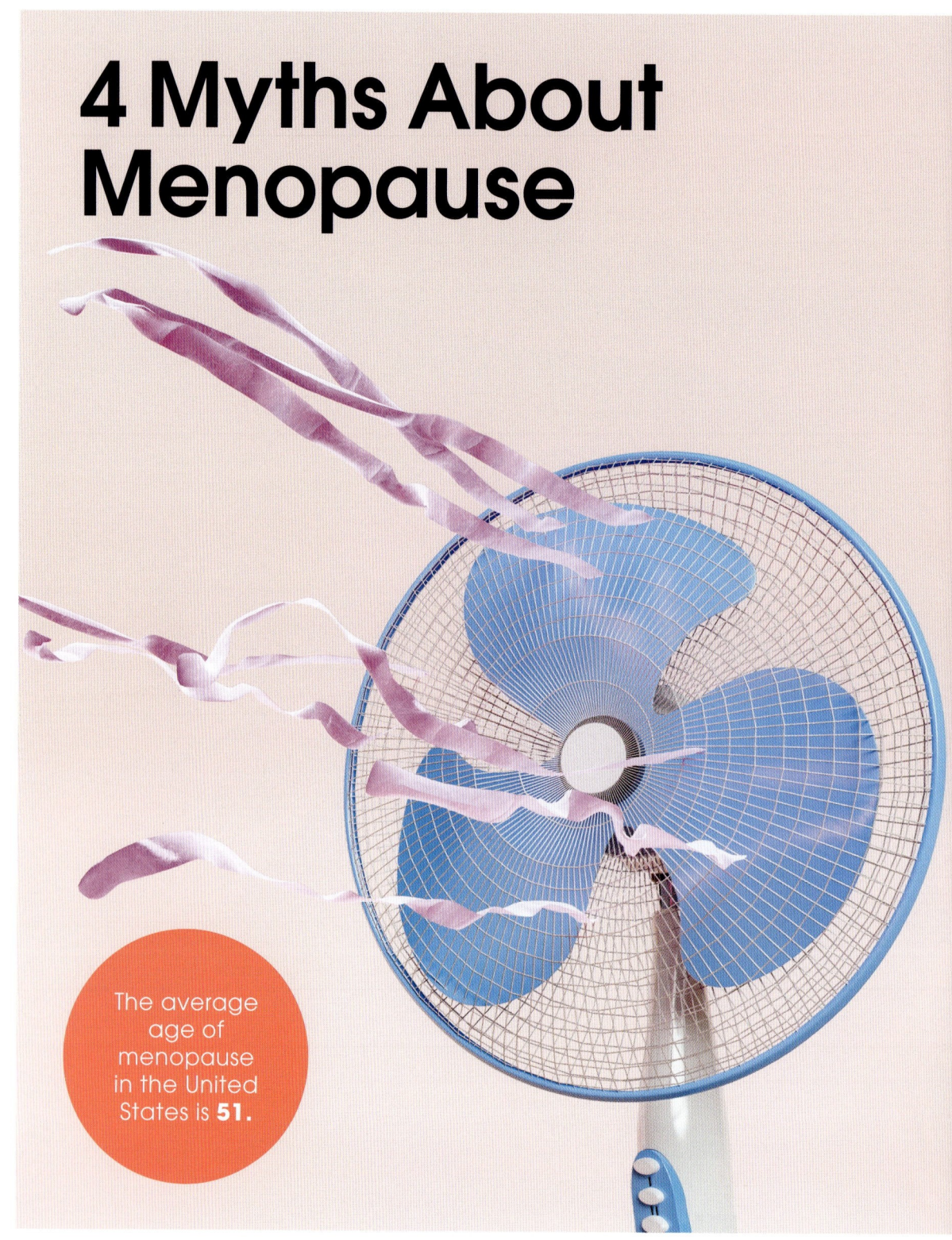

The average age of menopause in the United States is **51.**

1 MENOPAUSE SYMPTOMS DON'T LAST LONG

The menopausal transition is an extended journey, and symptoms can last as long as eight years. The good news is that some of the worst ones (like hot flashes, night sweats, and sleep disruptions) get better over time and usually go away as the body adjusts to lower levels of estrogen and progesterone, says JoAnn E. Manson, M.D., a professor of medicine at Harvard Medical School and chief of the division of preventive medicine at Brigham and Women's Hospital in Boston. Vaginal dryness and bladder issues can persist if they're untreated but they usually improve with medication, specifically vaginal estrogen, says Mary Jane Minkin, M.D., a clinical professor of obstetrics, gynecology, and reproductive sciences at the Yale School of Medicine.

3 SEX ALWAYS HURTS

While half of women say menopause has impacted their sex lives, 43% say they're having the same amount of sex as usual and 50% say sex is never painful, according to Bonafide Health's State of Menopause survey. And many symptoms that make sex less enjoyable can be treated. Hormone replacement therapy may boost libido, and "vaginal estrogen, vaginal dilators, and a good lube can help treat painful penetration, vaginal dryness, and bladder issues," Sherry Ross, M.D., women's sexual health expert and author, says. If continuing to have sex is important to you, she recommends that you "give your vagina a voice so you can continue to have a healthy sexual relationship during perimenopause and menopause." (See more on p. 92.)

2 THE SYMPTOMS ARE AWFUL

Menopause may not be a joyride, but it isn't an automatic trip to hot-flash hell either. About 85% of women have symptoms during menopause, but those vary widely in frequency and intensity, and some of them go away in five or sometimes fewer years, according to the Cleveland Clinic. For example, "night sweats wake some women up and they can't go back to sleep. Others stick a fan on themselves and sleep through the night and they're fine," says Natasha Diaz, M.D., founder of Roots Health DPC in Oak Park, Illinois. Only about 20% of women will have hot flashes and night sweats so disruptive that they will need to ask their doctors for prescription medications, says Dr. Manson. Dr. Diaz encourages women to tell their health-care providers about any bothersome menopausal symptoms (including bladder problems and vaginal dryness, which can lead to painful sex) because many medications, therapies, and lifestyle changes—often simple ones—can go a long way in easing symptoms. "Women don't have to live with those things," she says.

4 NATURAL REMEDIES ARE JUST AS EFFECTIVE AS MEDICATIONS

They are not. The research on their effectiveness is mixed, and some supplements, like evening primrose oil and kava, can be downright dangerous. A few, however, could prove beneficial or at least harmless. For one, melatonin supplements can help with certain sleep problems, according to the Mayo Clinic, and the herb black cohosh has shown some ability to help with hot flashes, the Menopause Society reports, though people with liver problems shouldn't take it. Many supplements in the U.S., however, are poorly regulated, so talk to your doctor first.

Three More Common Symptoms of Menopause

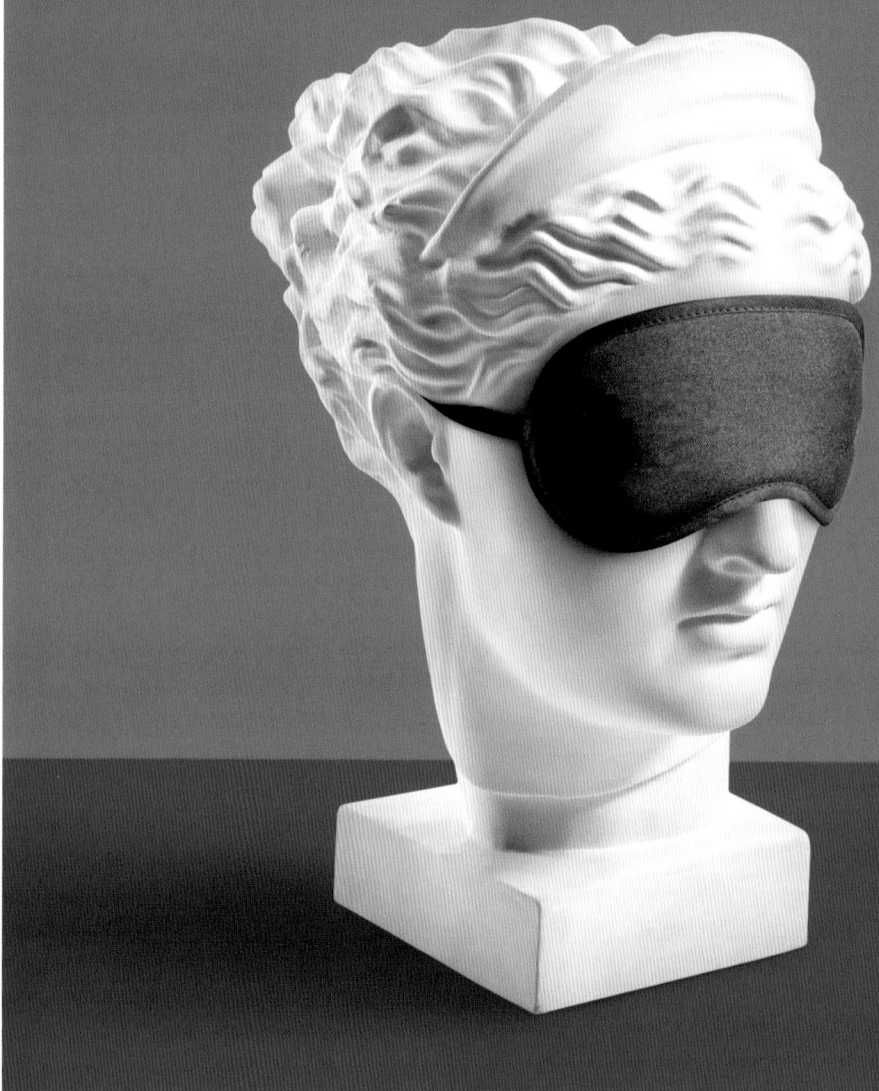

THE EFFECTS
OF DECLINING
ESTROGEN CAN
include thinning hair, heart palpitations, dizziness, and brain fog, as well as hot flashes and vaginal dryness, which we've discussed on the previous pages. Here are three more common menopause symptoms and how you can cope with them.

A BIGGER BELLY

Yes, your body may look different in your 50s than it did in your 30s. The bodily changes you are experiencing are real—even if you don't put on pounds, weight is often redistributed to your midsection. Menopause may contribute to this: As estrogen levels decline during perimenopause, your body starts shifting and fat may move to your belly rather than your hips and thighs, explains Stephanie S. Faubion, M.D., M.B.A., medical director of the Menopause Society and director of the Mayo Clinic Center for Women's Health. This is concerning because fat around the midsection is a risk factor for heart disease (the number one killer of women) even for those whose weight is in the normal range. If you're concerned about your weight or an accumulation of fat around your middle, increase your physical activity and follow a healthy eating plan to help.

MOOD CHANGES

Studies suggest that up to 68% of perimenopausal women report heightened depressive symptoms (compared with around a third of premenopausal women). Some women may become mildly irritable, while others suddenly feel sad or anxious or experience full-blown depression even if they've never had mental health struggles before. If you're feeling depressed or anxious, let your doctor know. The Menopause Society guidelines recommend psychotherapy and/or antidepressants and note that for some women HRT may help.

SLEEP PROBLEMS

About half of women going through perimenopause complain of poor sleep. Cooling pajamas and sheets could make night sweats more bearable, and a meditation app might be the ticket to deeper, sleep-inducing relaxation. Your doctor may recommend a prescription medication, HRT, or over-the-counter supplements like melatonin, but don't take anything on your own unless you run it by your health-care provider.

Is There Such a Thing as Male Menopause?

▶ In a word, no. The phrase is sometimes used to describe the slow decline in testosterone levels that occurs in men over many decades. But unlike women, for whom the ability to reproduce grinds to a halt at menopause, older men often have testosterone levels that are high enough to father children in their 70s or 80s.

UTIs and Uncomfortable Vaginal Changes? Yes, They're Treatable

▶ The genitourinary syndrome of menopause (GSM, for short) is a common affliction, consisting of a constellation of symptoms brought on by declining estrogen levels during the menopausal transition. The term GSM was adopted in 2014 to replace what used to be called vulvovaginal atrophy.

Symptoms of GSM may include vaginal dryness, burning, and irritation; sexual discomfort due to lack of lubrication and dry genital tissues, urinary urgency, pain during urination, or recurrent urinary tract infections. These can be treated with hormonal interventions, nonhormonal oral medications, and other nonhormonal remedies (such as vaginal moisturizers and lubricants).

The HRT Confusion

IN RECENT DECADES, PUBLIC OPINION ABOUT hormone replacement therapy (HRT) has swung in both directions, making it an utterly confusing issue for many women and even some doctors. Some of this stems from the conflicting information that's been circulating regarding the risks versus benefits. And some of the confusion relates to evolving scientific findings about HRT.

One of the things that sparked widespread fear of HRT was the original Women's Health Initiative (WHI) study, which was designed to evaluate the benefits and risks of hormone therapy in terms of its potential to prevent chronic age-related diseases. It was not designed to examine the use of hormone therapy to ease menopausal symptoms. In 2002, part of the WHI study was halted early because women who were taking HRT (estrogen and progestin) were found to have an increased risk for heart disease, breast cancer, stroke, and other scary health conditions. After that, many women avoided HRT even if their symptoms were driving them mad. Those findings were later disputed when researchers drilled down and discovered that they applied only to older women (age 65 and up), a key detail that got lost in the messaging.

Thanks to additional research, it is now widely accepted that for healthy women under age 60 or who are fewer than 10 years out from menopause, the risks of HRT are low, and it can safely provide relief from menopausal symptoms like hot flashes, night sweats, and vaginal/bladder issues (also called GSM, see page 93), says Sherry Ross, M.D., an ob/gyn and author of *She-ology: The Definitive Guide to Women's Intimate Health*. When it's used for the shortest possible time at the lowest effective dose, Dr. Ross adds, "the benefits of HRT often outweigh the risks when it comes to quality of life." HRT can help minimize estrogen-deficiency-affected health issues such as osteoporosis, dementia, and heart disease. On the other hand, women with a history of blood clots, heart disease, liver disease, or certain cancers may be advised to avoid HRT. Every woman should speak to her doctor to evaluate her individual risk factors.

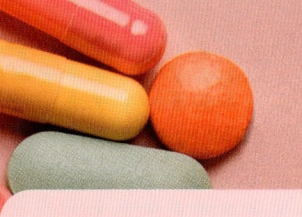

What's the Deal with Hot Flashes?

▶ **Millions of perimenopausal and postmenopausal women tough it out because they're worried that treating hot flashes with HRT is dangerous and they're convinced the flashes won't last long. Here's a reality check:**

How Long Do Hot Flashes Last?

Hot flashes last longer than was previously thought—some women experience them for seven to 10 years. And emerging evidence shows that hot flashes may not be harmless but may be associated with potentially life-threatening heart damage. In a 20-year study of more than 3,000 menopausal women, those who had frequent or persistent hot flashes had a dramatic increase in factors associated with heart disease, which may explain why stroke risk doubles in the 10 years after menopause.

How Do Hot Flashes Affect My Heart Rate and Blood Pressure?

Every time you have a hot flash, your heart rate and blood pressure increase. In other words, hot flashes make your heart work harder. It also appears that they cause

an inflammatory response, which can damage blood vessels. Add to this a hot-flash-induced elevation of LDL ("bad" cholesterol), and it's no wonder multiple studies show that women who have hot flashes are far more likely to have damaged blood vessels than those who don't, even when other risk factors are considered.

What Can I Do to Ease a Hot Flash?

If you're one of the 80% of perimenopausal or postmenopausal women who are experiencing hot flashes and you're concerned about your heart, it's important to lose excess weight, keep exercising, don't smoke, and eat healthily. But you also may want to rethink the "tough it out" approach to hot flashes. Since there are safe, effective hormonal and nonhormonal options that can ease them (see below), there's no reason to suffer—and there are now

compelling reasons to reduce the heat. Try these methods:

- **Estrogen therapy**
  This can be oral or transdermal (patches, gels, creams, sprays).

- **Nonhormonal Rx options**
  Veozah is a hormone-free treatment for moderate/severe hot flashes and night sweats. Paroxetine (Brisdelle) is an oral SSRI (selective serotonin reuptake inhibitor) that's been approved by the FDA for menopause-related symptoms. Other meds used off-label for hot flashes include gabapentin (an antiseizure med), clonidine (a blood pressure med), and oxybutynin (a bladder drug).

- **Natural remedies**
  There's some evidence that isoflavones (phytoestrogens) such as S-equol supplements can ease hot flashes.

Managing Menopause

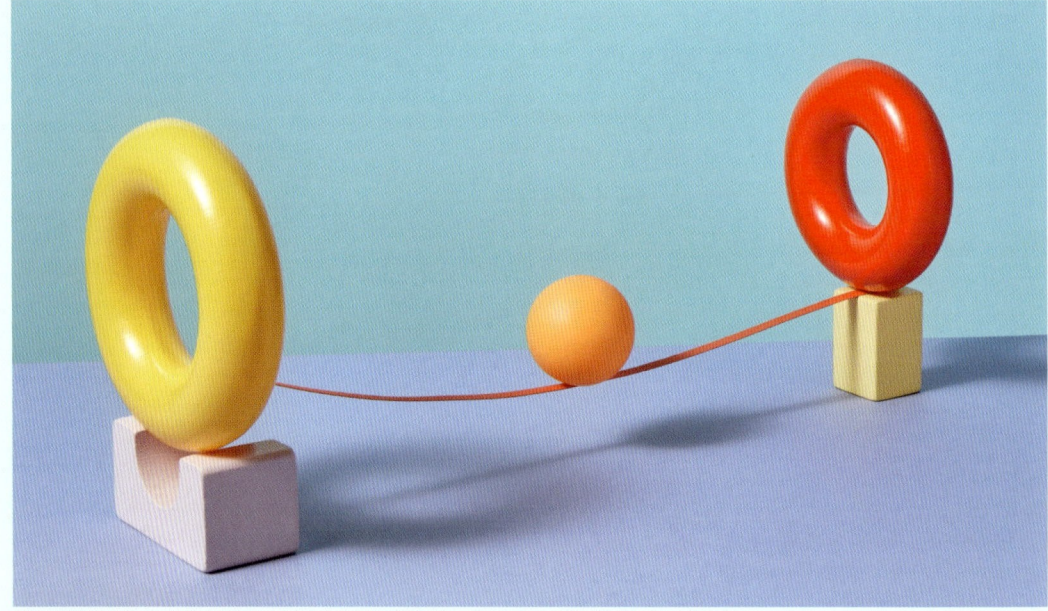

MENOPAUSE ITSELF ISN'T TREATED, BUT the symptoms can be treated successfully," says women's health expert Jennifer Wider, M.D. "Finding the right treatment depends on the symptoms and sometimes a little trial and error."

Some women choose to forgo treatment, either because their symptoms are not severe enough to require it, or they dissipate on their own. But others may choose medication, lifestyle changes, physical activity, natural and herbal remedies, or a combination thereof. "These options are not always easy," says Ann Cha, M.D., a board-certified ob/gyn in Johns Creek, Georgia. "For example, if you practice mindfulness or self-care, those aren't as easy as taking a pill." But she notes that lifestyle changes like these have other long-term benefits aside from symptom relief. "When you take care of yourself, you improve your long-term health," she says.

Here are some of the most common treatment options. Ask your doctor which options may be the best—and safest—for you:

MEDICATIONS
Hormone replacement therapy (HRT) You know by now that taking estrogen or a combination of estrogen and progesterone via pill, vaginal insert, or skin patch helps stabilize your hormone levels, and can help alleviate hot flashes, vaginal dryness, night sweats, insomnia, and other

symptoms, as well as lessen your risk for osteoporosis, heart disease, and dementia. However, those aren't the only options. Some doctors also prescribe low-dose testosterone, especially to perimenopausal women whose testosterone levels are way out of balance with estrogen. And hormone therapy isn't for everyone. It may come with an increased risk of certain types of cancer, blood clots, heart attack, and stroke. Here are some other options.

Low-dose antidepressants (selective serotonin reuptake inhibitors, or SSRIs) These medications may help reduce the frequency and severity of hot flashes while also helping with mood swings.

Vaginal estrogen Applying topical estrogen to the vagina via a ring, tablet, or cream may help remedy vaginal dryness and reduce urinary tract infections.

NATURAL REMEDIES

Supplements Adding calcium and vitamin D supplements to your daily nutritional regimen can help keep your bones strong.

Lubricant An over-the-counter lube can help with vaginal dryness.

Acupuncture Research is inconclusive, but many women find that this ancient practice alleviates menopausal symptoms such as hot flashes, insomnia, and mood swings.

Cognitive behavioral therapy (CBT) Dr. Wider recommends therapy for any mood issues. Studies also note that CBT may reduce depressive feelings and improve sleep.

LIFESTYLE ADJUSTMENTS

Prioritizing sleep Good sleep habits may increase the chance of getting adequate, restful slumber even if you're affected by symptoms like night sweats.

Relaxation techniques Deep-breathing practices, meditation, and other mindfulness practices may help alleviate menopausal symptoms, such as anxiety, irritability, and depression.

Exercising regularly Physical activity helps prevent weight gain and protects against osteoporosis. It also can help improve your mood and alleviate anxiety.

REMEMBER: It's important to discuss your personal and family health history with your doctor before choosing any treatment.

The Upside of Menopause

▶ There are many benefits associated with reaching the north side of this reproductive milestone. Some women are thrilled to say goodbye (for good!) to monthly cramps, mood swings, irregular bleeding, and hormonal headaches. And some are delighted to no longer worry about accidentally becoming pregnant.

There's even something called menopausal zest, as cultural anthropologist Margaret Mead noted in writings—a state that may involve a surge of energy and/or creativity, a newfound sense of liberation, or enhanced wisdom and clarity, among other perks. So consider this new change as an opportunity to thrive.

Skincare for the Ages

TIME HAS A WAY OF CHANGING JUST ABOUT everything—including our complexions. In our 20s and 30s, our skin has needs that are very different than it has when we are over 40. And while the thought of sifting through all the products promising to be the fountain of youth might be overwhelming, there are simple strategies you can use to keep your skin healthy through the years.

"It's good to understand the skin's natural aging process and what ingredients can help maintain and boost your skin's natural glow through each decade," explains Nazanin Saedi, M.D., F.A.A.D., a board-certified laser surgery and cosmetic dermatologist.

You'll find that your skin routines need to evolve as you get older, starting with prevention of problems and moving to rejuvenation, then to minimizing the visual

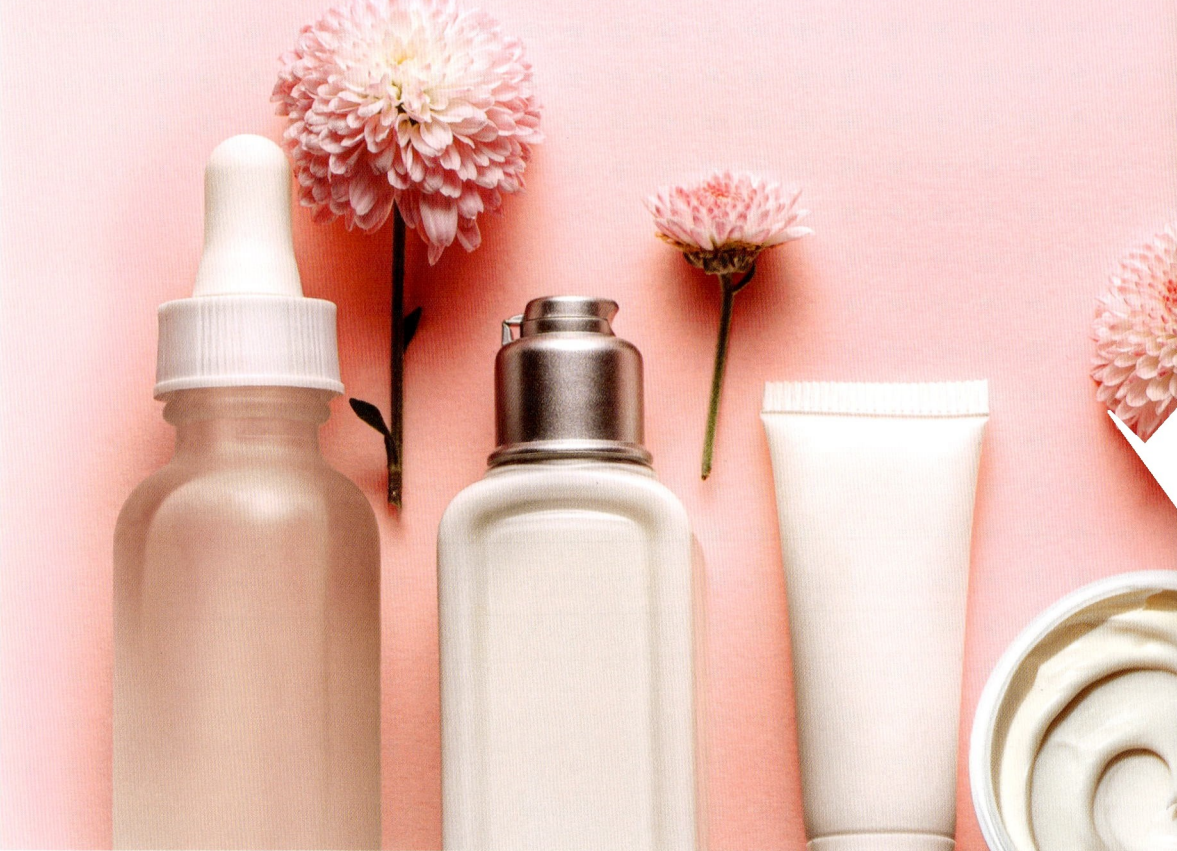

effects of aging. In addition to washing your face twice a day, consider adding these elements into your routine, if you haven't already.

IN YOUR 40S

Prevention and rejuvenation

No matter your age, the best way to avoid or delay skin issues such as skin cancer, wrinkles, dryness, and loss of firmness is to wear sunscreen every day to protect against UV damage (the main cause of both skin cancer and visible signs of aging), Dr. Saedi says.

(See Practice Safe Sun on page 103 for more on SPF.) It's also important in your 40s to introduce a retinol or a retinoid to your routine if you haven't yet. These vitamin A derivatives "will help increase cell turnover and collagen production," Dr. Saedi adds.

"Our 40s are when we usually first notice loss of firmness and elasticity in the skin, due to the drop in collagen production," says Karan Lal, D.O., F.A.A.D., a double board-certified dermatologist based in Scottsdale, Arizona. "This is a good time to start

The Nail File: Fixing Brittleness

▶ Like skin, nails get drier with age, which can lead to brittle, peeling, or splitting nails. What to do? Steer clear of alcohol-based hand sanitizers, which can be dehydrating, and avoid acetone-based polish removers. Wear gloves when you're washing the dishes, and apply a hand cream that contains lanolin, lactic acid, or urea after washing your hands. Taking a biotin supplement (2.5 mg) on a daily basis may improve brittle nails.

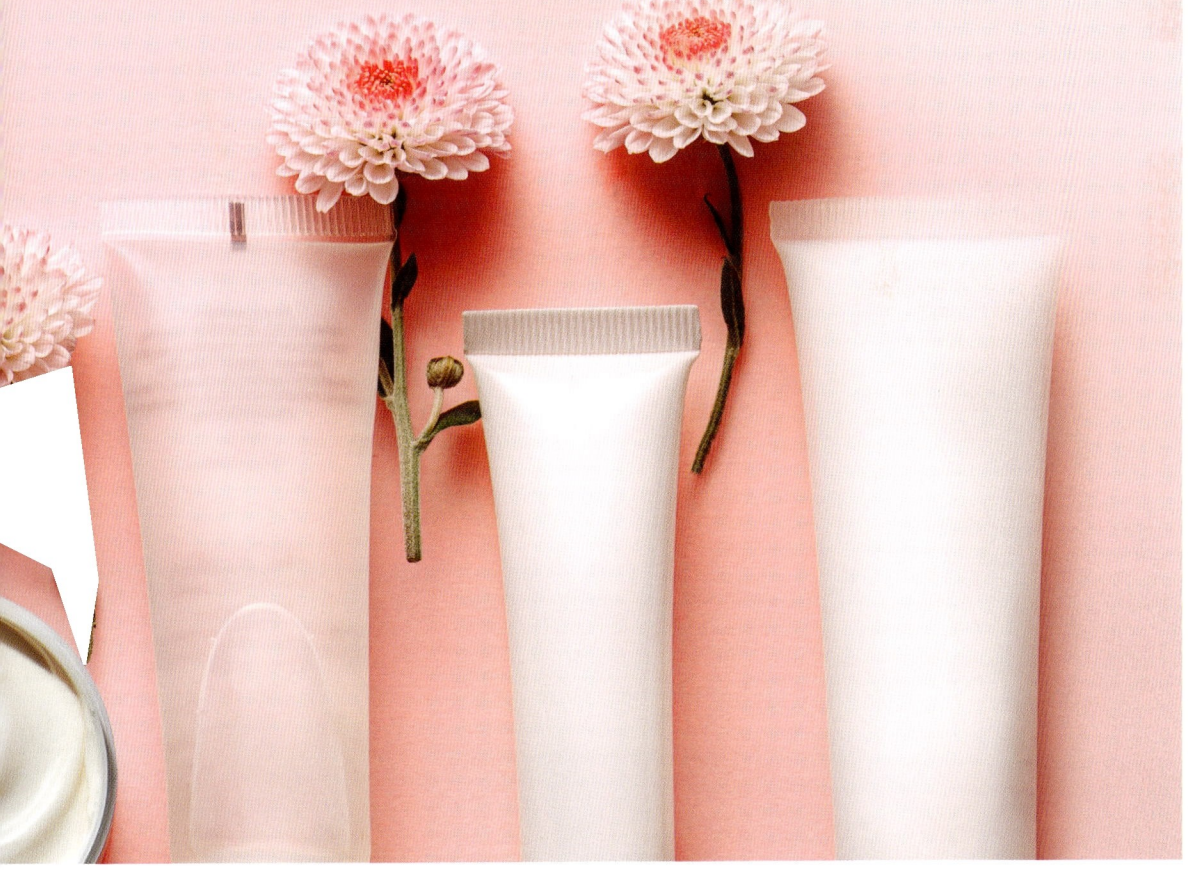

using products with growth factors to help rejuvenate and renew the skin." Growth factors are proteins that help support collagen production, which can help firm as well as tighten skin.

Repairing

New skin issues that appear in your 50s include dullness, age spots, and hyperpigmentation, says Dr. Lal. Good news: A quality vitamin C product will address all these concerns while contributing to a brighter complexion. Vitamin C is a powerful antioxidant that "fights free radical damage and hyperpigmentation and is overall very reparative for the skin," Dr. Lal says. These products tend to be most potent and stable in serum form, especially when combined with ingredients like vitamin E and ferulic acid. For best results, continue to use growth factors while introducing vitamin C.

During these years, skin also tends to skew more toward the sensitive end of the spectrum for many women due to slower estrogen production, Dr. Saedi adds. Use gentle products and ingredients that work for you.

Try an At-Home Facial Massage

▶ Add some pampering to your skincare routine, relieve tension in your face, and give yourself a healthy glow by treating yourself to a feel-good at-home facial massage.

Facial massage is a general term that refers to rubbing and manipulation of the skin and muscles of the face, says Joshua Zeichner, M.D., associate professor of dermatology and the director of cosmetic and clinical research in dermatology at Mount Sinai Hospital in New York City. "This can be done with your fingers or different types of tools or electronic devices."

Massaging can improve blood circulation in the skin, says Ramya Garlapati, M.D., board-certified dermatologist from California. "By stimulating blood flow, you can promote the appearance of a more glowing complexion."

Here are a few techniques, according to expert tutorials, you can try at home as you create your favorite facial massage routine:

- **Use your palms and fingertips to massage the sides of your face, starting at your chin and moving up toward your forehead. Then slide your hands back down.**

- **Use your index and middle fingers to press under your cheekbones. Start at the center of your face and move toward your temples.**

- **Use a circular motion to rub your fingers into your temples.**

- **Press and glide your ring fingers into your brow bone. Move from the inner** to the outer corner. Then do the same movement underneath your eyes.

- **Using your thumb and first finger, start at the outer corners of your eyebrows. Gently pinch your eyebrows as you move to the inner corner.**

- **Press your fingers into the center of your brows. Glide them up toward your hairline. Then move your fingers toward your temples.**

- **Press into your jaw as you move your fingers from the outside of your jaw toward your chin.**

- **Use the outside of your pinky fingers to press into your neck, starting at the top and moving downward.**

IN YOUR 60S AND BEYOND

Hydration

After age 60, skin is less efficient at retaining moisture and tends to appear drier because of lower estrogen levels. "Over time, your oil glands will produce less oil. This oil, called sebum, helps protect and moisturize your skin," explains Dr. Saedi, who recommends focusing on hydration at this age.

For optimal skin hydration and a boost of moisture, look for products that contain hyaluronic acid. This powerhouse ingredient "helps hydrate your skin by attracting water into it," Dr. Lal says. "It's going to give your skin that plump, youthful look."

Skincare Essentials at a Glance

▶ **When choosing skincare products, look for these active ingredients:**

Hyaluronic Acid
Benefits: Moisturizing

Niacinamide
Benefits: Brightening, eases inflammation, can minimize pores

Peptides
Benefits: Firming, smoothing, can reduce fine lines, can improve elasticity

Retinol
Benefits: Can reduce fine lines and wrinkles, smoothing

Vitamin C
Benefits: Brightening, smoothing, can reduce fine lines, eases sun and pollution damage

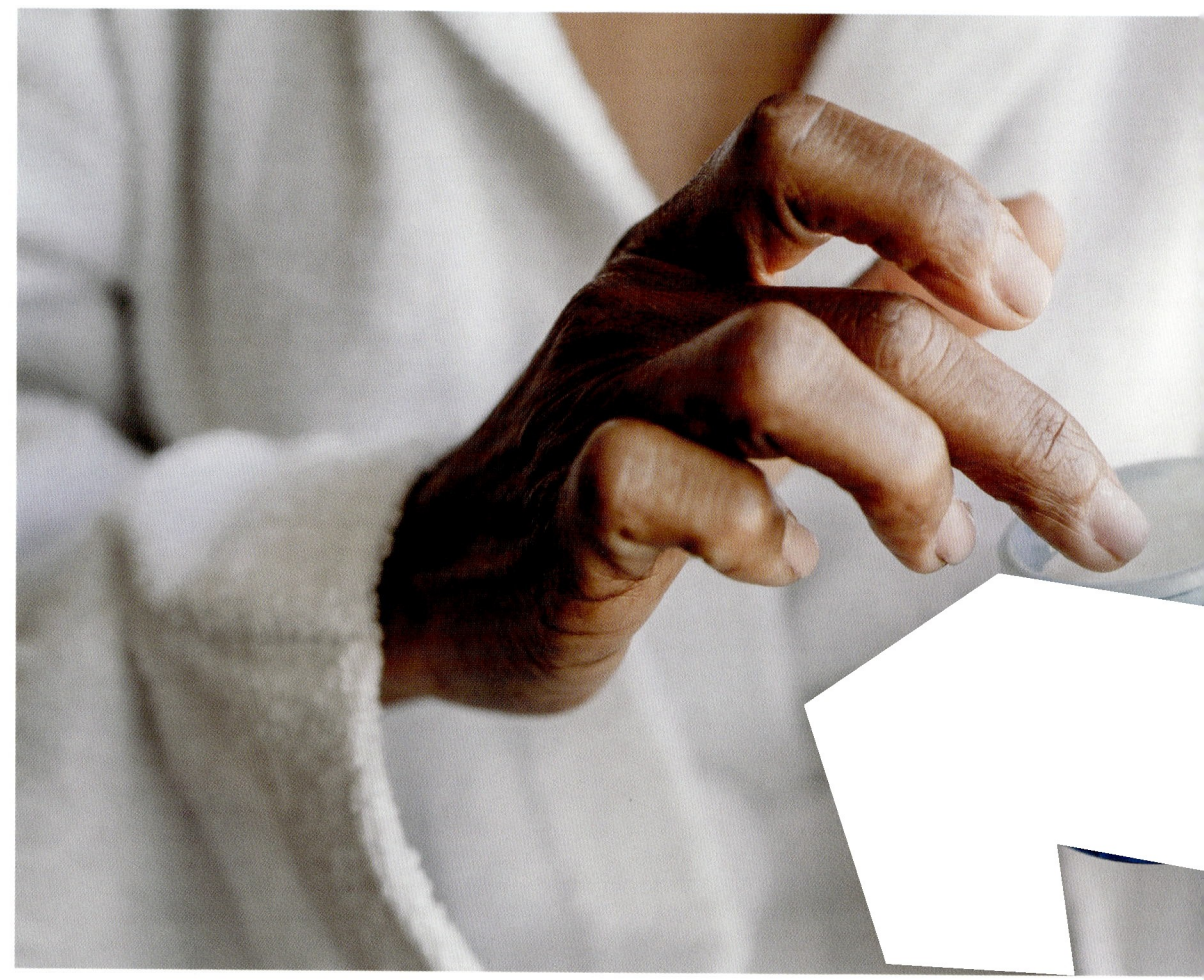

Get Resilient Skin

AS WE GET OLDER, CELLS IN THE THREE MAIN LAYERS OF skin—the epidermis, dermis, and hypodermis—don't clear out damage and make repairs the way they used to. By our mid-40s, our skin tears more easily and forms wrinkles.

"If we don't invest in fixing the machinery that turns over the skin, it goes to sleep," says Abigail Waldman, M.D., medical director of the Mohs and Dermatologic Surgery Center at Brigham and Women's Hospital and an assistant professor at Harvard Medical School. Here's how to wake up your skin again.

BUILD MORE RESILIENT SKIN

The primary method for restoring skin's natural resilience is actually to injure it by using retinoids and processes like microneedling to stress skin and instigate cell turnover.

Retinoids, typically used in facial creams, essentially reawaken your skin's cellular-turnover machinery, which can then strengthen the skin's protective function, limit moisture loss, and protect collagen.

Procedures like chemical

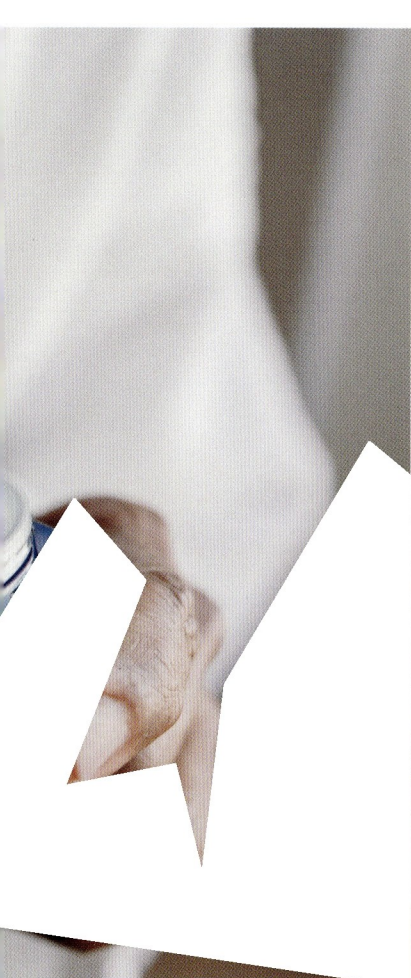

peels, microneedling, and microdermabrasion lead to tiny injuries in the outer layers of the skin, creating more collagen and elastin. It's like exercise, Dr. Waldman says: "To build muscle strength, you're creating tiny injuries your body will fix and make stronger."

PRACTICE SAFE SUN

Applying sunscreen seems like it should be a no-brainer. Slather it on and repeat every few hours. Easy peasy, right?

Turns out, there is a *right* way to apply sunscreen so that it's effective. When you do use it correctly, you'll protect your skin from the sun's harmful UV (ultraviolet) rays, reducing your risk of sunburn, skin cancer, and premature signs of aging. No wonder Claire Chang, M.D., a board-certified cosmetic dermatologist at UnionDerm in New York, says that sunscreen and SPF is "the most crucial step of your regular skincare routine."

CHOOSE THE RIGHT SUNSCREEN

"The best sunscreen is the one that you will use regularly and remember to reapply," says Dr. Chang. Here are the things to look for:

SPF 30 or higher No amount of SPF (sun protection factor) can filter out 100% of UV rays, says Dr. Chang, but she recommends a minimum of SPF 30 and ideally, SPF 50 or higher—especially if you're spending lots of time outdoors.

"Broad spectrum" on the label Broad spectrum indicates that a sunscreen protects the skin from both UVA and UVB rays. "UVA is primarily responsible for tanning and premature skin aging while UVB can cause sunburns," Dr. Chang says. However, both UVA and UVB exposure can lead to skin cancer, so it's crucial to choose a "broad spectrum" sunscreen that protects against both.

Water-resistant formulas If you'll be swimming or sweating a lot, go for a water-resistant sunscreen. "It stays effective for 40 minutes in the water and should be reapplied every 40 minutes," Dr. Chang says. "'Very water-resistant' sunscreen stays effective for 80 minutes in the water, at which time it should be reapplied."

Mineral blockers Both Dr. Chang and Orit Markowitz, M.D., F.A.A.D., a board-certified dermatologist and founder of OptiSkin, recommend mineral over chemical sunscreens because they're less likely to cause irritation and they're effective immediately upon application. (Chemical sunscreens need some time to be absorbed into the skin before they're fully effective.)

Mineral blockers typically contain zinc oxide or titanium dioxide, which sit on the skin and act as barriers that block UV rays. Chemical sunscreens, on the other hand, contain filters like octisalate or avobenzone, which penetrate the skin and protect it by absorbing UV rays.

Other products containing SPF Plenty of products, like moisturizers and lip balms, contain SPF. Experts agree that sunscreen offers the best protection, but products with SPF 30 can be good options.

SPF Indoors— Really?

▶ Yes, many skincare experts recommend wearing SPF even when you're inside or in a car. Harmful UV rays can come through windows, and research has linked blue light from screens with skin aging.

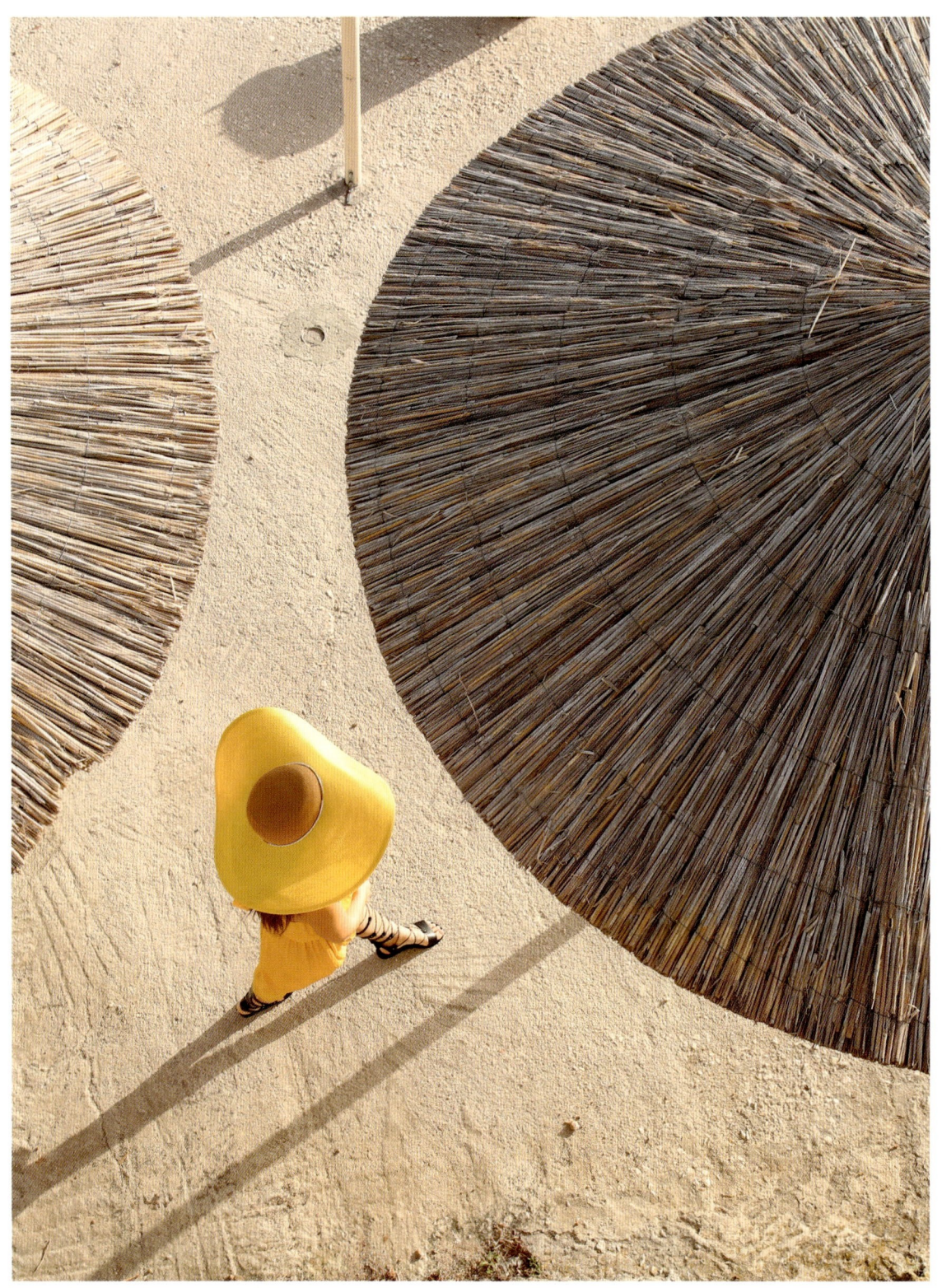

HOW TO APPLY SUNSCREEN

1 **Start with a thick base layer on any skin exposed to sun.**
As a rule of thumb, the Skin Cancer Foundation recommends using a shot glass-size amount of sunscreen to cover the entire body, which equates to about a half-teaspoon dollop to protect the face and neck specifically.

2 **For your face, apply sunscreen at the right time.**
Sunscreen should be the last step in your morning skincare routine before you apply makeup. That means you want to put it on right after you've applied serum and moisturizer.
To simplify your routine, you can opt for a face moisturizer with SPF—just make sure it's at least SPF 30 and carefully apply it the same way you would sunscreen.

3 **Spread it out evenly.**
Use more than you think you'll need, Dr. Chang says, and make sure to spread it evenly.

4 **Cover often-forgotten areas.**
Be sure to protect your hairline and part line, your hands, neck, the tops of your feet, around your eyes, ears, and lips. Lip balms with SPF 30 and above can protect lips too.

5 **Let it sink in before sun exposure.**
This is especially true for chemical sunscreens, which need time to be absorbed before they're fully effective. Wait 15 to 30 minutes before stepping outside.

6 **Reapply often.**
"Sunscreens lose their efficacy with time," Dr. Chang says. You need to reapply at least every two hours—or every 90 minutes, if you can. Same goes for SPF moisturizers. To avoid applying lotion over makeup, try an SPF compact powder.

7 **Seek shade when possible.**
Even if you wear sunscreen and are diligent about reapplying it, that alone won't protect you from 100% of UV rays, which is why Dr. Chang says "it's important to wear sun-protective clothing, wide-brimmed hats, and seek shade during peak sun hours."

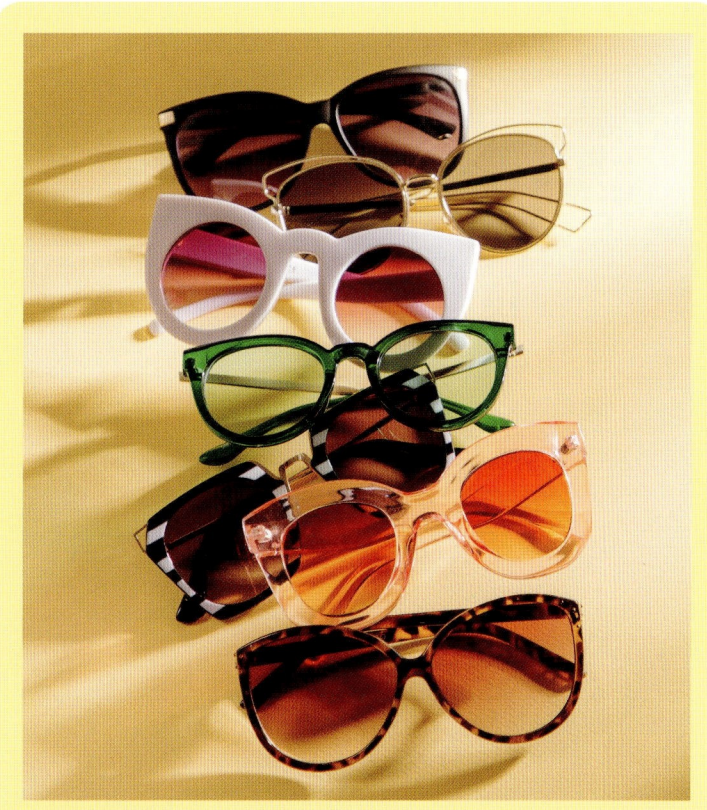

Protect Your Peepers
▶ Don't forget that your eyes are also susceptible to sun damage. Ultraviolet radiation from the sun can cause cataracts, macular degeneration, and even skin cancers like melanoma. To protect your eyes, it's essential to wear sunglasses with UV protection—ideally, shades that block 99% to 100% of both UVA and UVB light—all year long whenever you're outdoors.

Why Does Hair Turn Gray?

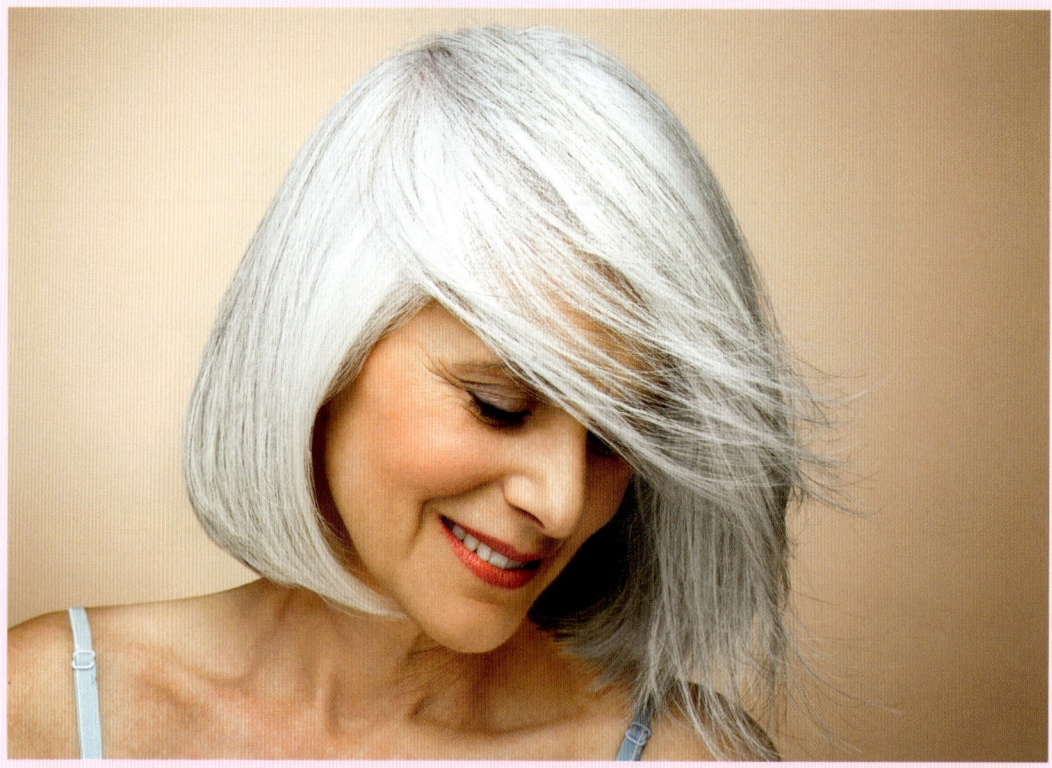

WE'VE ALL HEARD THAT STRESS CAUSES GRAY hair, and in fact, studies suggest a link between the two. Does that mean stressing less can help prevent gray hair? It's possible, and finding ways to de-stress can do wonders for your whole body—not just your hair. (See tips on de-stressing on page 150.)

But there are so many other reasons why your locks might be getting lighter. General aging has a lot more to do with your silver strands. And underlying health conditions like nutrition issues or alopecia (an autoimmune disorder) could also be a factor.

"Gray hair is really hair with less melanin, [a pigment that] gives skin and hair color," explains Azadeh Shirazi, M.D., a board-certified dermatologist. "White hair completely lacks [melanin]. With aging, there's a gradual decline in the number of stem cells that mature to become melanin-producing cells. These cells may wear out, become damaged, or lose the support systems [that] keep them working."

"There is a genetic component," explains Janiene Luke, M.D., a board-certified dermatologist at Loma Linda University Faculty Medical Group in California. "However, hair growth and hair pigmentation are highly regulated processes with multiple genes and cell-signaling molecules involved, where any disruption of these processes can lead to gray hair."

What's on our scalp, or rather, on the hair bulb (the base of the follicle, under the skin), also plays a part, according to Marisa Garshick, M.D., F.A.A.D., a board-certified dermatologist. "As we age there is a buildup of hydrogen peroxide in the hair bulb, which can destroy the pigment-producing cells, leading to decreased melanin and gray hair."

Is It Possible to Reverse Gray Hair?

▶ There isn't much you can do to stop graying when it is part of the normal aging process, explains Dr. Luke. "Early on in the process, however, if there are reversible causes leading to graying (such as smoking or nutritional deficiencies), people can try to make lifestyle modifications such as quitting smoking and maintaining a healthy diet packed with nutrients and antioxidants to help protect the cells involved in hair pigmentation."

But, Dr. Shirazi thinks that the future might hold some additional options: "New studies show that by stimulating stem cells back into action, pigment-producing cells can be revitalized to reverse gray hairs." The research still has a way to go before you can count on preventing or reversing grays.

Which means there is no quick fix...yet. So, be wary of any drug or product that claims to restore your colored hair. "Be careful about any non-FDA-approved medications or supplements claiming to reverse hair graying by potentiating melanocyte stem cells," says Oma Agbai, M.D., board-certified dermatologist and director of multicultural dermatology and hair disorders at the UC Davis Medical Center.

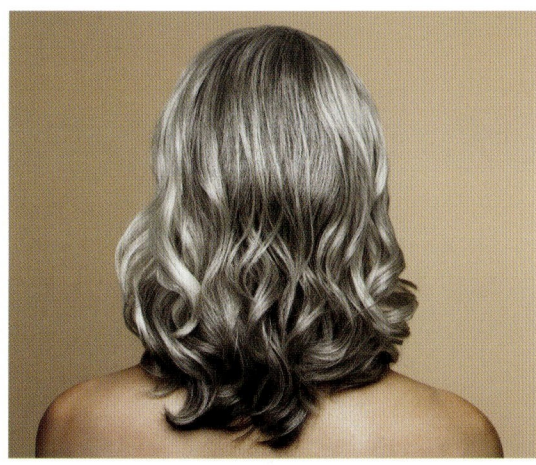

Embrace the Look

▶ Thanks to celebrities who tout their grays (we're looking at you, Andie MacDowell and Helen Mirren), embracing gray hair is more in than ever—and the trend is not leaving anytime soon.

In the opinion of celebrity hairstylist Michael Dueñas, a cultural shift has already occurred. "Gray hair is not necessarily a look," he says. "It's a mindset." In other words, as long as you're confident, you'll rock it no matter what.

Surprising Reasons You May Be Losing It (Hair, That Is)

IT'S NORMAL TO SHED A CERTAIN AMOUNT OF HAIR ON A DAILY BASIS. But when a brush quickly becomes tangled with strands, or handfuls of hair clog the shower drain, it can make you wonder if you're losing too much.

The truth: "On average, we lose 50 to 100 hairs a day," says Francesca Fusco, M.D., a New York City–based board-certified dermatologist who specializes in hair loss. "That's just hair going through its cycles, and there will be a new one to replace it." Experts say the average number of hairs shed

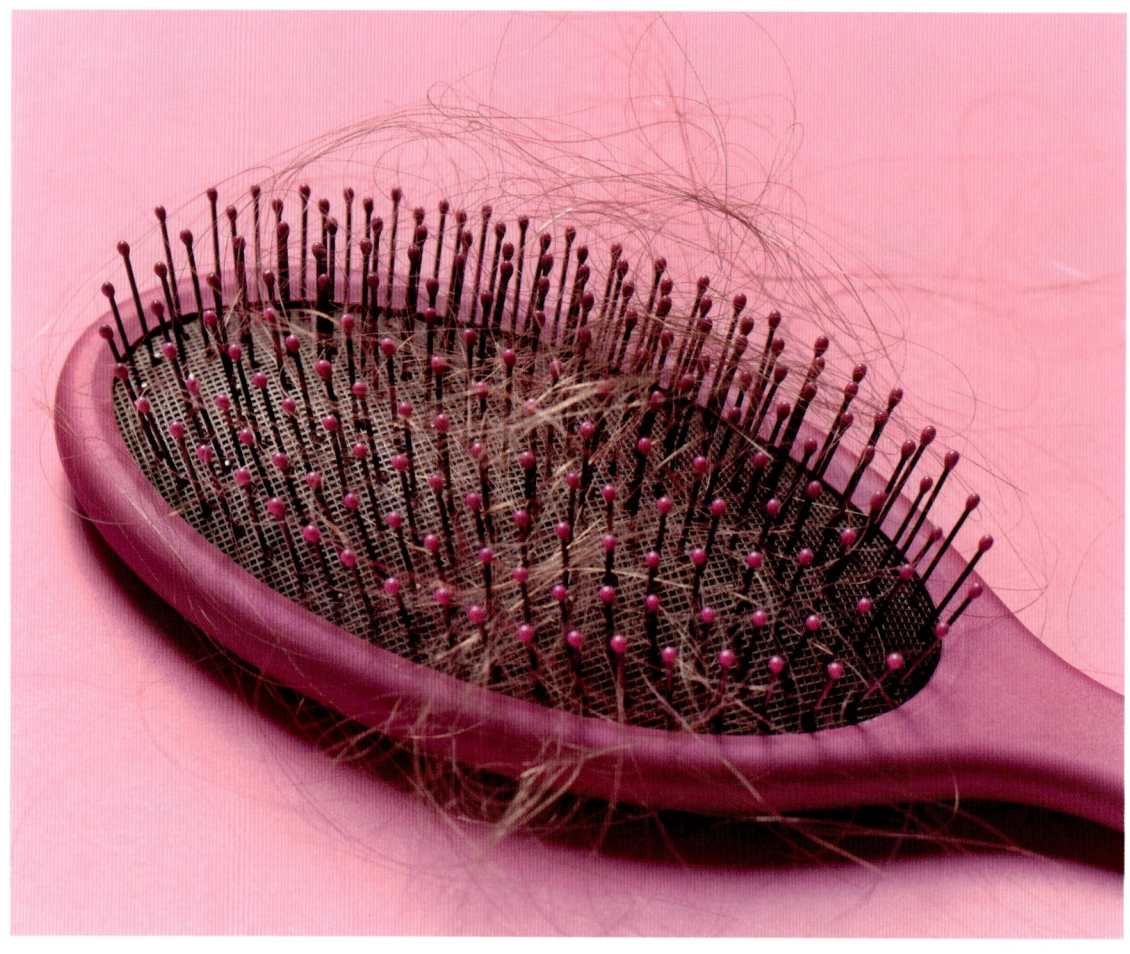

by men and women per day is about the same.

However, as people get older, "the rate of hair growth slows, and hair becomes thinner," says Usha Rajagopal, M.D., board-certified plastic surgeon and medical director of San Francisco Plastic Surgery and Laser Center.

REASONS BEHIND THE LOSS

There are various causes of excessive hair loss, including some medical conditions (such as a bad case of COVID, thyroid disorders, or anemia), certain medications (including chemotherapy as well as some antidepressants and hypertension drugs), and certain lifestyle factors (such as stressful events or certain hairstyles and treatments). Genetic factors often contribute to hair loss, and they can be passed down from either side of your family. In addition, deficiencies in iron, zinc, vitamins A and D, and other essential nutrients can contribute to hair loss, and hormonal fluctuations related to pregnancy, childbirth, menopause, and perimenopause can cause hair loss.

Hair loss is often hereditary. In fact, by the age of 50, at least half of all white men have thinning hair (white men, followed by West Asian and Afro-Caribbean men, are the most likely to experience male pattern baldness, while Native American men do not experience male pattern hair loss).

You're in Good Company

Intense emotional stress can cause hair loss, typically two to three months after a triggering event, as Melanie, an advertising executive, discovered eight years ago when a bald patch suddenly appeared on her head. When her dermatologist examined her scalp and asked what was happening in her life, Melanie mentioned that a new supervisor had taken over her department and was making work incredibly stressful. The diagnosis: telogen effluvium, a form of temporary shedding that can be sparked by stress or trauma. "That's when I started planning my exit strategy," recalls Melanie, now 45. "Work was miserable enough, but the fact that it was causing me to lose my hair was the final straw." Within a few months, she found a new position in a more congenial, supportive environment and her hair began to gradually grow back over time.

WHAT TO DO?

If the extent of your hair loss is upsetting you, schedule a visit to a dermatologist, who will examine your scalp and check for possible underlying causes for the hair loss. If a medical condition is the culprit, treating it directly, perhaps with medication, may help restore hair growth. If a nutrient deficiency—involving iron, vitamin D, or protein—is to blame, taking specific supplements may remedy the situation.

Minoxidil—which comes in an oral prescription or an over-the-counter topical solution that's applied directly to the scalp—has been shown to be effective in treating certain types of hair loss in both men and women. Another option: Nutritional supplements like Viviscal and Nutrafol are designed to reduce

shedding and enhance hair growth, though they haven't been well studied and are expensive. If these approaches don't help sufficiently, ask your dermatologist about stronger treatments such as laser and light therapy treatments or a hair transplant.

Nourish Your Tresses

▶ The three most important vitamins for healthy hair growth are vitamins A, C, and B7. You can find them in strawberries, eggs, lentils, fatty fish, spinach, nuts and seeds, sweet potatoes, carrots, yogurt, and red bell peppers. See the nutrition information starting on page 112 for more healthy foods.

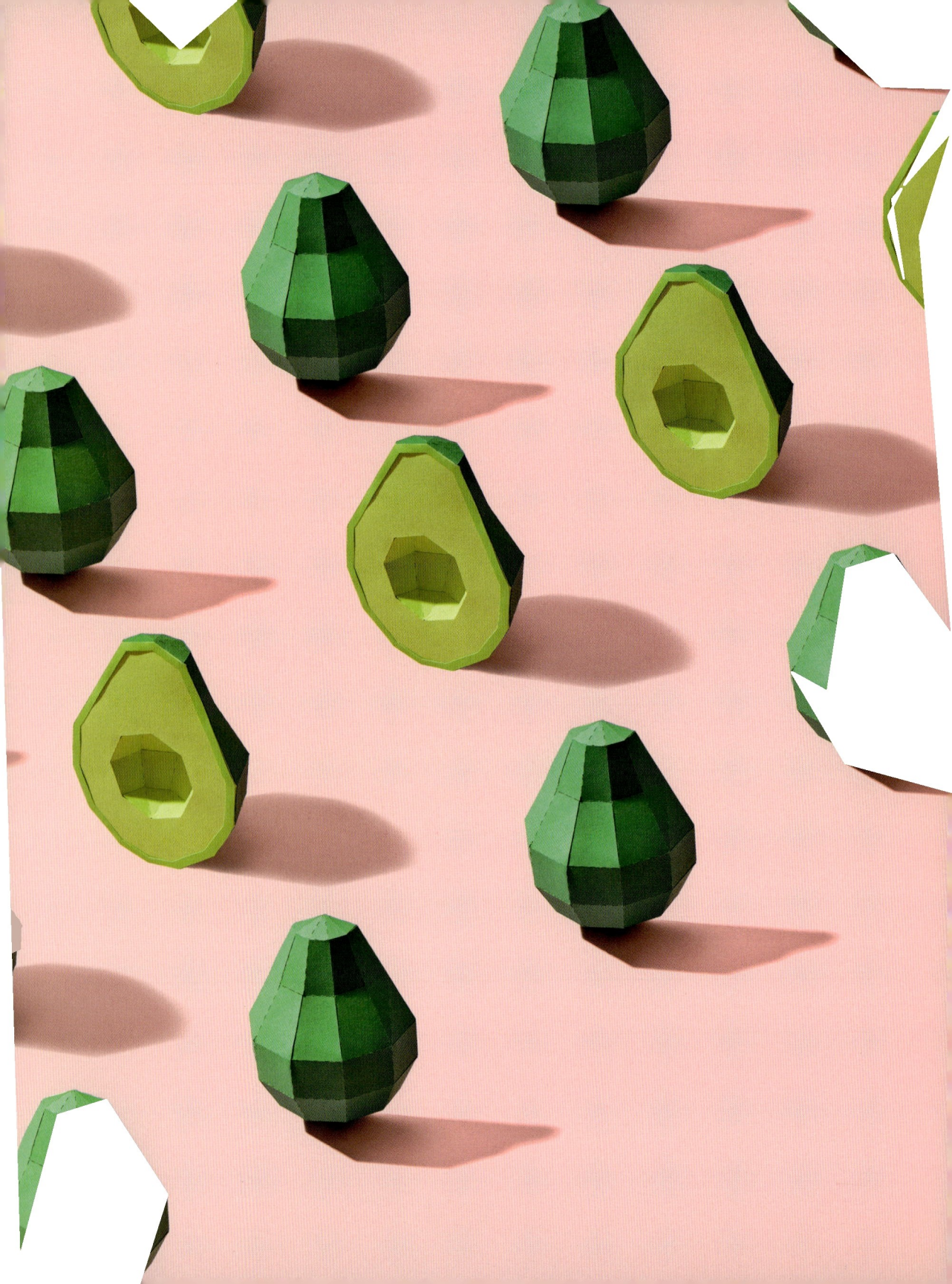

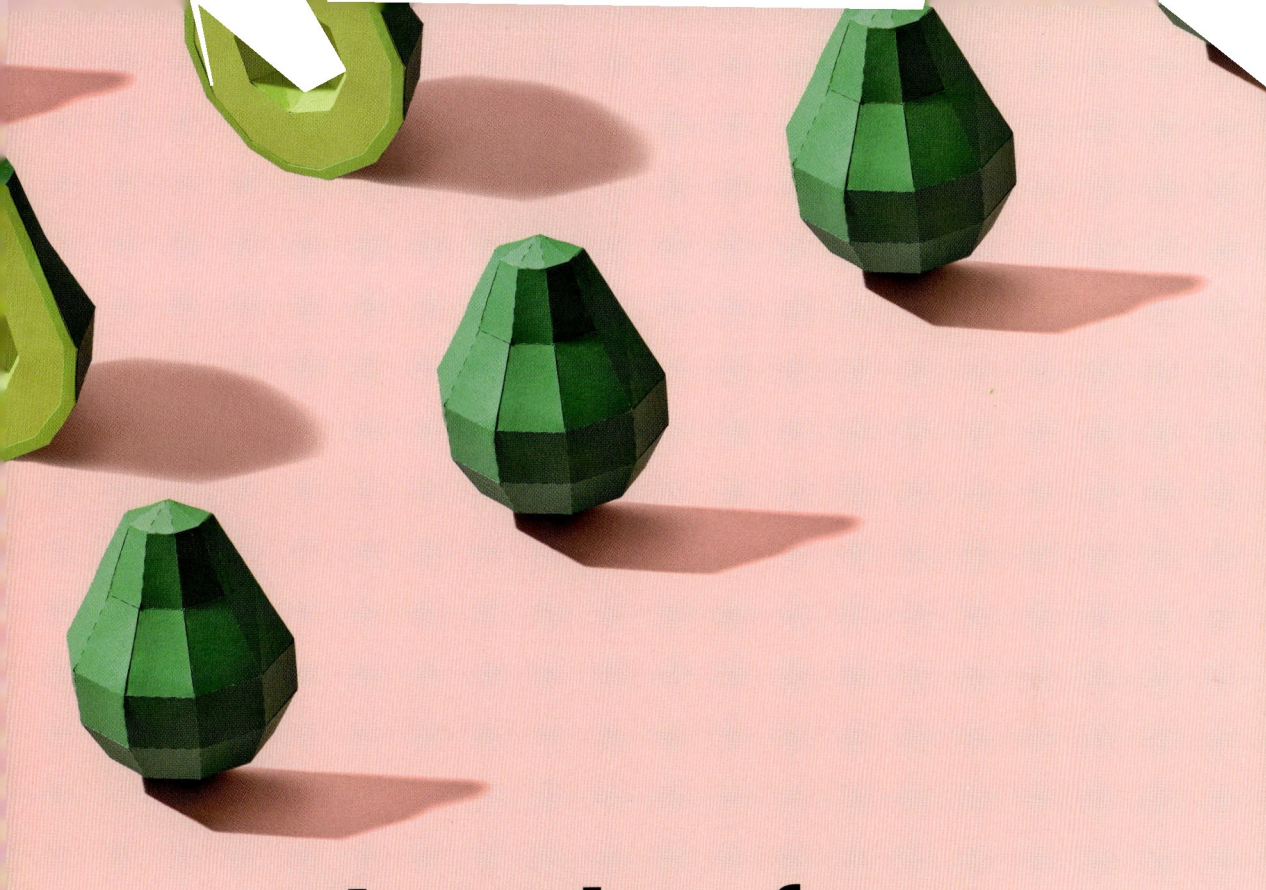

chapter four

SHIFT YOUR LIFESTYLE

Along with genetics, lifestyle is the most important influence on your longevity and health span. Eating well, exercising, getting sufficient rest, and managing stress can make a tremendous difference in how you experience your older years.

You Are What You Eat

YOU ARE WHAT YOU EAT" TURNS OUT TO BE TRUE. Eating healthy foods helps you have a healthy body. Beyond your physical health, your diet also influences your mood and emotional health. These factors can all influence the length and quality of your life.

Several delicious, nutritious eating plans have been shown to improve health and possibly also lifespan. In recent years, the Mediterranean diet and the DASH diet have consistently led the pack when it comes to the healthiest diets on the planet. These diets emphasize fruits, vegetables, beans, nuts, whole grains, lean protein, low-fat dairy products, and healthy fats while limiting foods with added sugars or simple starches.

They're easy to follow, and both have been shown to reduce the risk of heart disease, improve brain health, and decrease systemic inflammation, which is a major contributor to heart disease, high blood pressure, type 2 diabetes, some cancers, neurodegenerative diseases, and many other conditions.

Here's a closer look at how these eating plans compare:

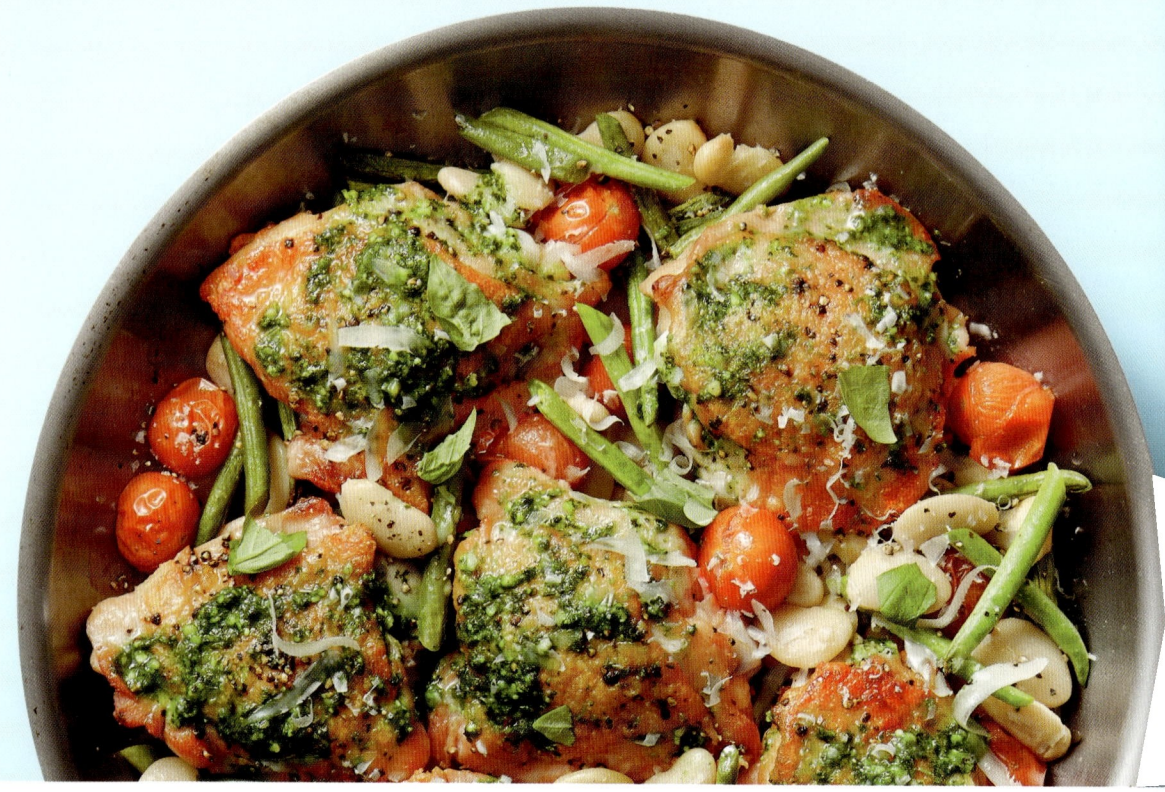

THE MEDITERRANEAN DIET

Year after year, the Mediterranean diet is ranked as one of the top diets, and an overwhelming amount of research shows it can lead to sustainable weight loss, improve heart health and brain function, and even help prevent chronic conditions like diabetes and cancer.

Additionally, research has found that replacing saturated fats like butter, mayonnaise, and dairy fat with olive oil, a feature of this diet, could have benefits for your heart health, increase longevity, lower your risk for cancer, and improve cognitive functioning. Plus, the American Heart Association recently released new heart-healthy guidelines that include a diet that mirrors the Mediterranean diet.

The Mediterranean diet isn't about restricting calories, but nor is it about eating only pasta, pizza, and drinking wine. The Mediterranean diet is actually more of a style of eating. There aren't any major rules about counting calories or sugar intake; it simply encourages enjoying whole foods in moderation.

Ultimately, the Mediterranean diet is a plant-based eating plan with fish, poultry, and dairy like milk, cheese, and yogurt occasionally thrown into the mix. You'll eat plenty of colorful fruits and vegetables, fresh herbs, fish and other types of seafood two to three times per week, olive oil, nuts and seeds, beans and legumes, and whole grains like brown rice, quinoa, and oats.

You'll limit your intake of refined grains and oils, red meat or deli meats, processed or packaged foods, and foods high in added sugar, such as pastries or candies.

Unlike many fad diets, an abundance of legitimate studies back up the benefits of the Mediterranean diet. Here are some highlights:

Heart health Alongside the DASH diet, the Mediterranean diet is known to protect your ticker. One large study of more than 30,000 women found that adherence to the eating plan over a 10-year period led to lower risk of heart attack, stroke, and heart failure. In

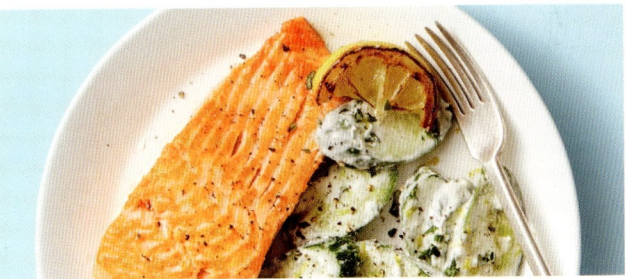

Your Mediterranean Menu

▶ To reap the impressive benefits that come with this approach to eating, here's what to aim for.

Daily
- Fruits and vegetables
- Herbs and spices
- Legumes
- Nuts and seeds
- Olive oil
- Whole grains

Several times a week
- Fish and shellfish (two to three times a week)
- Poultry (without the skin)
- Eggs
- Cheese
- Unsweetened yogurt

Occasionally
- Red or processed meat
- Refined grains
- Packaged or highly processed snacks
- Butter
- Soda and sugary drinks
- Sweets and desserts

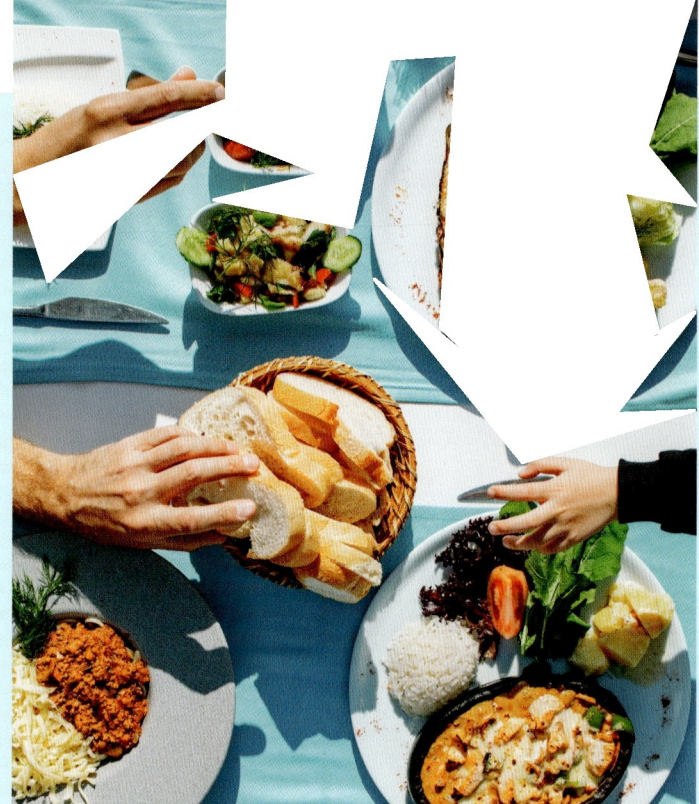

another study, participants had lower blood pressure after following the Mediterranean diet for just six months. Researchers attribute these positive outcomes to the abundance of heart-healthy nutrients found in the diet—and the absence of highly processed foods and added sugars.

Cancer risk A comprehensive scientific review found that people living in the Mediterranean region have lower rates of cancer than those in Northern Europe or the United States, and the authors credit this to following a Mediterranean diet. Research also found that loading up on foods that are staples of the Mediterranean diet can decrease the levels of inflammatory markers that are associated with tumor growth.

Brain function Scientists also suggest that polyphenols—compounds in plant-based foods that have antioxidant and anti-inflammatory properties—may benefit brain health. For example, polyphenols can influence neurotransmitters in the brain that have anti-depressant properties. In addition to regular exercise, quitting smoking, and maintaining a healthy weight, the World Health Organization recommends following a Mediterranean diet to decrease your risk of developing dementia

as it is "the most extensively studied dietary approach in relation to cognitive function."

THE DASH DIET

If you want a doctor-recommended eating plan that creates healthy, sustainable habits, and also gives your heart health a boost, look no further than the DASH diet.

DASH stands for Dietary Approaches to Stop Hypertension, and was developed to help lower blood pressure without medication. It focuses on the foods you should be eating, without cutting out any major food groups. It's all about having delicious meals that nourish your body and developing healthy habits you can sustain for the long haul.

Much like the Mediterranean diet, the DASH diet emphasizes fish, poultry, whole grains, fiber-rich veggies and fruits, low-fat or nonfat dairy, legumes, nuts, vegetable oils, and seeds. The diet suggests limiting sugar-sweetened beverages, sweets, and saturated fats, like fatty meats, full-fat dairy products, and tropical oils.

What makes the DASH diet specifically great for people with hypertension is that it caps sodium at 2,300 milligrams a day and encourages sticking to 1,500 milligrams per day—which is in line with the American Heart Association's recommendations.

The success of the DASH diet took off when the National Heart, Lung, and Blood Institute funded research on the benefits of the eating plan and found that it significantly lowered blood pressure and reduced the risk of heart disease in study participants. Because of this, U.S. News & World Report has consistently ranked the DASH diet as one of the top diets to follow for overall well-being.

Time and time again, research backs the DASH diet. In a meta-analysis published in the journal *Advances in Nutrition*, researchers found the plan significantly improved blood pressure numbers in adults with and without hypertension.

The DASH diet can also enhance overall heart health and help you maintain a healthy weight. There's even some research that points to the DASH diet as a veggie-forward option to protect against cancer risk. A study published in the journal *Annals of Epidemiology* suggests a higher diet quality, like that of the DASH diet, could lower risk for high-aggressive prostate cancer.

Your DASH Diet Menu

▶ **The foods you'll eat on the DASH diet can lower your blood pressure as well as improve insulin sensitivity and reduce triglyceride levels (a type of fat in the blood). Following are some of the foods encouraged on the plan:**

- Whole grains, such as brown rice, quinoa, farro, and freekeh
- Fruits, including berries, apples, oranges, and pears
- Vegetables and legumes
- Low-fat or nonfat dairy
- Lean meats, fish, and poultry
- Nuts and seeds
- Healthy fats, like extra-virgin olive oil, avocado, nuts, and seeds

The DASH diet doesn't cut out any types of food. But certain foods should be enjoyed in moderation. Here's a list of foods to limit to occasional treats or special occasions:

- Foods high in salt, like processed foods or restaurant meals
- Foods high in saturated fats such as fatty meats, full-fat dairy, and tropical oils such as coconut, palm kernel, and palm oils
- Sweets (including artificial sweeteners, sugar-sweetened beverages, and sugar-free candies)
- Excessive alcohol (no more than one drink a day for women and two a day for men)

The MIND Diet

▶ The Mediterranean-DASH Intervention for Neurodegenerative Delay (MIND) diet is a combination of the DASH and Mediterranean diets. It centers on foods that improve brain health with the overall goal of lowering your risk of Alzheimer's disease and mental decline.

The diet focuses on foods like leafy greens, nuts, and berries, and is naturally low in carbohydrates. "It tends to be low in sodium and high in potassium, encouraging followers to choose healthy fats and lean protein sources," says Jessica Cording, R.D., the author of *The Little Book of Game Changers*.

One study found that a pool of people aged 58 to 98 who self-reported closely following the MIND diet for an average of 4.5 years had a 53% decrease in the risk of Alzheimer's disease.

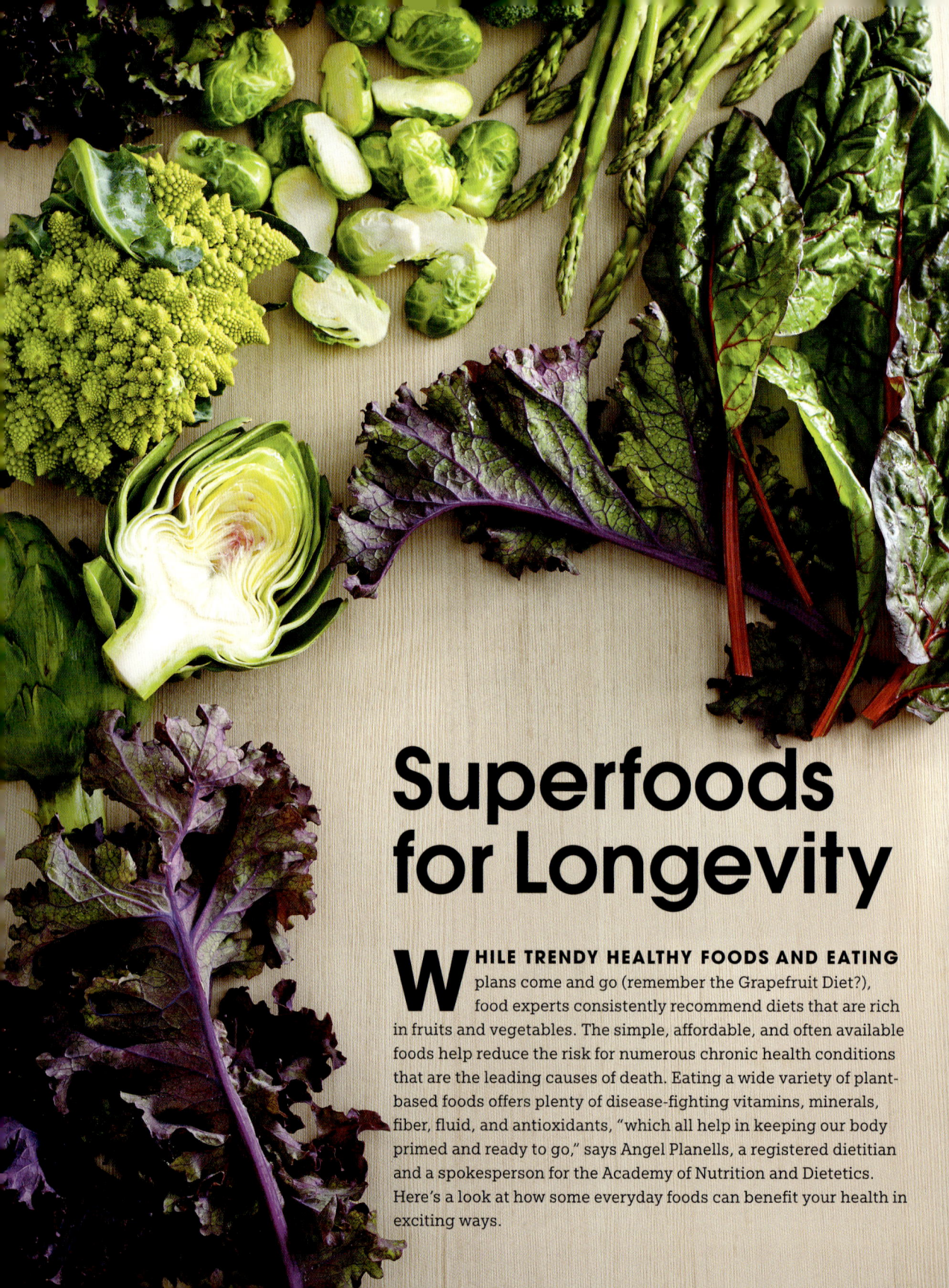

Superfoods for Longevity

WHILE TRENDY HEALTHY FOODS AND EATING plans come and go (remember the Grapefruit Diet?), food experts consistently recommend diets that are rich in fruits and vegetables. The simple, affordable, and often available foods help reduce the risk for numerous chronic health conditions that are the leading causes of death. Eating a wide variety of plant-based foods offers plenty of disease-fighting vitamins, minerals, fiber, fluid, and antioxidants, "which all help in keeping our body primed and ready to go," says Angel Planells, a registered dietitian and a spokesperson for the Academy of Nutrition and Dietetics. Here's a look at how some everyday foods can benefit your health in exciting ways.

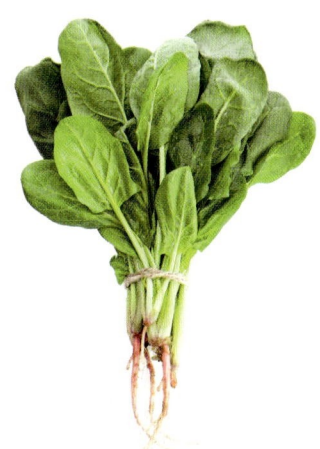

Fight Infection

CARROTS

The same nutrient that makes carrots healthy for your eyes— vitamin A—can help your body fight infection. People who are deficient in vitamin A experience an increased risk of infections even before they notice other symptoms of vitamin A deficiency, such as dry eye.

MUSHROOMS

Edible mushrooms are a good source of selenium, which improves the body's ability to fight infection by increasing white blood cell production. Mushrooms also contain vitamin D (as long as they're grown in sunlight), which may play a crucial role in immune system regulation.

SPINACH

This leafy green is a good source of riboflavin and folate, which are B vitamins that alert the immune system to fight infection. An Australian study found that bacteria and yeast synthesize B vitamins in the body, creating by-products that trigger immune cells to recognize and fight infection.

Lower Cholesterol

ARTICHOKES

One cooked artichoke has a significant amount of soluble fiber, which is important for lowering cholesterol. "Soluble fiber creates a gel-like substance that can bind with cholesterol to help excrete it," says Shelly Wegman, a registered dietitian at UNC Health Rex in Garner, North Carolina. Research shows that increasing dietary soluble fiber by 5 to 10 grams per day can lower cholesterol by 5%.

SESAME OIL

This oil is rich in heart-healthy compounds called phytosterols. "They help block the absorption of harmful LDL cholesterol," says Judy Fulop, a naturopath at Northwestern Memorial Hospital in Chicago.

WHOLE OATS

"Old-fashioned" oats are a rich source of a soluble fiber called beta-glucans. "Think of beta-glucans as long strands that tangle as they move," says Daniel Gallaher, Ph.D., a food science and nutrition professor at the University of Minnesota. The strands "catch" cholesterol as they exit your body. Oatmeal also contains soluble fiber, which helps reduce your low-density lipoprotein (LDL), the "bad" cholesterol.

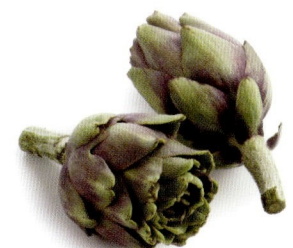

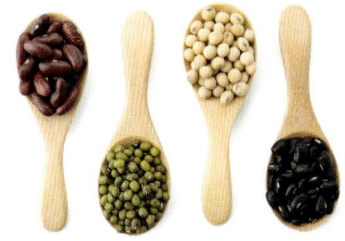

Steady Blood Sugar

AVOCADOS

Avocados have both fat and fiber, which help balance blood sugar, and they slow down digestion and metabolism. This makes them a perfect addition to a meal with carbs (enter avocado toast!).

BEANS

"Beans offer both fiber and plant-based protein, two blood sugar–stabilizing nutrients that you want to focus on," says Lauren Twigge, M.C.N., R.D.N., L.D., founder of Lauren Twigge Nutrition. Beans also contain resistant starch, a type of fiber that has been found to improve blood sugar levels and body weight.

BLUEBERRIES

A *BMJ* review found that adults who ate blueberries had up to a 26% lower risk of developing type 2 diabetes than those who didn't. Often considered the best anti-aging fruit, it is also high in antioxidants, which are natural compounds that help fight cell-damaging free radicals.

LENTILS

This legume is high in protein and fiber, which slows the body's process of turning carbohydrates into glucose in the blood, helping to prevent a spike in blood sugar levels.

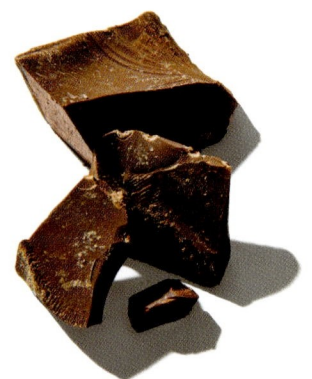

Lower Blood Pressure

ARUGULA

This leafy green is one of the richest sources of healthy nitrates. Nitrates are converted into nitric oxide, which can widen blood vessels and ease blood flow, lowering blood pressure.

DARK CHOCOLATE

This treat is an excellent source of flavonoids, which a *BMJ* study linked to reduced blood pressure. "Heart benefits of chocolate have been seen with as few as 10 chocolate chips a day," says Adrienne Youdim, M.D., a nutrition specialist and the author of *Hungry for More*. Opt for a one-ounce square of dark chocolate with at least 70% cocoa or add unsweetened cocoa powder to oatmeal.

MILK

We all know that milk is a great source of bone-strengthening calcium. But it also contains nutrients like potassium and magnesium that can lower blood pressure and decrease your risk of developing hypertension. It's so effective for maintaining heart health that skim milk is recommended as part of the official DASH diet.

Improve Liver Health

BRAZIL NUTS

Just one or two Brazil nuts provide more than your daily dose of selenium, a trace element that's crucial for liver health. "Selenium is required for glutathione peroxidase, a major detoxification enzyme and antioxidant, to work," says Diane Vizthum, a registered dietitian in Baltimore.

BRUSSELS SPROUTS

This vegetable is a good source of sulforaphane, which may help protect the liver. "Sulforaphane increases detox agents in the liver, boosting their function," says Judy Fulop, a naturopath at Northwestern Memorial Hospital in Chicago. "It also decreases enzymes that cause liver damage due to factors such as excessive alcohol consumption."

EGGS

Want to show your liver some love? Eat more eggs. The yolks are rich in choline, an essential nutrient that plays an important role in helping your liver metabolize fat. Just one has around 35% of the 425 milligrams of choline you need per day. (You can also find choline in Brussels sprouts and peanut butter.)

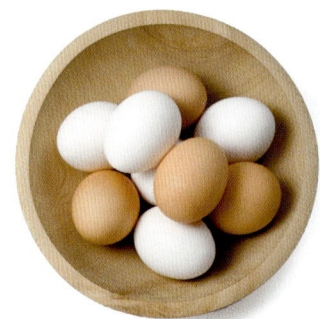

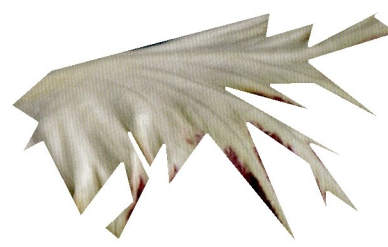

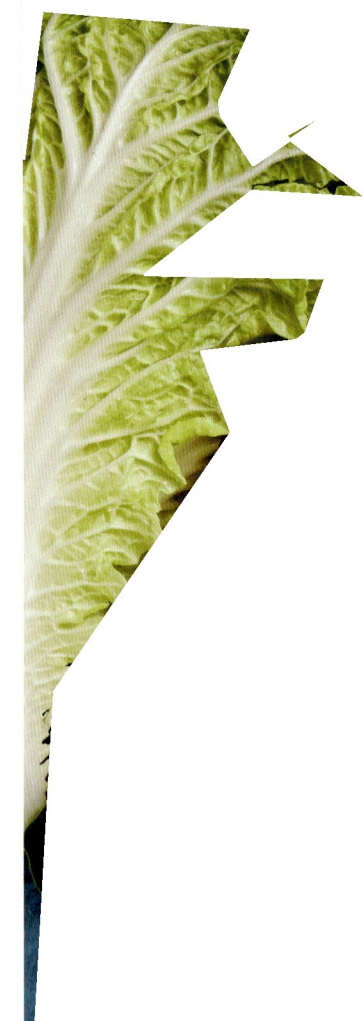

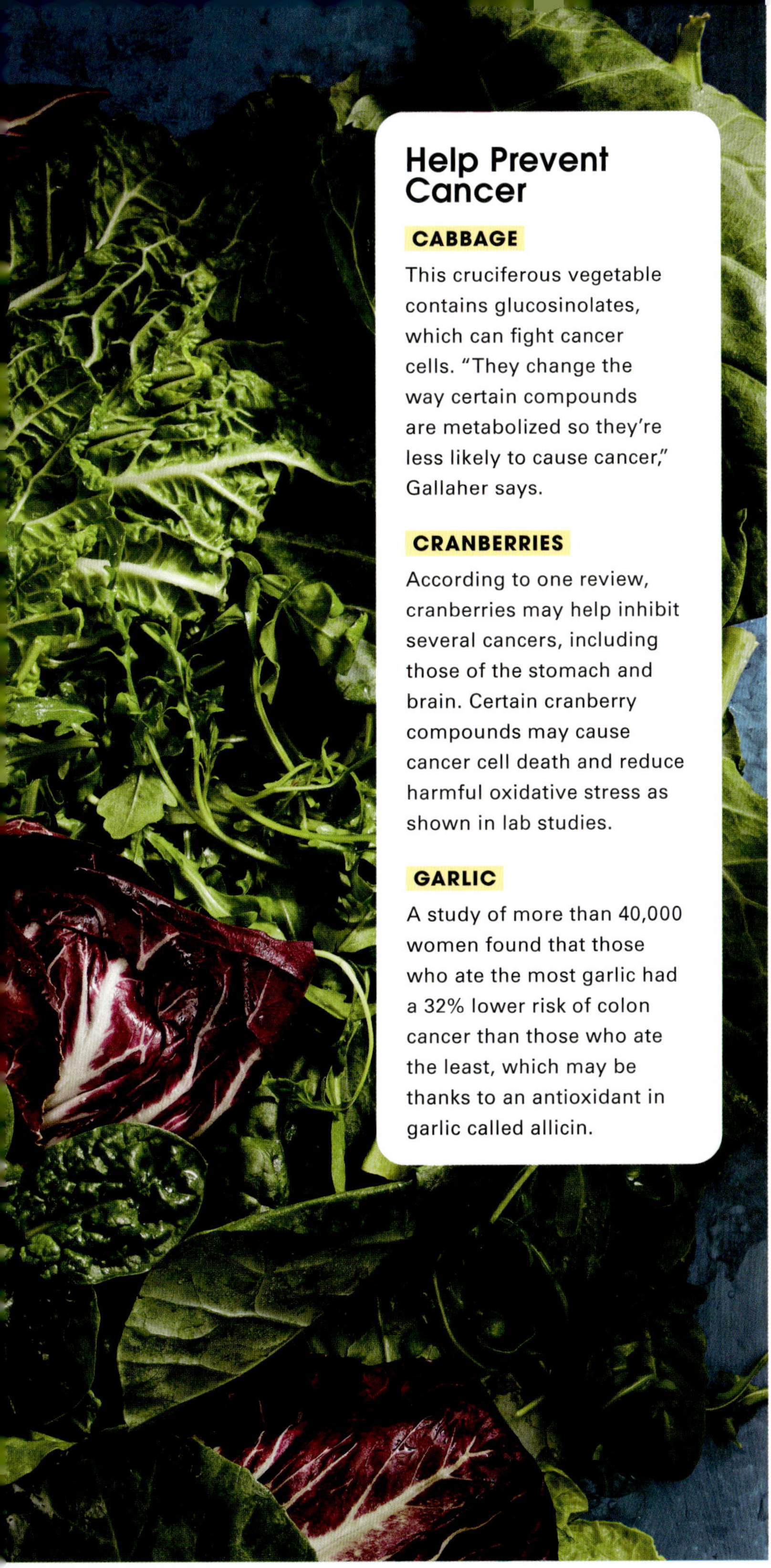

Help Prevent Cancer

CABBAGE

This cruciferous vegetable contains glucosinolates, which can fight cancer cells. "They change the way certain compounds are metabolized so they're less likely to cause cancer," Gallaher says.

CRANBERRIES

According to one review, cranberries may help inhibit several cancers, including those of the stomach and brain. Certain cranberry compounds may cause cancer cell death and reduce harmful oxidative stress as shown in lab studies.

GARLIC

A study of more than 40,000 women found that those who ate the most garlic had a 32% lower risk of colon cancer than those who ate the least, which may be thanks to an antioxidant in garlic called allicin.

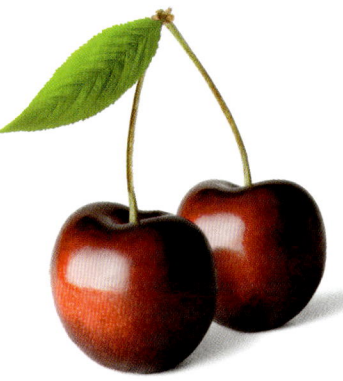

Ease Inflammation

TART CHERRY JUICE

Oregon Health & Science University researchers found that women who drank tart cherry juice twice daily for three weeks had significantly less inflammation than those who drank artificial juice. Tart cherries are rich in antioxidants, which combat inflammation.

EGGPLANT

Purple and blue foods like eggplant get their hue from anthocyanins, antioxidants consistently shown to reduce inflammation, Vizthum says. Other good sources of anthocyanins include plums, cherries, purple and red grapes, and red and purple cabbage.

WALNUTS

One review of studies published in the *Journal of Nutrition* found that antioxidant polyphenolic compounds in walnuts can reduce harmful inflammation in brain cells, potentially lowering the risk of cognitive decline. (Walnuts are heart-healthy too, with one *Circulation* study finding that just ½ cup of walnuts a day improved LDL cholesterol in healthy adults.)

Drink Up!

WATER IS THE ULTIMATE HEALTH ELIXIR— and its benefits only increase as we age. Our parents and grandparents barely gave a thought to water—they would just fill a glass and drink it down on a hot day. Today we're practically obsessed with the stuff, and for good reason: Water is the most important thing we consume.

Water is the most prevalent element in the human body, and depriving your body of water will deprive it of its necessary functions, says David Cutler, M.D., family medicine physician at Providence Saint John's Health Center in Santa Monica, California. It's important to avoid dehydration in your daily life that could lead to larger health concerns in the future. "There's a wide range of adequate water intake levels to achieve optimal health," he adds.

HOW MUCH WATER DO YOU NEED?

The bottom line is that there is no specific required amount of daily water intake for adults. The National Academy of Medicine generally recommends women consume an average of approximately 2.7 liters (91 ounces) of total water—from all

beverages and foods—each day, and men average approximately 3.7 liters (125 ounces), but there's a range of normal. About 20% of a person's water intake comes from food, such as fruit, vegetables, and soups; the rest is from the liquids they drink.

Pay attention to your body's signs of thirst and dehydration. Here are some important questions to consider, according to Dr. Cutler:

- **Are you thirsty?**
- **Are you not sweating when you're hot?**
- **Is your pee getting darker?**

"Pay attention to these signs, and when those happen, drink more water," says Dr. Cutler.

DEHYDRATION AND AGING

Dehydration can lead to all sorts of health issues, such as fatigue, muscle cramps, lightheadedness, even chills, in the short term. Recent research shows that staying properly hydrated can significantly impact your health long-term, and even longevity.

A study published in the journal *eBioMedicine* in 2023 tested the hypothesis that optimal hydration may slow down the aging process in humans. Using health data gathered from 11,255 adults over a 30-year period, researchers analyzed links between levels of salt in the blood—which go up when fluid intake goes down—and various indicators of health.

The researchers found that adults with salt levels at the higher end of a normal range were more likely to develop chronic conditions and show signs of biological aging than those with salt levels in the lower ranges. Adults with higher salt levels were also more likely to die at a younger age.

"The results suggest that proper hydration may slow down aging and prolong a disease-free life," said Natalia Dmitrieva, Ph.D., a study author and researcher at the National Heart, Lung, and Blood Institute, in a press release.

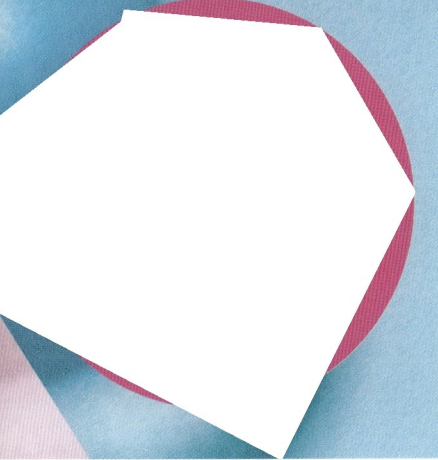

Hold the Wine (or Go Easy)

▶ Recent research about alcohol and life expectancy has overturned some previous thinking about alcohol's effect on our health. Suddenly that second round of margaritas doesn't sound as enticing.

The sobering data comes courtesy of Tim Stockwell, Ph.D., a scientist at the Canadian Institute for Substance Use Research: Unfortunately for frequent imbibers, if a person were to drink seven alcoholic beverages a week (beer, wine, or spirits), they risk cutting their life expectancy by two and a half months. The numbers get even bleaker when the amount of alcohol consumed per week increases: A person who drinks 35 alcoholic beverages a week is looking at shaving two years off their life, according to the research.

Stockwell notes that these numbers are averages, and some people could end up luckier than others, but he disputes the notion that alcohol is good for you, even in moderation.

Meanwhile, many people don't realize that both men and women develop an increased sensitivity and a decreased tolerance to alcohol as they get older. As a result, having one martini or margarita in your 60s or 70s could affect you the way two or three of these cocktails did in your 20s or 30s. This is largely because the amount of water in the body decreases as people get older: Alcohol is a water-soluble substance, which means that if you drink the same amount at 60 as you did at 30, your blood alcohol level will be much higher and it will be eliminated from the body more slowly, thereby increasing the risks associated with drinking.

You're in Good Company

In her mid-50s, Louisa noticed that her nightly glass or two of wine just wasn't serving her as well as it once had. Instead of feeling relaxed she just felt…sleepy. And while she fell asleep quickly, she found herself waking several times through the night. In the mornings she felt groggy and slow moving. After talking to her doctor, she decided to try Dry January. Within a few weeks, she found she was waking up less during the night and felt more refreshed in the morning. While she missed the nightly ritual, she found that a mocktail or sparkling water was just as relaxing without the downsides. Now, four years later, she drinks a glass of wine on special occasions but loves that she can take it or leave it.

Do You Need Probiotics?

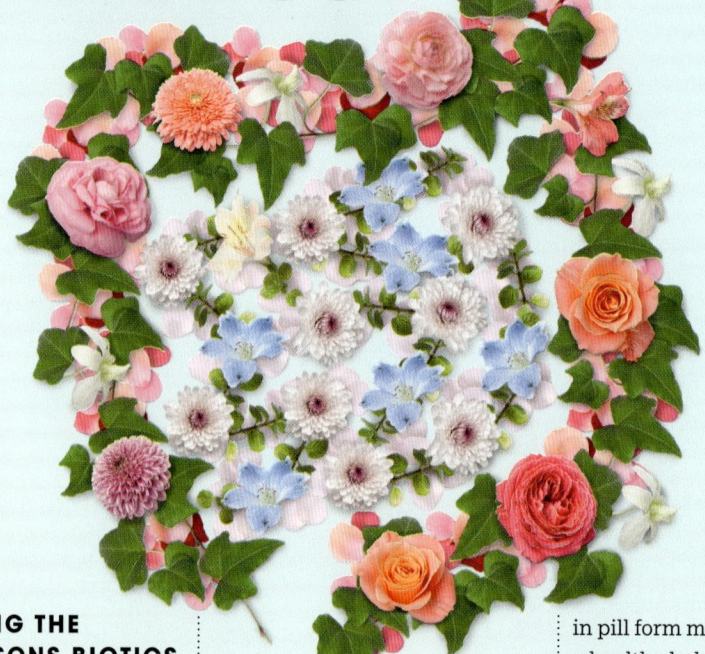

AMONG THE REASONS BIOTICS MATTER: THE trillions of bacteria, fungi, parasites, and viruses that live inside the gut, collectively known as the gut microbiome, play a huge role in our overall health as well as the health of our digestive systems. The microbiome is so intricate that distinct colonies reside in different parts of the GI tract, says Eran Elinav, M.D., Ph.D., head of the systems immunology department at Israel's Weizmann Institute of Science. Scientists don't yet know the ideal mix of

organisms, but having an imbalanced microbiome has been linked to numerous illnesses including diabetes and childhood asthma. The food we eat, which becomes the food the microbes in our guts feast on, is a crucial component in fostering a diverse microbiome. "Of the many environmental factors that impact our gut microbes, nutrition is probably the most important," Elinav says.

You've probably heard about probiotic supplements—they are nutrients and microorganisms

in pill form meant to help keep a healthy balance of bacteria in your gut, which confers a host of benefits. But you can get these and the other "Ps" in food form. Here's what you should know about feeding your gut:

PROBIOTICS

These good-for-you live microorganisms, such as bacteria and yeast, live peacefully in your body, providing numerous health benefits and protecting you against harmful organisms. You can increase the ratio of good to bad bacteria in your gut through food. The best sources of probiotics are fermented dairy products such as yogurt and kefir, which usually boast multiple strains of bacteria. Though you may have heard that other fermented products such as kimchi and sauerkraut also contain probiotics, that's not exactly true, according to the National Institutes of Health; they *do* contain live bacteria, but these beneficial bugs lack sufficient strength and number to qualify as probiotics.

PREBIOTICS

As helpful as probiotics are when you eat them, they pass through the digestive tract, so they work their magic only until you poop them out. If your goal is to improve your long-term gut health by growing more good microbes in your gut, consider prebiotics, the majority of which are essentially carbohydrates we can't digest, such as fiber. These healthy carbs are like fertilizer for friendly gut bacteria. The best way to load up on prebiotics is by eating fiber-rich plant foods, especially bananas, asparagus, whole grains (such as oats and barley), onions, garlic, and soybeans. "One advantage to getting prebiotics from foods is that you can get many different types of fiber, and that in turn promotes a more robust and varied population of beneficial microbes," says Monica Reinagel, L.D.N., C.N.S., owner of Nutrition Over Easy in Baltimore.

POSTBIOTICS

If probiotics and prebiotics had a baby, it would be called postbiotics, substances your body produces after it feeds on prebiotics and probiotics. These include B vitamins, enzymes, amino acids, and short-chain fatty acids such as butyrate. You can get them from food with a probiotic- and prebiotic-rich diet, which can help you produce your own internal postbiotic supply. And while kimchi and kombucha may not contain sufficient probiotics, they *do* provide your body what it needs to produce postbiotics, as do yogurt, kefir, and other pickled vegetables.

The Truth About Your Maturing Metabolism

▶ You've probably heard that it's easy to gain weight as you get older and harder to lose it. And you may have heard that this happens because your metabolism simply and inevitably hits the brakes as you age.

Not exactly. Experts long believed that metabolism—the process through which the body converts food into energy—progressively slows with age, resulting in near-inevitable weight gain. But now, landmark research published in the journal *Science* has shown that's not the case. Our metabolisms actually hold steady from ages 20 to 60, found a 40-year study of some 6,500 people. And while this internal engine does start to slow after age 60, the change is subtle, happening at a rate of just 7% per decade.

That might come as a welcome surprise: When it comes to sticking to a healthy weight, your body *isn't* working against your efforts after all! So how do we explain that age-related weight gain happens? It is true that the average American adult puts on 1 to 2 pounds per year through age 55, *Journal of the American Medical Association* findings show. That's because our habits change with age, which makes it easier to add fat, says metabolism researcher Herman Pontzer, Ph.D., coauthor of the *Science* study and author of *Burn*.

In other words, our metabolism isn't slowing because we're older, it's slowing because we move less, which leads to more body fat and less calorie-burning muscle. But you can keep your metabolism humming by—you guessed it—staying active. If you feel you need to lose weight, talk to your doctor.

The Importance of Movement

REGULAR MOVEMENT IS VITAL TO YOUR health. It can improve everything from your weight, blood pressure, and cholesterol to your balance, energy, mood, and memory, explains Danine Fruge, M.D, A.B.F.P., former medical director at the Pritikin Longevity Center.

You begin to experience age-related muscle loss called sarcopenia, losing on average 3% to 5% of your muscle mass per decade, as early as your 30s, explains Dr. Fruge. But regular movement can help mitigate that muscle loss, protect you from falls, and even increase your longevity.

Regular physical training can improve your cognitive function and even reduce the risk of dementia. Exercise can help support your mental health by boosting endorphins and lowering cortisol levels caused by stress.

"Many health issues crop up in higher numbers as we age, like heart disease, cancer, arthritis, and Alzheimer's. Having a tool as simple as walking 10 minutes or more a day is an incredible weapon to help fight disease," says David Sabgir, M.D., a cardiologist and Walk With a Doc founder.

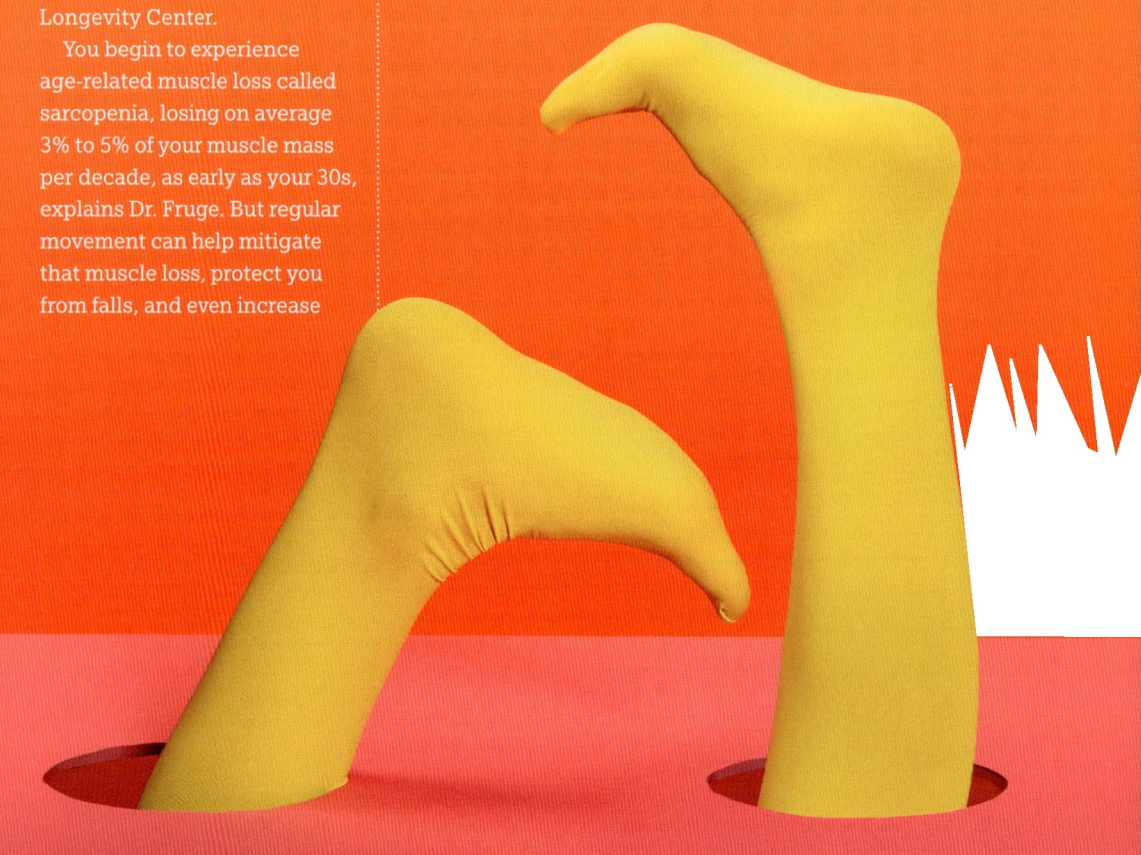

The Centers for Disease Control and Prevention recommends doing strength-building activities twice a week and a minimum of 150 minutes a week of moderate-intensity aerobic activity. It can feel daunting to squeeze in those extra minutes of movement with other daily responsibilities, but one study found that a minimal amount of physical activity each day could have some serious health perks.

The study published in the journal *JAMA Internal Medicine* set out to see if physical activity could increase the longevity of adults in the U.S. Researchers used data from 4,850 participants in the National Health and Nutrition Examination Survey who were 40 to 85 years old. Researchers estimated that approximately 110,000 deaths per year could be prevented if adults in this age group increased their moderate-to-vigorous physical activity intensity by just 10 minutes per day.

Seema Bonney, M.D., functional medicine doctor at the Anti-Aging and Longevity Center of Philadelphia, suggests 10 minutes be a starting point. From there, gradually increase physical activity to 20 or 30 minutes per day.

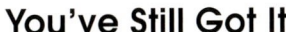

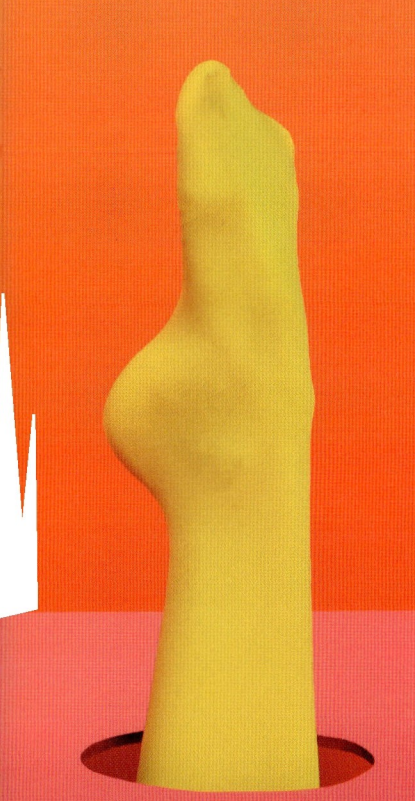

You've Still Got It

▶ It's not a myth: Muscle memory is a real thing, but it may not be exactly what you thought it was. When scientists and exercise physiologists talk about muscle memory, they're referring to a phenomenon in which previously trained muscles gain strength and volume much faster after a period of not being used than never-trained muscles do when starting from square one.

This means that if you were once fit but you've been inactive for a while, you can regain your former level of fitness with retraining, whether it's with aerobic exercise or strength training. How quickly you get there depends partly on your age, how fit you were before the hiatus, and how long the break lasted. The key is not to overdo it or ramp things up too soon, which could lead to injury.

After a substantial exercise break, start at a level below what you were accustomed to doing then gradually increase it in terms of duration, frequency, and intensity with aerobic exercise, advises Cedric Bryant, Ph.D., president and chief science officer at the American Council on Exercise. With strength training, start with a weight that you can comfortably lift for two to three sets of 10 reps. Then after two to three weeks, gradually increase the weight if you feel like you could do more reps.

The take-home message: You can reclaim and regain your previous fitness level after a period of inactivity. But be smart about how you do it.

Functional Fitness Is Your BFF

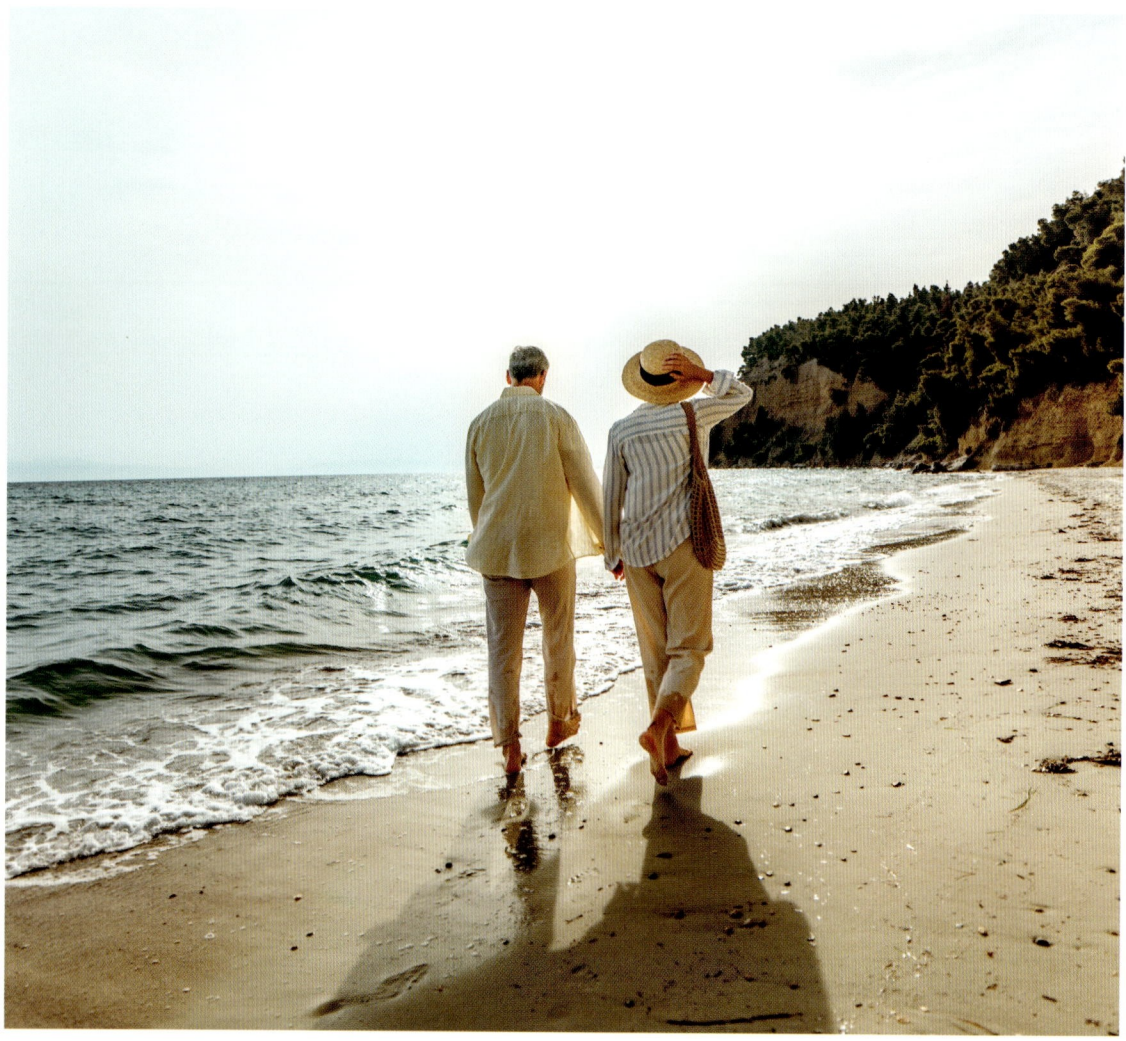

WHEN YOU WERE YOUNGER YOU MAY HAVE TAKEN your ability to run or lift things overhead for granted. As you get older, however, physical functionality becomes something you value. Whether you want to run a half marathon or chase a toddler, roll out of bed in the morning without pain or mow the lawn, place a book on a high shelf or pick something up from the floor, your physical functionality—which reflects the interplay between flexibility, strength, balance, and aerobic endurance—keeps you moving through life.

While all of the body's systems work together to keep you alive and mobile, the muscular, nervous, and skeletal systems contribute most to movement, while the cardiovascular and circulatory systems bring oxygen to the cells in your body, allowing you to have the endurance to participate in daily activities as well as take hikes, play pickleball, or even just walk to your mailbox.

When any of these systems are out of whack, they affect your physical functionality—that is, your ability to participate meaningfully in life in a physical way.

Some of these components naturally start to decline in the third and fourth decades of life, says Marco Brotto, Ph.D., M.Pharm., director of the Bone-Muscle Research Center at the University of Texas at Arlington. These declines can lead to pain and a lack of independence, and diseases such as osteoporosis and depression, and when your mobility is limited, you're more likely to become sedentary. The more sedentary you are, the more your mobility deteriorates, creating a downward spiral.

The good news is that declines in mobility can be prevented and even reversed. But to build more physical resilience, it's important to act now; whether you are 40 or 80, it's never too late to start.

Read on to explore the importance of four of the key elements of physical functionality—balance, flexibility, strength, and aerobic endurance. You'll discover tools to gauge where you currently stand and exercises to help you keep these fitness factors in top-notch shape.

You're in Good Company

Five years ago, Maddy nearly gave up tennis after suffering a bad ankle sprain and a broken wrist when she fell during a tennis match. "My orthopedic surgeon told me that I'd come to the point in my life where I had to think about body maintenance—I couldn't just run out the door and play sports anymore," says Maddy, a business consultant in her late 40s. After her injuries healed, she started doing yoga to enhance her flexibility and resistance training to build muscle strength. The combination made a difference in helping her stay injury-free after returning to tennis, a sport that she plans to continue to play long into the future.

The Value of Mixing Up Your Workout

▶ Research from Johns Hopkins Medicine shows that exercise may be the closest thing we have to a fountain of youth. Besides lowering your risk of various diseases, it can even prevent some age-related changes in your DNA. There are many ways to stay active, but mixing up your workout routine is crucial to your health. One study in *British Journal of Sports Medicine* examined data from nearly 100,000 participants in a prostate, lung, colorectal, and ovarian cancer screening trial. After adjusting for demographic and lifestyle risk factors, researchers found that after years of follow-up, those who reported cardiovascular activity and weightlifting once or twice a week had up to 47% lower risk of dying compared with those who did not exercise. Researchers noted that this number increased the more often the participants lifted weights, and those who performed aerobic exercises but did not lift weights had a 32% lower risk of dying prematurely.

What does Mixing It Up Look Like?

▶ To bring your joints through their full range of motion, do a mix of strength, cardio, balance, and stretching. First, let's take a look at flexibility (on the next page).

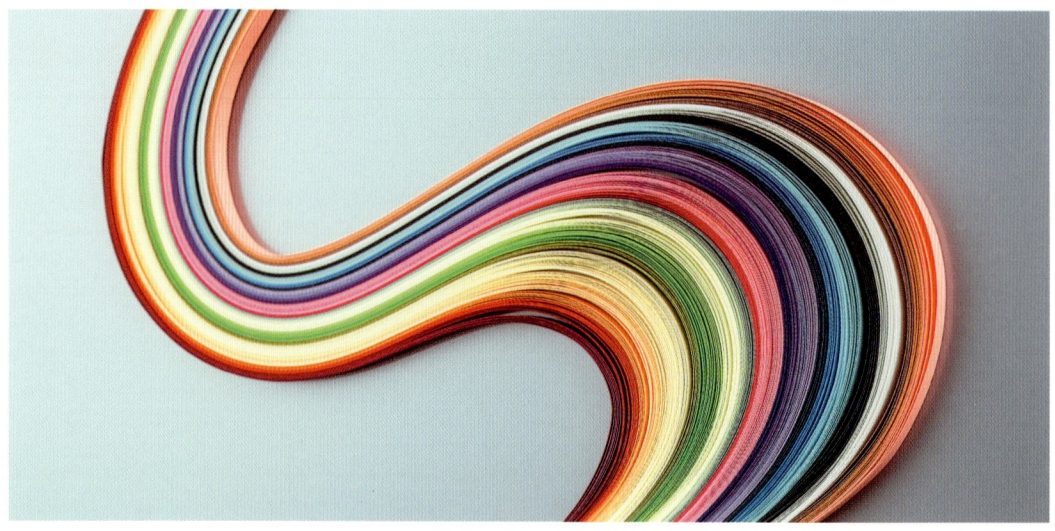

Flexibility

FLEXIBILITY KEEPS MUSCLES MOVING AND FEELING better, and is crucial for injury prevention. "Muscles only work well when they are full length and elastic," says physiotherapist Sally Roberts.

There's also new evidence that being flexible could help you live longer. That's the major takeaway from a study in the *Scandinavian Journal of Medicine & Science in Sports*. Researchers analyzed data from more than 3,100 people over age 28, looking at how flexible they were and how long they lived.

The researchers specifically looked at data from clinical exams that gave patients a "Flexitest" that checked how flexible they were in 20 body joint movements. Overall, the researchers found that people with higher flexibility levels had higher survival rates for deaths from natural or non-COVID causes, particularly in women. Women with lower flexibility scores had a 4.78 times higher risk of dying compared to their more flexible counterparts.

TEST YOUR FLEXIBILITY

You can gauge your lower-body flexibility at home with the sit-and-reach test. Spend a few minutes warming up your muscles by walking or doing jumping jacks. Then, take off your shoes and sit on the floor with your legs extended in front of you and your feet about 6 inches apart. Place a tape measure between your legs with the end toward your crotch and the 15-inch mark lined up with your heels.

Stack your hands on top of each other, hinge forward at the hips, and reach your hands as far as you can. Hold the position for two seconds and notice where your fingertips are on the tape measure.

How did you do?

If your fingertips reached to 12 inches or less, your flexibility needs some work.

If your fingertips reached between 13 and 19 inches, that's good.

And if you reached 20 inches or farther, that's great.

Simple Everyday Stretches

Before starting, keep these best practices in mind:

Breathe Begin with a few minutes of deep breathing.

Push yourself, but not too hard Aim for a 70 on a scale of 1 to 100.

Listen to your body "Normal" discomfort feels like tightness or stiffness as you begin a stretch. Sharp or burning pain is a warning that something is wrong.

Genie Twist

1. Stand with your legs hip-width apart and parallel, your back straight, and your abdomen tight.
2. Bend your knees softly. Lift your arms to chest height, palms down. Fold your arms at shoulder height, fingertips to elbows.
3. Without moving your pelvis or hips, twist to the right (**A**). Stay in the twist, and turn your head to the left (**B**), with your chin toward your left shoulder. Then twist and turn your head to the right, with your chin toward your right shoulder. Repeat the left and right head-turning twice.
4. Untwist, returning to center. Switch the top arm, then repeat all steps.

TIP:
Try adding "micro walks" to your day. Walking between 10 and 30 seconds at a time breaks up long periods of sitting or inactivity.

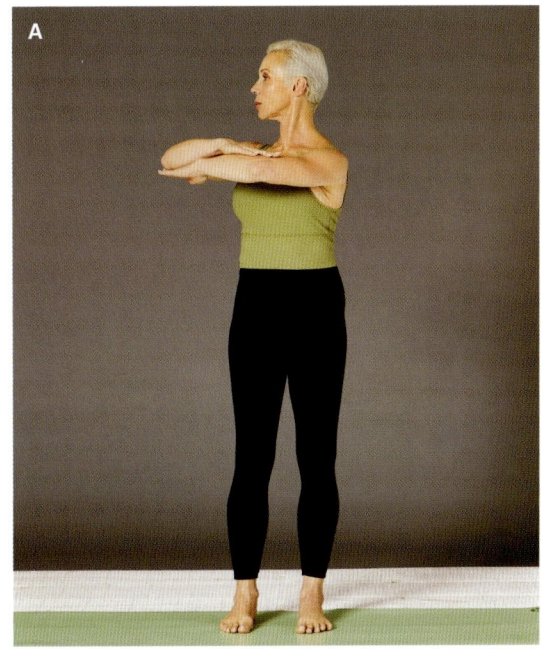

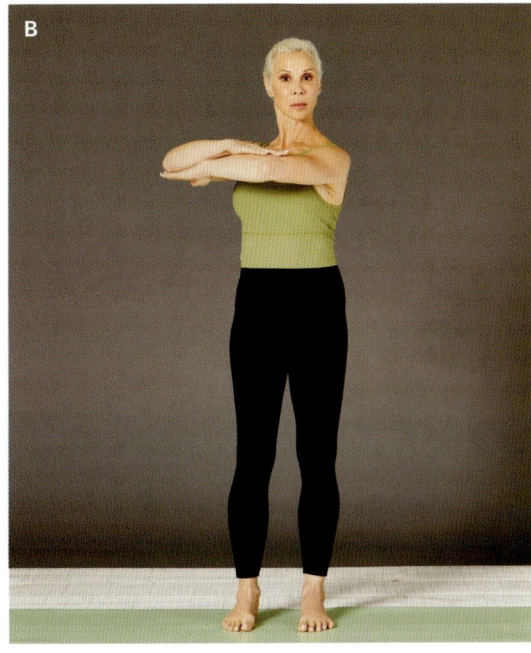

Thigh and Hip Stretch

1. Grab a chair and sit upright with your shoulders over your hips and your legs a little more than sit-bone width apart. Bend your knees at a 90-degree angle, with your knees over your heels. Point your feet forward.
2. Slide over in the chair so your right sit bone is off the side of the chair. Position your shoulders over your hips.
3. Pull your right foot straight back until your knee is under your hip; your heel will be lifted. Straighten your right leg, and push your right heel back. Hold the stretch for three counts.
4. Return to the starting position, and repeat the stretch on the left side.

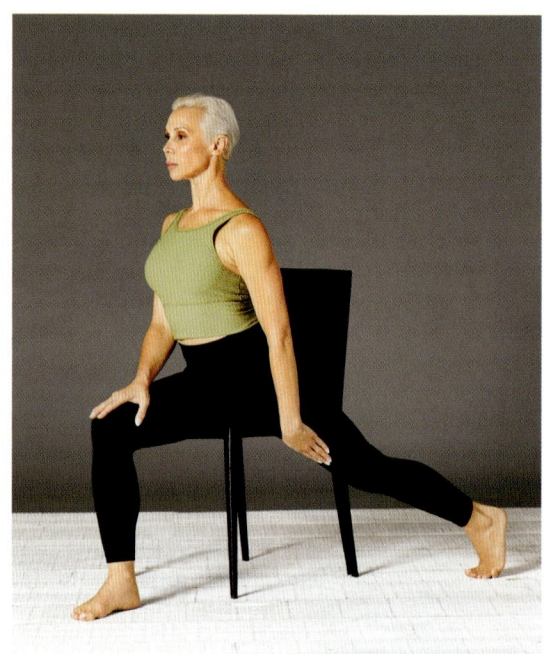

The Roll Down

1. Stand with your legs hip-width apart and parallel, your back straight, and your abdomen tight.
2. Bend your knees softly, and place your hands on your thighs. Pull your abdomen in. Inhale, and lower your head.
3. Exhale, and gradually roll your spine down, your hands sliding down your legs as the upper and lower back stretch. Pull your abdomen in.
4. Reverse the action, and roll up. Repeat twice.

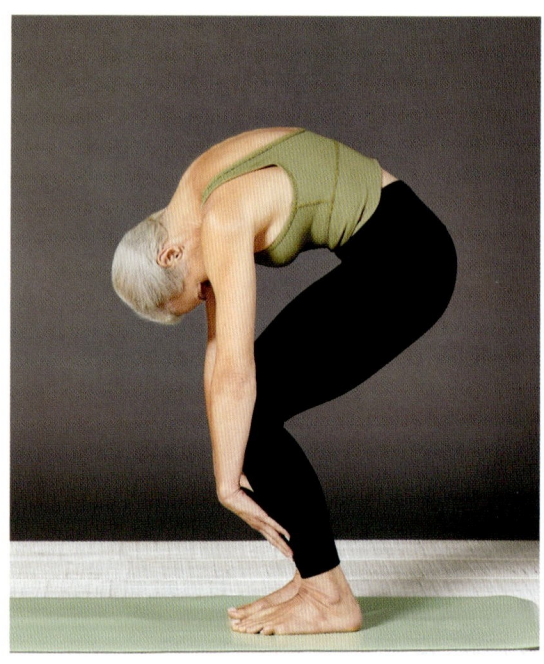

Extended Cat

1. Begin this stretch standing facing the chair, your hands on the seat in front of you and in line with your shoulders. Keep your elbows soft and pointed toward your ribs and your palms flat with your fingers pointing forward. Your legs should be hip-width apart and parallel.
2. Walk your feet slowly and carefully backward, keeping a straight back as much as you can, without moving your hands. Your body should be in an inverted-L position—shoulders in line with your wrists, arms straight, and elbows soft. Point your fingers and toes forward, legs hip-width apart.
3. Inhale, and round your spine like a scared cat. Bring your gaze to your navel (**A**).
4. Exhale. With your abdomen pulled in to protect your spine, lift your chest, and gently arch your back into the cow position (**B**). Repeat the cat and cow postures three times. End in the cat position.

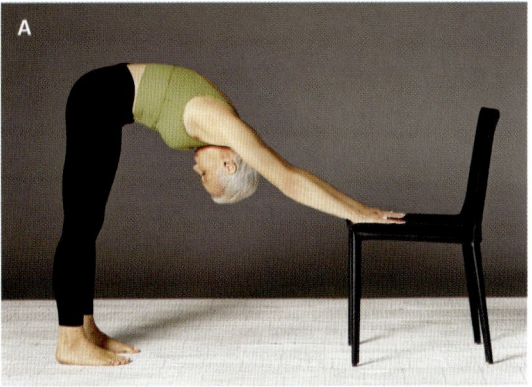

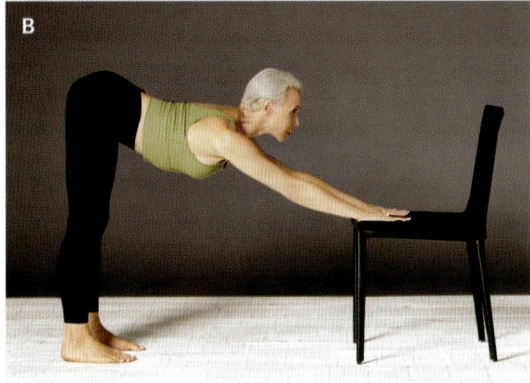

Foot Towel Stretch

1. Spread a towel on the floor. Sit upright with your shoulders over your hips, legs hip-width apart, your knees bent at 90 degrees, and your feet on the towel.
2. With your right foot, lift and spread your toes, then lower them. Grasp the towel with your toes, and pull it toward your heel. Relax your right foot.
3. Repeat with your left foot. Complete three times, alternating feet.

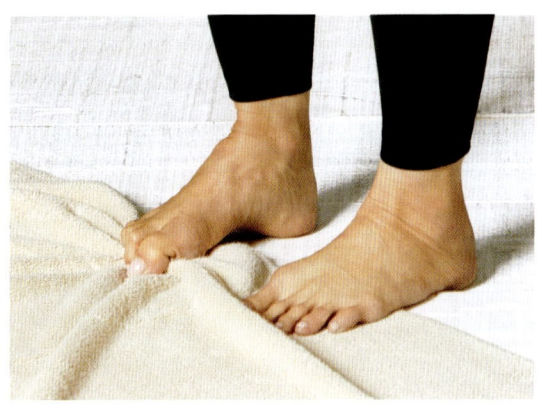

Balance

STANDING AND STAYING UPRIGHT MIGHT SEEM LIKE a simple act to pull off, but it takes teamwork from three major systems: your vision, your inner ear, and your internal sense of limb position and movement, called proprioception.

Poor balance can negatively affect your life in many ways, from making it more difficult to navigate daily activities to being an adverse indicator of longevity: One study showed that middle-aged and older adults who cannot balance on one leg for 10 seconds are nearly twice as likely to die from any cause in the next 10 years.

Most of our daily activities require flexibility and balance, so keeping these elements sharp helps us perform these tasks and also avoid injuries and falls, says Melissa Prestipino, P.T., D.P.T., owner of Maize & Blue Rehab in Sparta, New Jersey.

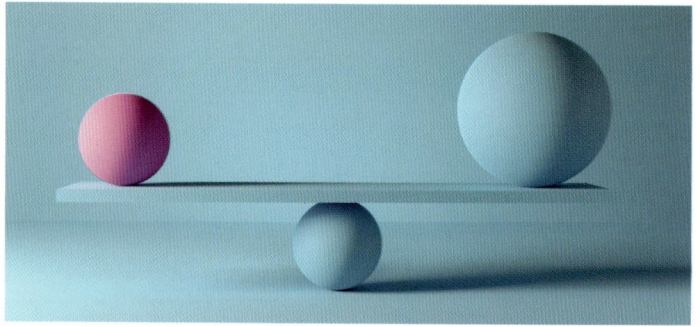

TEST YOUR BALANCE

Try these three stability challenges to find out where your balance falls right now.

Test 1 Stand still with your feet lined up heel to toe.

Test 2 Stand on one foot, raising the other so it hovers a few inches off the floor.

Test 3 Hold the position in test 2, then close your eyes.

For each challenge, how easy was it for you to stay upright for at least 10 seconds?

Simple You didn't sway or touch your foot to the floor. Your balance: GREAT

Fairly easy You may have wobbled slightly. Your balance: NORMAL

A little tricky You needed occasional support (like a countertop) to balance. Your balance: OK

Difficult You couldn't maintain the pose, even with support. Your balance: POOR

Balance Boosters

Working on your balance throughout life will mean that by your older years, when balance gets rockier, you won't be starting from a deficit. Do these simple stability exercises daily to get steadier:

Stand on one foot while brushing your teeth or waiting in line at the grocery.

Walk as if you were on a balance beam, putting the heel of your leading foot to the toe of your standing foot and continuing for 20 steps when going to get the mail or heading to your car.

Stand on your tiptoes while washing dishes or blow-drying your hair.

The Better-Balance Workout

These exercises engage your whole body as they fine-tune your balancing skills. **Bonus:** They'll also tone and strengthen your lower body and core.

Skater Taps

Stand with your feet wider than hip-width apart, with your hands on your hips, and sink into a squat. Hold the squat, then tap your left leg straight out to the side, shifting your torso as little as possible. Bring your leg back to center and repeat with your right leg. That's 1 rep—do 10.
Pro tip: When doing squats, make sure your knees don't extend beyond your toes.

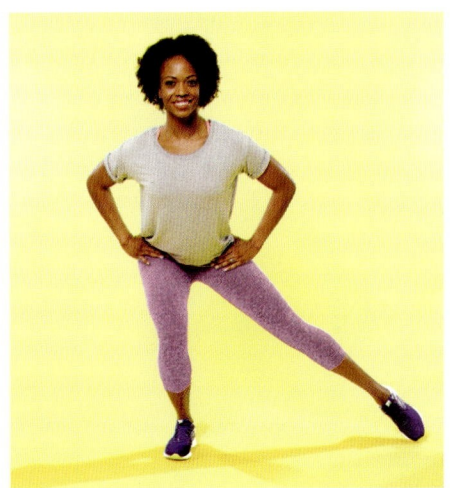

Single-Leg Dead Lift

Stand with your feet hip-width apart. Raise your right knee toward your chest. Bend your left leg slightly, hinge forward, and extend your right leg behind you, reaching your hands toward the floor. Hold a moment, then return to start. Repeat 10 times, then switch legs.

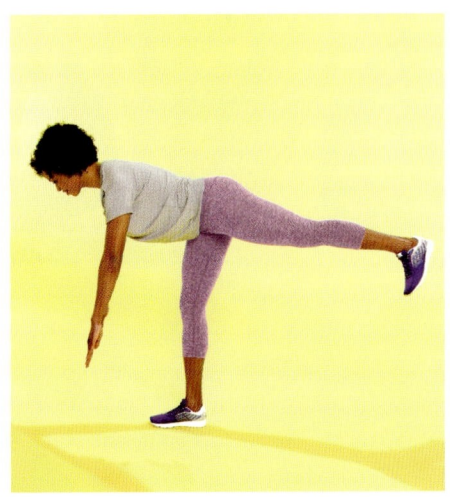

TIP:
In addition to 150 minutes of formal cardio each week, it's also wise to move all day long. Every movement counts: sweeping the kitchen, taking the stairs, grabbing a jump rope, playing with your dog, or dancing to your favorite song between work calls (might as well make it fun!).

One-Foot Hop

Stand with feet hip-width apart, then lift your right leg slightly out behind you, keeping your foot off the floor. Place your hands on your hips, then take a small hop forward. Regain your balance, then hop forward again. Do 10 hops on one leg, then switch sides.

Pro tip: If hopping forward is too challenging, hop in place instead.

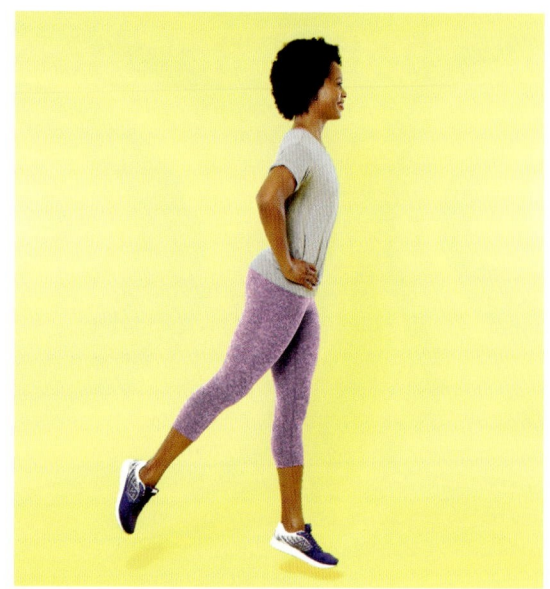

Pillow Stance

Stand with both feet in the center of a pillow, your hands on your hips. Lift your right leg to hip height with the knee bent 90 degrees. Hold as long as you can without lowering your right leg, then switch legs. Repeat twice for each leg.

Pro tip: Focusing on a spot a few feet in front of you can help you stay steady.

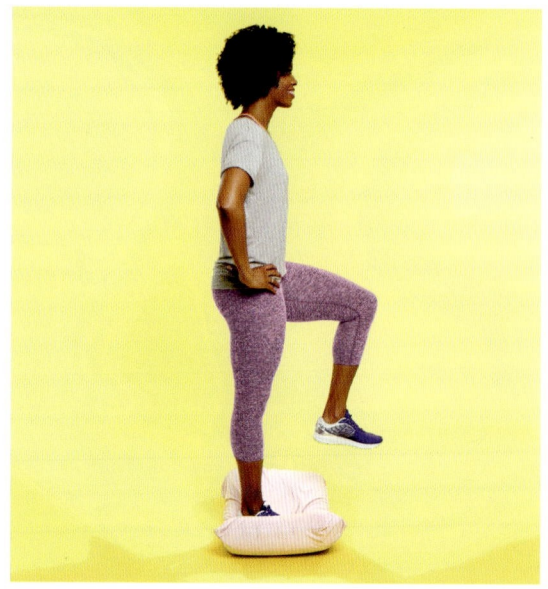

Semicircle Sweeps

First, stand on your left foot, with your hands on your hips, and extend your right leg in front of you at the 12 o'clock position. Then, while keeping your leg straight, sweep the foot around in a semicircle to the 6 o'clock position, then bring it back to 12 o'clock. Repeat 10 times; switch legs.

TIP:

When you're working to make physical activity a habit, try to avoid going more than two consecutive days without doing some form of exercise (unless, of course, you're sick or injured).

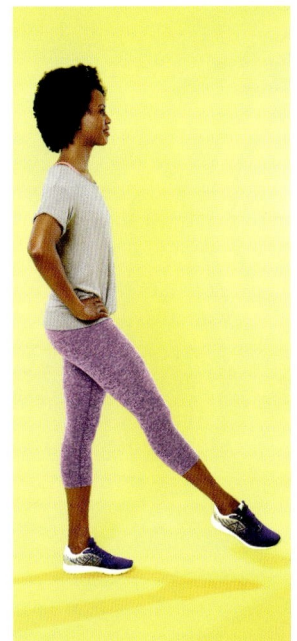
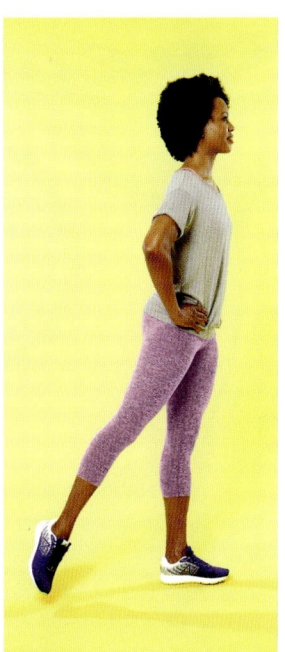

Should I Do Cardio Before or After Lifting Weights?

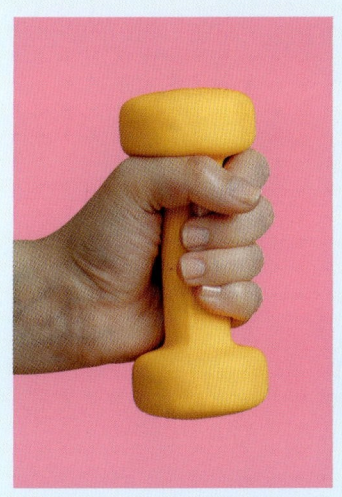

▶ The American Council on Exercise (ACE) created a guide to help people decide a fitness routine order that's best for them, depending on their goals. According to the ACE:

- If your main goal is endurance (i.e., distance running), **do cardio first.**

- If your main goal is weight loss, **strength train first.**

- If your main goal is to get stronger and build muscle, **strength train first.**

- If you are focused on upper-body strength training, **do either cardio or weights first.**

- If you are focused on lower-body strength training, **strength train first.**

- If your fitness goals are general with no aim for strength or endurance, **choose your preferred order.**

Strength

YOU DON'T NEED TO BECOME A POWER LIFTER TO become stronger. All you need is one pair of light dumbbells to make a powerful difference for your health. You can build lean muscles, ease achy joints, lower chronic-disease risks, and lose weight—no matter where your fitness is right now. A weightlifting program using light weights is an excellent way to build up the strength of your core (a.k.a. midsection) to give you a solid, steady foundation.

The benefits of increased core strength are no joke. A strong core helps you move more fluidly and avoid falls and injuries related to sudden movement. Plus, light weight training improves bone density, supports heart health, boosts your mood, and reduces risk of injury.

STRENGTH TEST

How is your strength? Try these at-home strength tests to get started.

Stand from Sitting Build thigh and core strength by getting out of a chair then sitting back down without using your hands—in reps of 10. Stand and lower yourself in a controlled fashion with your gaze straight ahead. Once this becomes easy, try doing it on one leg with the other foot lifted, then switch legs. After doing these exercises at least three times a week for a month, try the sit-to-stand test.

Stand from the Floor Test

Start by sitting on the ground cross-legged. Without using your hands or any other part of your body for support (though reaching your arms out in front of you can help you steady yourself), push yourself into a standing position. Once you reach a standing position, lower yourself back to sitting cross-legged on the floor, without using your hands.

If you can't do it on the first try, don't give up. Work up to it by building your strength through squats and chair stands.

Your ability to stand from a seated position without using your hands may have big implications for your longevity. In one study involving more than 2,000 adults ages 51 to 80, those who couldn't perform the sit-to-stand test without using support had higher mortality rates (from any cause) over a six-year period.

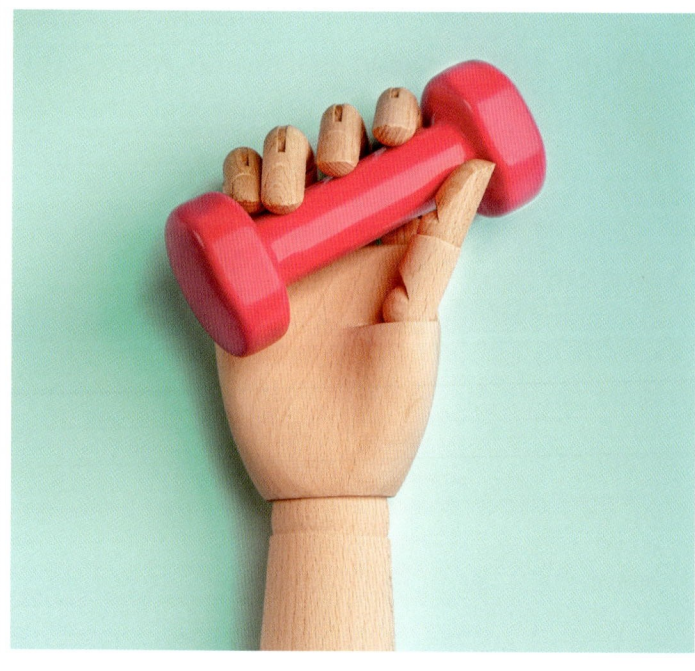

No Equipment? No Problem!

Pilates is a low-impact form of exercise that will boost your strength, balance, and mobility to help you move through life safely and with minimal joint pain. The best part? You can fit in a great workout in just 10 minutes a day! **Perform each exercise for 45 seconds, resting for 15 seconds in between moves. End there or repeat the circuit again.**

Side Plank Hip Drop

Start on your side with your top foot crossed in front of the other, then prop yourself up on your bottom elbow, staying in line with your shoulder. Keep your left forearm perpendicular to your trunk, your palm flat on the floor, and your head in line with your spine. Inhale, expanding through your ribs and core, then exhale and lift your hips and torso off the floor as you pull your core in, keeping your hips stacked. Slowly lower yourself to the floor.

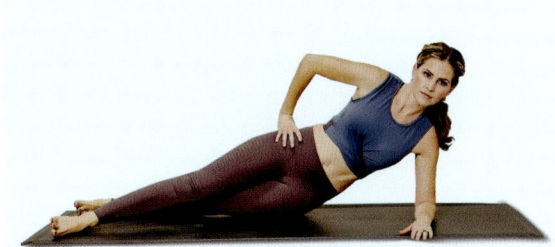

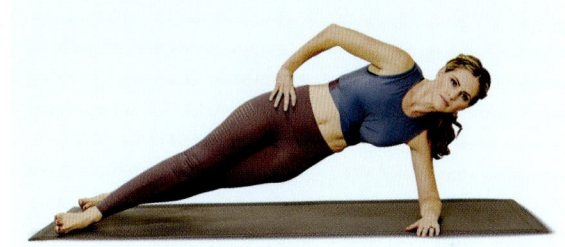

Live Longer by Strength Training 30 Minutes a Week

▶ Strength training has already been linked to health perks like better bone density and lean muscle mass, but it's also associated with living longer. That's the major takeaway from a meta-analysis in the *British Journal of Sports Medicine*. For the analysis, researchers looked at data from 16 studies of nearly 480,000 people between the ages of 18 and 98.

The researchers discovered that people who did 30 to 60 minutes per week of resistance-, strength-, or weight-training had a 10% to 20% lower risk of early death from all causes. They also had a lower risk of developing heart disease (46%) or cancer (28%). The researchers even discovered that people who did up to 60 minutes a week of muscle-strengthening activities had a lowered risk of developing diabetes.

Front Plank Body Saw to Pike

Begin in forearm plank position. Inhale as you slightly shift your weight forward, then exhale as you hike your hips up to the ceiling. Bring your head between your elbows and squeeze your abs to pull your torso toward your thighs.

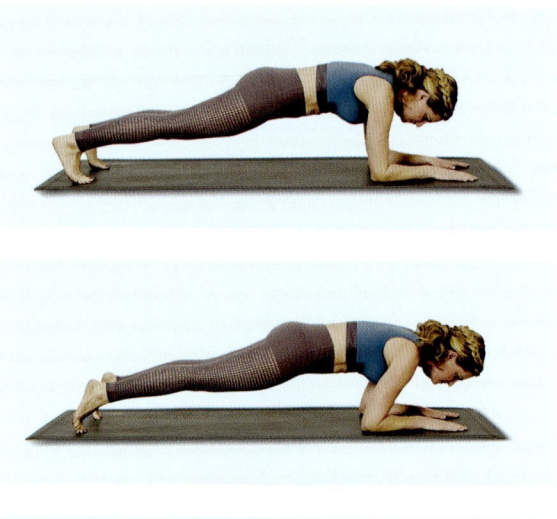

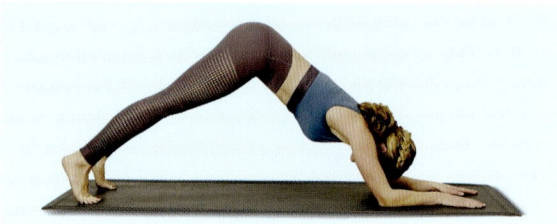

Pilates Hundred

Start on your back. Bend your knees and lift them until they are parallel to your hips. Lift your shoulders off the mat and pulse your arms up and down. Inhale for 5 pulses, then exhale while doing 5 more. Continue this pattern until your 45 seconds are up.

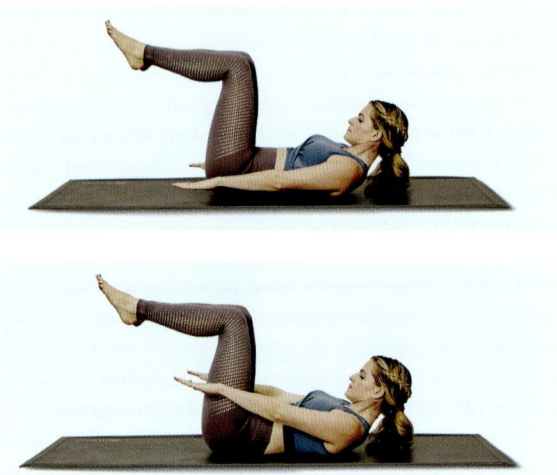

You're in Good Company

When Janine, a lawyer and dedicated runner in her 50s, began taking Pilates Reformer classes, she was focused on developing strength in her core. "I've always had weak abs, and I know core strength is especially important as we get older," says Janine. Within a few months, she began to notice a difference in her core strength and tone, but she also gained a surprising benefit. "For the first time, I can lift my suitcase into the overhead compartment on a plane without assistance," she says.

Plank Singles

Begin by lying on your stomach. Prop yourself up in a sphinx position with your elbows directly beneath your shoulders, forearms anchored to the floor. Brace your core to avoid overarching your lower back, and keep your neck in line with your spine. Breathe in and, as you exhale, draw the navel to the spine and lift your hips, then your knees. Hold for one count, then return to the ground.

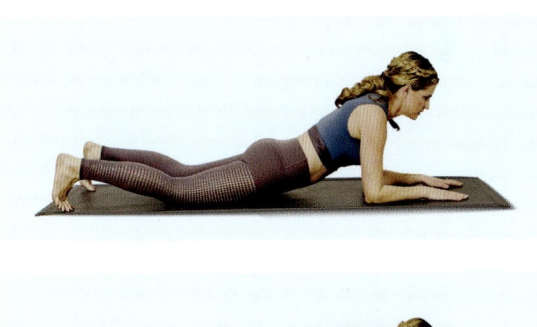
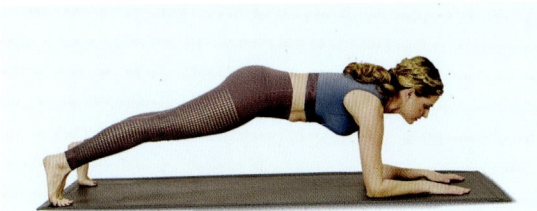

TIP:
Adding five additional minutes of exercise to your daily routine can reduce blood pressure and may lower your risk for heart disease, according to research in *Circulation* in 2024.

9 Moves for Strength and Health

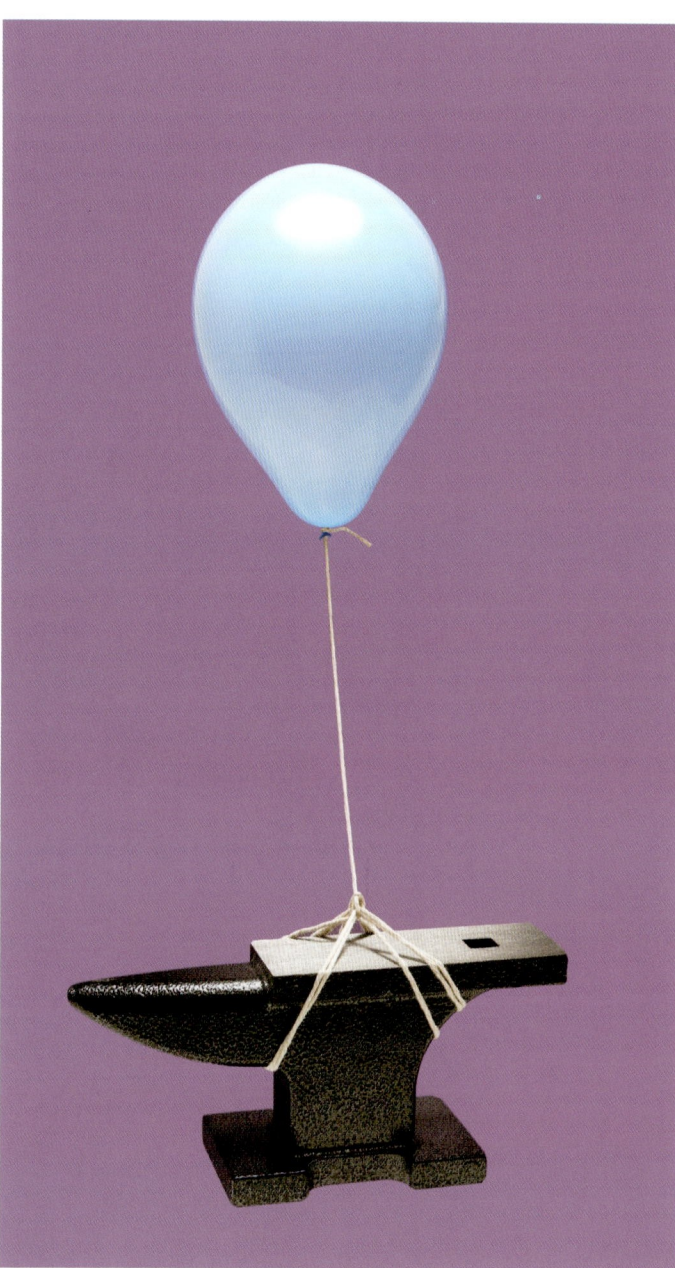

IN THIS WORKOUT, YOU'LL DO EIGHT STRENGTH MOVES. Your final move is a HIIT move, the one that brings a little extra magic (actually, science!) to the whole thing. HIIT stands for high-intensity interval training and provides a totally doable workout boost. You simply add extra bursts of energy to a small section of your workout. Yes, you'll really sweat during those 30 or so seconds, but the perks far outweigh the temporary strain.

Studies have shown that HIIT workouts bring a host of benefits: The method improves cardiac function, muscle function, and memory faster than regular exercise. A specific aging-related benefit is that HIIT routines have been shown to lengthen the ends of your telomeres, which keeps you healthy a lot longer. (See page 19.)

You can do this workout no matter what your fitness level. The best thing about this workout is that it's easy to start and just as easy to make more challenging as you get stronger!

THE MOVES

Do these nine exercises once and be proud of yourself! But do them as a full workout per the guidelines below to truly reap the strength, cardio, and longevity benefits.

- Do 8 to 12 reps of each exercise. For the first eight exercises, focus on your form, not on speed. For the squat toe tap jumps (page 145), make sure you keep moving as you go from one rep to the next. Your heart rate will go up!

- Complete three to four circuits of all nine moves. Start with two circuits, and add more as you get stronger.

- Rest for two to three minutes between circuits.

- Add weights when you're ready. This routine is effective without dumbbells, but to continue to challenge yourself (crucial for strength, weight loss, and longevity), add 5- to 15-lb. weights as you continue to follow this routine.

Sumo Squat with Drag

1. If using dumbbells, hold one horizontally in front of your chest.
2. Stand with your feet a little wider than hip-width apart, toes facing out. Bend your knees and squat, pushing your butt back and keeping your knees over your ankles.
3. As you return to standing, drag your right leg behind your left leg so the right foot ends up slightly behind and to the left of your left foot.
4. Step your right leg back into starting position and repeat the sumo squat, followed by the drag with the left foot.
5. Continue alternating sides to complete at least four reps on each side.

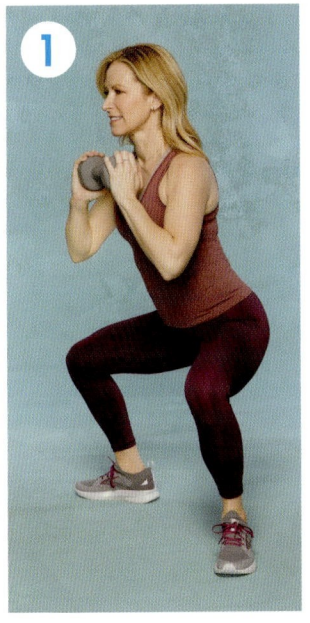
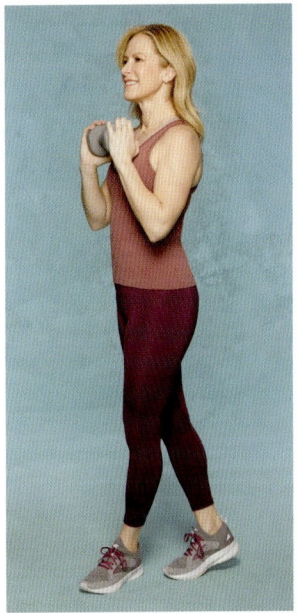

Overhead Triceps

1. If using dumbbells, hold one in each hand. Raise your left hand over your head while resting your right hand (and dumbbell) on your hip.
2. Bend your left elbow to lower the dumbbell behind your head. Keep your elbow tight beside your ear.
3. Straighten your arm and repeat for at least four reps.
4. Repeat with your other arm.

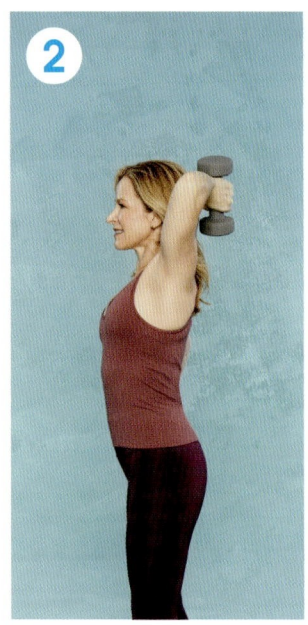
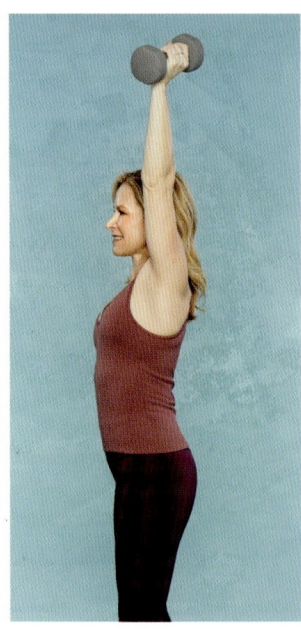

Squat to Lunge

1. If using dumbbells, hold one horizontally in front of your chest or two facing each other over your shoulders.
2. Stand with feet hip-width apart, toes facing forward. Sit into your heels and bend your knees into a squat.
3. Return to standing and lunge backward with your left leg. Bring your left leg back to starting position.
4. Repeat the squat, this time lunging back with your right leg.
5. Continue alternating sides to complete at least four reps on each side.

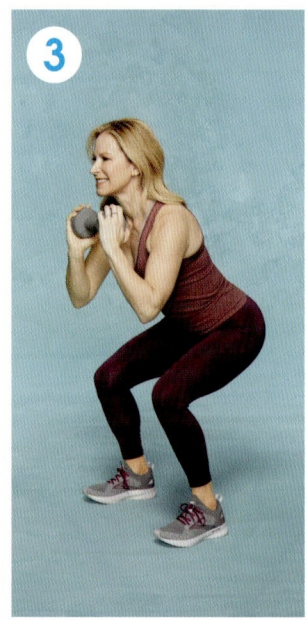
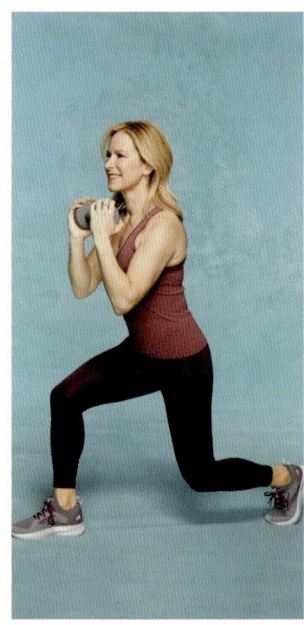

Core Toe Taps

1. Lie on your back with your knees bent in tabletop position (thighs perpendicular to the floor, knees bent, calves parallel with the floor).
2. Place your hands behind your head and raise your shoulders from the floor.
3. Gently alternate tapping your right and left toes on the floor for at least four reps with each foot.

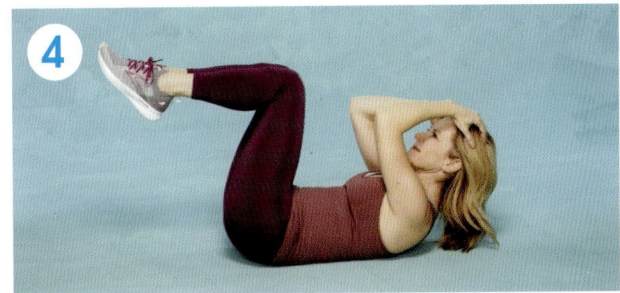

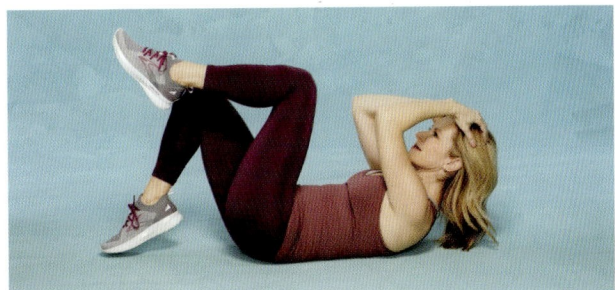

TIP:
Thirty minutes of strength training per week is easily achievable: It's just six minutes a day if you do it five days a week.

Push-Up with Reach Out

1. Start in push-up position, hands slightly wider than your shoulders. Keep your abs tight and knees bent, with pressure slightly above your knees.
2. Bend your elbows to lower your body to the ground.
3. Extend your arms and legs out in a V, keeping your head neutral.
4. Pull your arms and legs back into their original position and push your body up by straightening your arms and keeping your core tight.
5. Repeat 8 to 12 times.

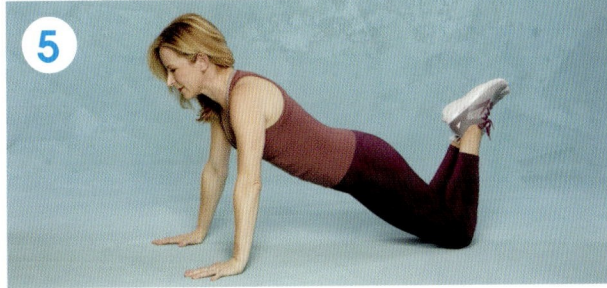

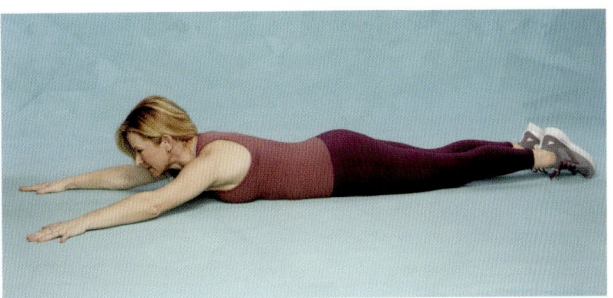

Stagger Biceps

1. If using dumbbells, hold one in each hand with your palms facing forward.
2. Stand with one foot a step behind you. Keeping your elbows tight to your body, bend your elbows to raise your hands to chest height.
3. Keeping your elbows tight to your body, raise and lower your arms three-quarters of the way up and all the way down.
4. Repeat at least four times.
5. Switch legs and perform the same number of reps on the other side.

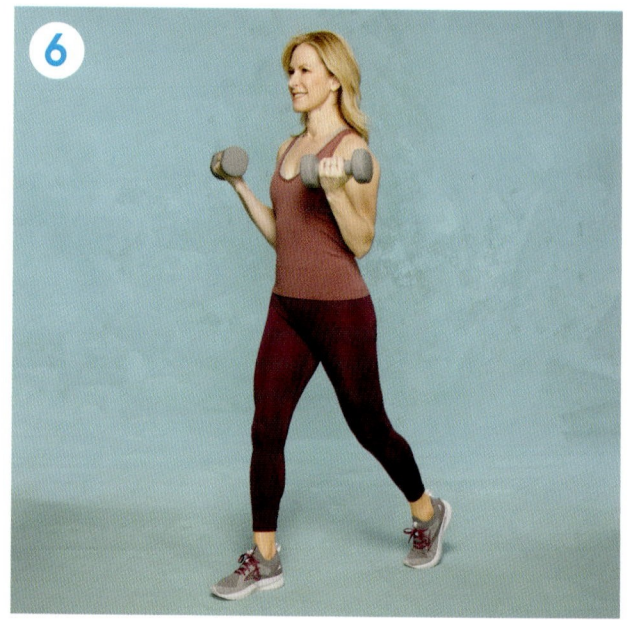

Bird Dog

1. Start down on your mat with your knees under your hips and your hands under your shoulders.
2. Bring your left knee and right elbow together below your chest.
3. Extend your left leg behind you, and your right arm in front of you.
4. Repeat with your right leg and left arm, then continue alternating sides to complete at least four reps on each side.

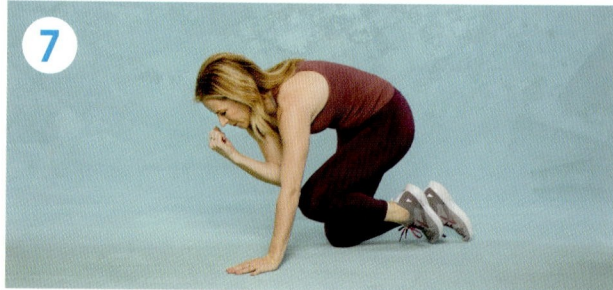

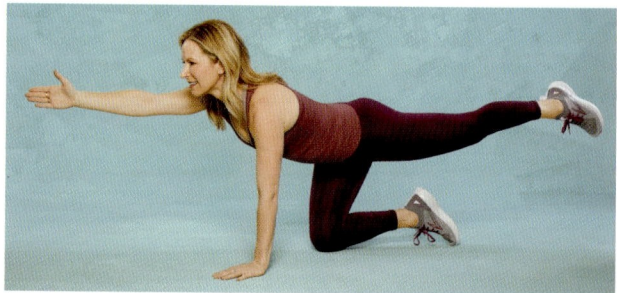

One Arm, One Leg Dumbbell Row

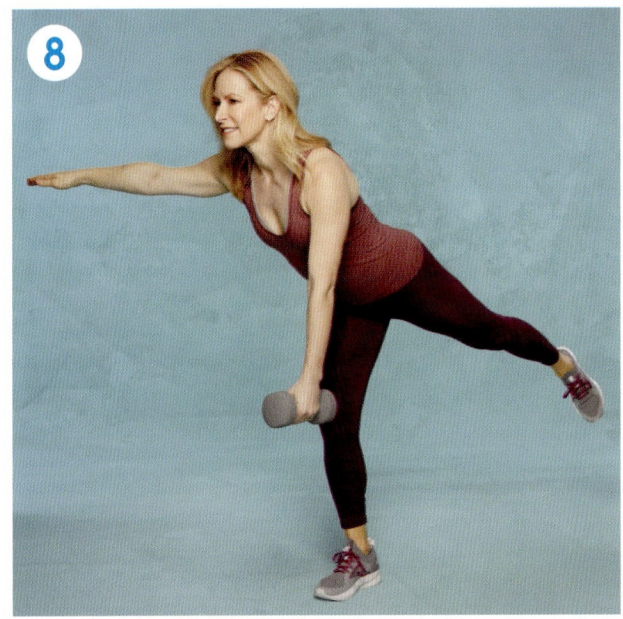

1. If using dumbbells, hold one in your left hand.
2. Stand with your feet hip-width apart, toes facing forward. With your right knee slightly bent, lean forward and raise your left leg behind you. Hold your right arm out to the side for balance.
3. Keep your body square to the front and your hips parallel to the floor, squeeze your glutes, and bend your left elbow to raise the weight to your body.
4. Lower the weight and return to starting position. Move the weight to your other hand and repeat.
5. Continue alternating sides to complete at least four reps on each side.

Squat Toe Tap Jumps

This is your HIIT move—get ready to sweat!

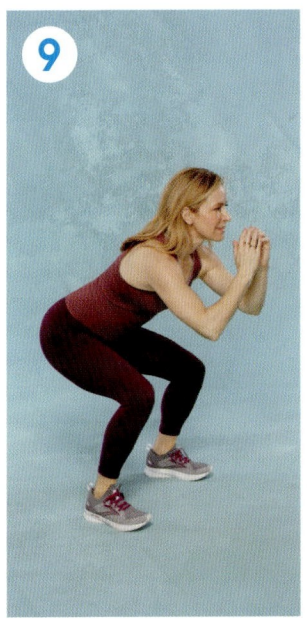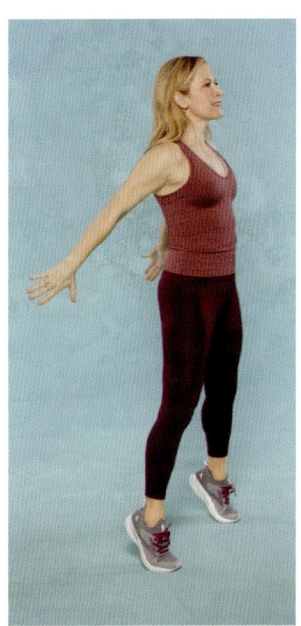

1. Start with your feet hip-width apart, toes facing forward. Bend your knees into a squat position, then straighten your legs and jump forward onto your toes.
2. Fall back into a squat and repeat 8 to 12 times.

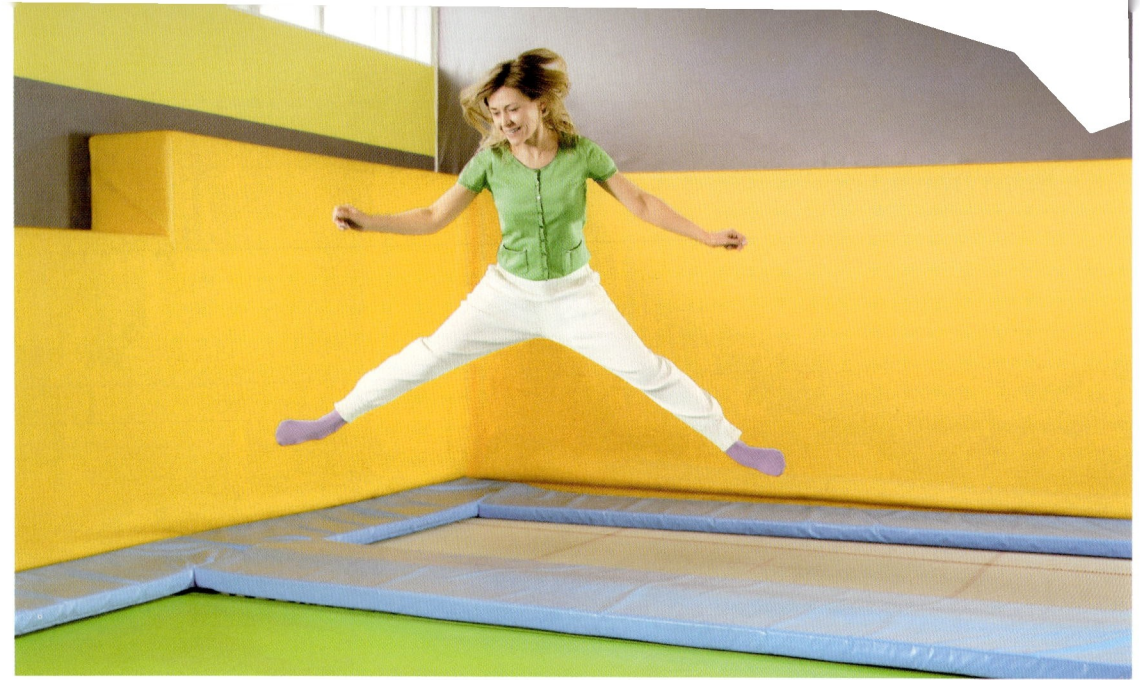

Cardio (a.k.a. Get Moving)

IT DOESN'T MATTER HOW YOU DO IT, AS LONG AS YOU MOVE YOUR BODY. Regular exercise keeps muscles strong to help us stay active in old age, and does even more for our health spans, including stimulating anti-inflammatory activity throughout the body and keeping cell-damaging insulin levels in check.

What's most important when it comes to a cardiovascular workout is to get in some kind of movement that gets your heart working hard for 150 minutes per week (or about 30 minutes a day, five days a week), says Nicole Weinberg, M.D., a cardiologist at Providence Saint John's Health Center in Santa Monica, California.

A cardio workout doesn't necessarily need to look like burpees and sprints (though it can if that's what you want it to be), it just depends on your goals and fitness level, says Marisa Hope, a certified personal trainer and owner of e(M)powered personal training.

Walking is a good starter form of exercise for people who aren't very active, and you can make tweaks to make it more challenging, like picking up your pace or walking for longer periods of time.

WORKING OUT CAN BE FUN

Think beyond the treadmill or neighborhood running routes. Exercise comes in all kinds of different forms. Try one of these as a fresh exercise motivator that involves a little trip down memory lane.

Trampolining

"Jumping on a trampoline is low impact, so it's kind to your bones and joints, and it's a good way to boost your fitness endurance and strengthen your cardiovascular health," says Latreal Mitchell, a personal trainer and the founder of MEI Wellness. Score some time on your kids' or grandkids' backyard trampoline, find smaller rebound trampolines (mini trampolines) that fit in the house or garage, or find a local indoor trampoline park.

Why We Love It
• Strengthens your core muscles

- Works out your lower body
- Gets your heart rate up for a great burst of cardio

Bowling

Whether you can roll a perfect strike or you still need the bumpers, bowling is a social way to stay active when you use proper form. "Bowling form is all about single-sided strength and overall dexterity," says Teddy Savage, national lead fitness trainer at Planet Fitness. "This is similar to exercises like curtsy lunges, wood choppers, and alternating front shoulder raises."

Why We Love It
- Improves stability and balance
- Strengthens upper body and core
- Engages hips
- Clocks steps

Roller Skating

Lacing up and wheeling around in an indoor roller rink is more than just nostalgic. "Besides getting your body in motion, it ties in traditional exercise principles that you practice when you do movements like lunges, squats, and resistance moves," says Savage. Skating smarts: Wear a helmet and wrist and knee pads to help protect you if you fall.

Why We Love It
- Supports good balance and coordination
- Promotes joint mobility
- Strengthens muscular and cardiovascular endurance
- Targets your entire lower body and core

Other fun fitspo? Boxing, virtual reality fitness games, and mini golf are all fun, social, and get your heart rate going!

Do the Talk Test

▶ In addition to measuring your heart rate using a heart-monitoring fitness tracker, using the talk test is a great option to ensure you're pushing yourself appropriately. "If you're doing cardio and you can have a full conversation without being out of breath," Hope says, "you're likely not pushing yourself hard enough." Aim to be a little breathless during conversation, and you'll likely be in a good spot for heart-healthy benefits.

In the Zone

▶ When it comes to cardio, your heart rate can be a good indicator of how hard you're working. To calculate your maximum heart rate (the rate you should never exceed) you can use the basic formula of 220 minus your age. Hope says this calculation is not an end-all-be-all, and many studies have suggested it's a little too general to be accurate. But it's a good baseline to work from to get an idea of where you'd like to be for a good cardio workout. You can measure your heart rate using a smart watch; some machines at the gym can also do this, albeit inexactly. Once you know your maximum heart rate, you can figure out where your heart rate should be using the three zones of exercise.

- **Zone 1** Known as the recovery zone; Hope says your heart rate will be between 65% and 75% of your calculated maximum heart rate.

- **Zone 2** To achieve an anaerobic workout, Hope suggests your heart rate will reach around 75% to 80% of your calculated maximum heart rate.

- **Zone 3** For a truly high-intensity workout, your heart rate will be between 80% to 90% of the calculated maximum heart rate for no more than 60 seconds at a time, Hope says.

For what cardiologists consider a cardiovascular exercise, Dr. Weinberg says you'll need to reach the third zone or about 85% of your maximum heart rate. She emphasizes that you do not need to have your heart rate at this level throughout your entire workout, but aim to achieve it periodically throughout your session for solid cardiovascular benefits.

"When your heart rate is at that threshold, you have flow changes throughout your arteries," she says. "Your heart is a muscle, so a lot of it is about working out that muscle, getting good blood flow, and having your heart expand and contract."

The Wellness Power of Walking

NO MATTER YOUR FITNESS LEVEL, WALKING CAN go a long way in boosting your overall health.

"Walking is an easy-to-do exercise that has so many benefits with very little risk of injury," says Adam Mills, M.S.E.d., R.C.E.P., registered certified exercise physiologist and cycling coach at Source Endurance. "Walking can reduce rates of chronic disease," he adds.

According to Melina B. Jampolis, M.D., author of *The Doctor on Demand Diet*, the key is to walk for at least 30 minutes a day to get maximum benefits. Studies have shown that walking regularly can lower blood pressure, improve cognition, and promote heart health.

Walking can seriously help you add years to your life too— and it doesn't take much to see results. In fact, people who completed the recommended 150 minutes of weekly exercise in at least 10-minute spurts had a 31% lower risk of premature death. Other research shows the faster you walk, the more your risk drops. The longer life benefit is believed to come from the cardiorespiratory workout walking provides.

HOW LONG IS LONG ENOUGH?

You've probably heard the 10,000-step goal thrown around, but should that number really be your goal every day?

A study published in *JAMA Network Open* found that 7,000 steps was associated with a lower rate of premature death for people ages 38 to 50. If that number of steps seems steep for you right now, another *JAMA* study found that just 4,400 steps a day lowered that premature death rate for older women (when compared with women who took just 2,700 steps).

So, if 10,000 steps is not feasible for you to reach today, remember that small gains still make a difference.

Aim for at least a half hour of walking per day, but it never hurts to do more, according to Mills. "Walking 30 minutes a day is good. Walking more than 30 minutes a day is better," he says. The more you walk, the more benefits you'll see over time.

IS IT BETTER TO WALK FASTER OR LONGER?

As it turns out, walking faster may be better for you and your long-term health. The faster a person walks on average, the lower their risk of both all-cause mortality and death linked to heart disease, says a study in the *British Journal of Sports Medicine*.

Another study in *Cancer Epidemiology, Biomarkers & Prevention* looked at more than 200,000 cancer survivors between the ages of 50 and 71 and found that those who walked at the slowest pace had more than double the risk of death from any cause, compared with those reporting the fastest walking pace.

How fast is fast enough? The optimal speed you should aim for is walking at least 4 miles per hour (mph), according to a *Mayo Clinic Proceedings* study. When it comes to the health benefits of walking, slow and steady does *not* win the race.

CHALLENGE YOURSELF WITH A WALKING WORKOUT

To determine the best walking workout for you, consider when

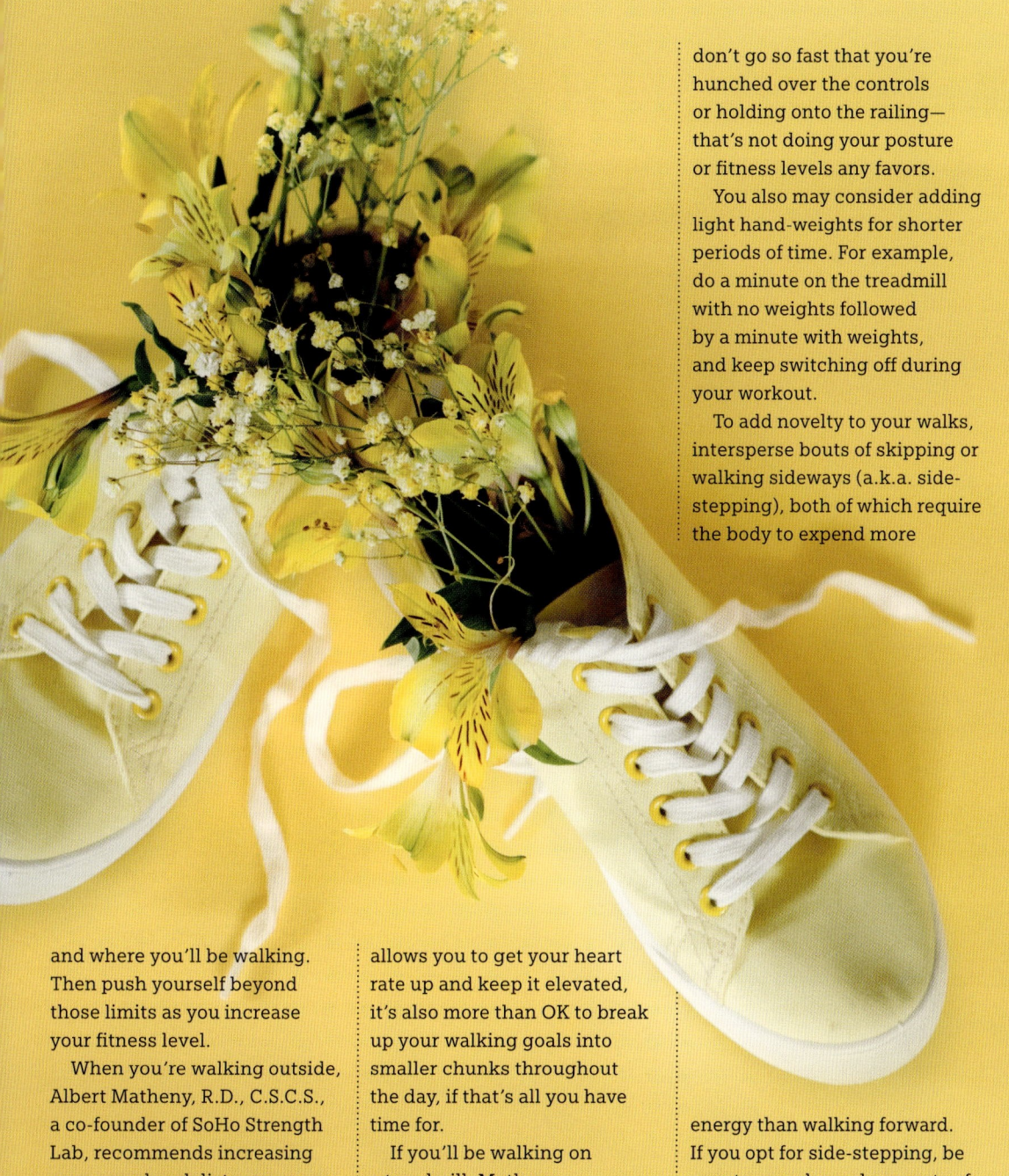

don't go so fast that you're hunched over the controls or holding onto the railing—that's not doing your posture or fitness levels any favors.

You also may consider adding light hand-weights for shorter periods of time. For example, do a minute on the treadmill with no weights followed by a minute with weights, and keep switching off during your workout.

To add novelty to your walks, intersperse bouts of skipping or walking sideways (a.k.a. side-stepping), both of which require the body to expend more

and where you'll be walking. Then push yourself beyond those limits as you increase your fitness level.

When you're walking outside, Albert Matheny, R.D., C.S.C.S., a co-founder of SoHo Strength Lab, recommends increasing your speed and distance as you start to feel more comfortable. Keep in mind that while walking a consistent distance over time

allows you to get your heart rate up and keep it elevated, it's also more than OK to break up your walking goals into smaller chunks throughout the day, if that's all you have time for.

If you'll be walking on a treadmill, Matheny recommends experimenting with the incline and speed to keep pushing yourself. Just

energy than walking forward. If you opt for side-stepping, be sure to spend equal amounts of time leading with each leg to develop greater muscle balance and coordination.

How Stress Ages You

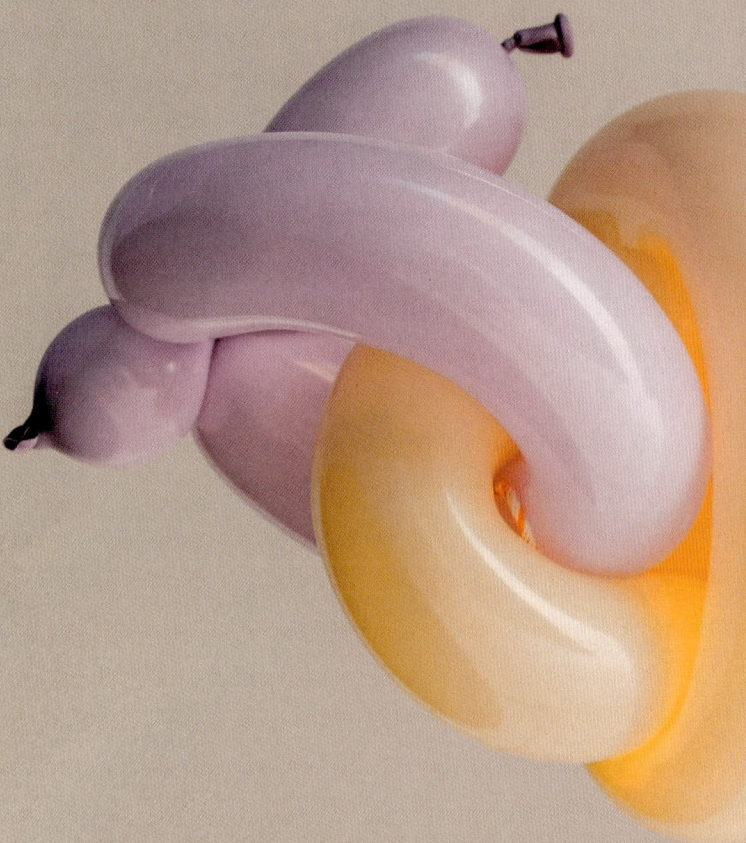

WHILE EVERYONE WORRIES FROM TIME TO TIME, feeling chronically stressed can speed up the aging process, says Elissa Epel, Ph.D., director of the Aging, Metabolism, and Emotions Center at the University of California, San Francisco.

The stress reaction stems from a powerful primal instinct—namely, the fight-or-flight response. "The amygdala, the brain's emotional center, is activated within a few seconds to respond to threats," says Rashi Aggarwal, M.D., an associate professor of psychiatry at Rutgers New Jersey Medical School. The hypothalamus then triggers the release of stress hormones such as cortisol and adrenaline, causing heart rate to speed up, blood pressure to rise, breathing to become more rapid, and muscles to contract.

When you're not in life-threatening situations and yet your brain responds to financial pressures, for example, by repeatedly signaling that you are in a dire crisis, health problems can occur. Studies show that long-term stress is linked with increased inflammation, which plays a role in conditions like rheumatoid arthritis, heart disease, chronic pain, high blood pressure, and depression. And chronic stress may hasten the wear and tear on your body over time—a phenomenon called "allostatic load"—accelerating the aging process.

Fortunately, you can manage your reaction to stress. In addition to eating nutritious foods, connecting with friends, and getting enough sleep—use the following tactics to keep your mind and body in a better state of balance.

GIVE YOUR BRAIN A BREAK

"When you're in overdrive, your brain is constantly seeking ways to stay safe—there's no respite," says Luana Marques, Ph.D., an associate professor of psychiatry at Harvard Medical School and former president of the Anxiety and Depression Association of America. It's important to give

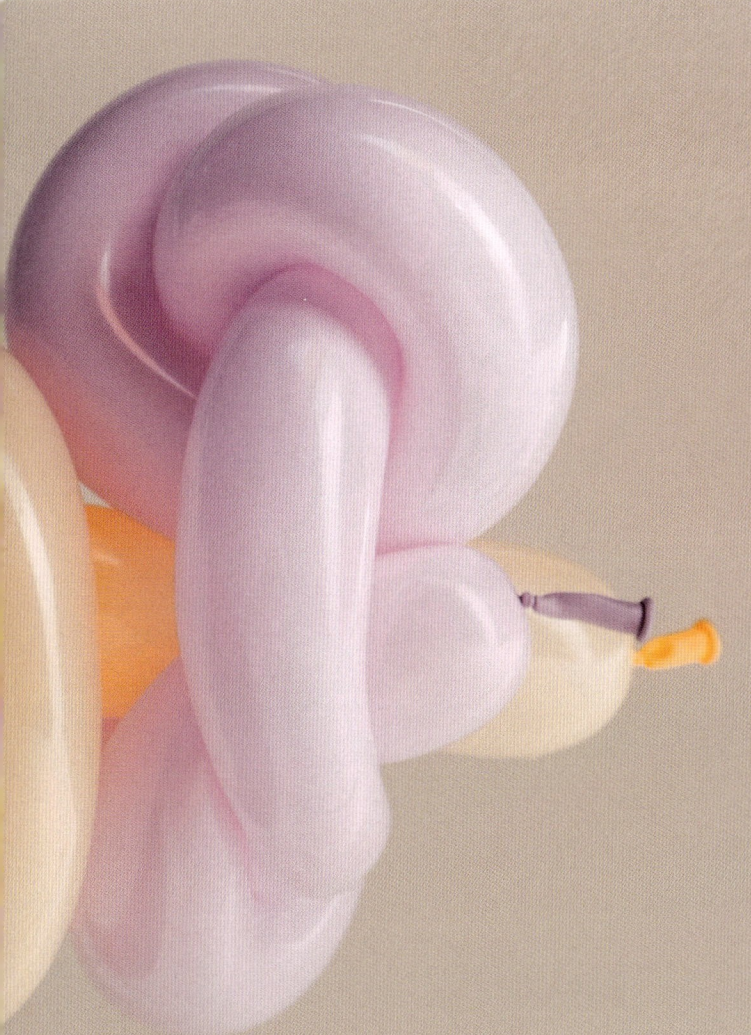

your brain time to shut off and recharge during the day.

For example, if the news is ramping you up, limit yourself to news sites once or twice a day instead of doomscrolling repeatedly. Likewise, set boundaries for social media and turn off unnecessary notifications.

Taking a short walk or even doing a few jumping jacks helps your brain hit the brakes, no matter what is kicking your stress response into high gear. Numerous studies have shown that physical activity releases positive chemicals (such as endorphins and serotonin) that have anti-inflammatory and antidepressant effects.

DO ONE THING AT A TIME

Multitasking seems efficient, but it often leaves people feeling frazzled and distracted. Instead, concentrate on a single task at a time. "One way to increase satisfaction in life in general is to practice focusing on the present moment," says Marques. Over time, you'll see that staying in the moment and not letting yourself get sidetracked is empowering. When walking outdoors, turn off electronics and observe what's around you. Play with your pet without turning on the TV or chatting with a family member. Tuning in to your senses of sight, sound, touch, and hearing for even a minute or two can settle your mind. Do this anytime, anywhere, to reduce your heart rate and blood pressure and soothe your jangled nerves.

TAKE A DEEP BREATH

One of the most powerful and scientifically proven stress-busting strategies is free, easy, and something that can be done anywhere: breathing. Taking a few deep, mindful breaths is an effective way to slow your heart rate and lower your blood pressure, and it can reduce anxiety within minutes. There are many types of breath work exercises to do, but being intentional is key. To start, practice mindful breathing by sitting and doing nothing but paying attention to your breath for one minute. If your mind wanders, it's OK: Note it and then return to focusing on your breathing. Surrender to

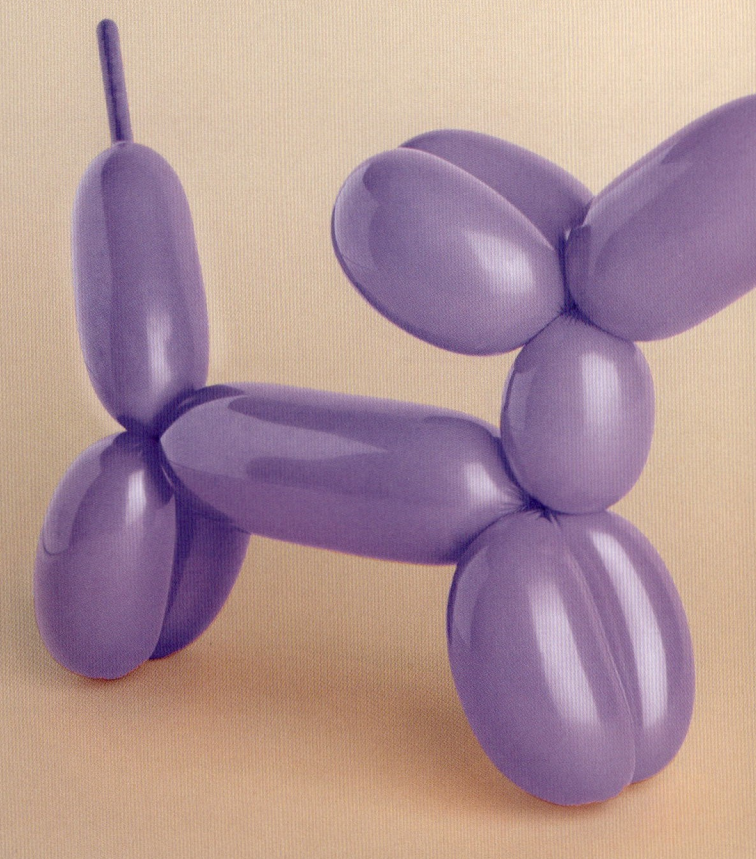

Good Stress vs. Bad Stress

▶The way many people talk about *stress*, it might as well be a four-letter word. But stress isn't all bad. In fact, there is such a thing as positive *stress*: It's called *eustress*, which is essentially stress without distress. With good stress—such as making a career-boosting presentation at work, throwing a party for people you love, or embarking on a new physical challenge on vacation—the challenge or stimulation often leads to feelings of personal fulfillment. The goal in life is to embrace opportunities for experiencing *eustress* and minimize those involving *distress*.

this simplicity with the goal of working up to three minutes, suggests Roberto Benzo, M.D., director of the Mindful Breathing Lab at the Mayo Clinic in Rochester, Minnesota.

REFRAME YOUR THINKING

Part of handling tough times well is the way you approach them. "We tend to push away negative experiences, but if we can work through difficulties, that's how we build resilience," says Neda Gould, Ph.D., director of the Mindfulness Program at Johns Hopkins University School of Medicine. "Try to come up with a more balanced way of looking at things. You may think *This is never going to end* or *I'm always going to feel this way*, but everything comes to an end eventually. In the meantime, what can you do to find one small joy every day?" While you're at it, remind yourself that you've overcome many other challenges in your life and you'll surmount this one too.

SCHEDULE SOME FUN

When you're stressed, even usually fun things may not seem delightful, but you can flip the script by penciling a pleasurable activity in on the calendar. Essentially, scheduling something you enjoy ahead of time gives your brain notice and tells it to pay attention because you're going to do something entertaining, Dr. Aggarwal explains.

Plan to see a movie or set up a recurring "family fun" night to play board games or make pizza. Arrange a backyard barbecue with neighbors. Make time for a craft project or schedule a phone call with a friend instead of texting. The idea is to set an intention to do something enjoyable.

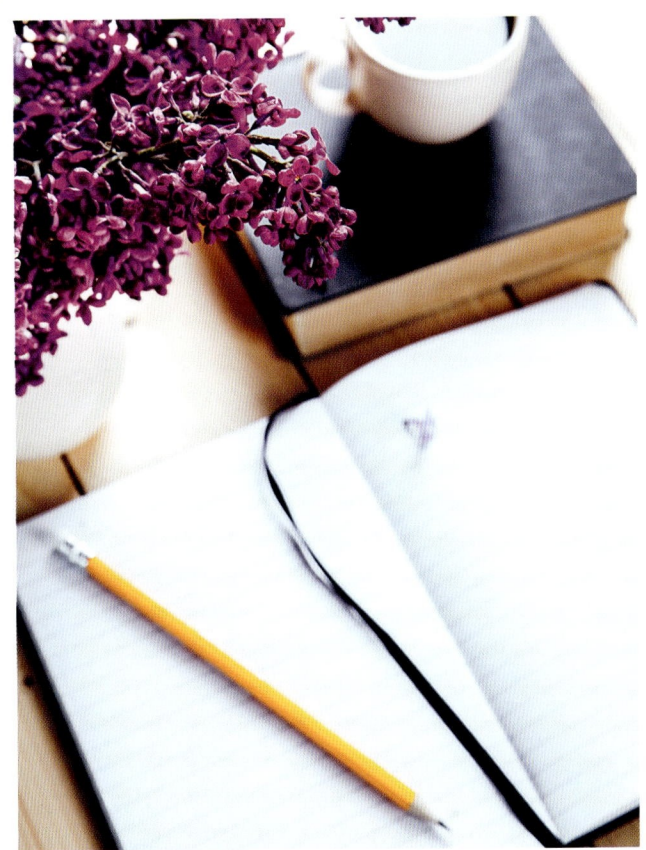

Thank Goodness for Gratitude

▶ Another powerful way to short-circuit stressful thoughts is to focus on what's good in your life. Studies have found that experiencing gratitude and appreciation is associated with a lower risk of depression, anxiety, substance abuse, and eating disorders. Other research shows that spending just a few minutes thinking about things you're thankful for can improve your mood. And there are many ways to count your blessings: Keep a gratitude list and write down five things you're grateful for every night before going to bed. Write a thank-you note to someone who has helped you. Or simply close your eyes for 30 seconds and think of all the people for whom you're thankful. "It's important to practice gratitude with intent, because the brain tends to focus on the negative during times of stress. We have to override it," says Neda Gould.

Beware of Burnout

IT'S NOT JUST YOU: RESEARCH SHOWS THAT AN INFLUX of people worldwide are experiencing symptoms of burnout. A Microsoft survey of 20,000 people globally found that 50% of employees and 53% of managers were feeling burnt out at work.

Charryse Johnson, L.C.M.H.C., N.C.C., a certified mental health counselor and founder of Jade Integrative Counseling and Wellness, often refers to burnout as "managing the invincible load." And without intervention, it can escalate into more serious mental health issues. "It is not just about alleviating symptoms, but understanding the ingredients that make us susceptible to [feeling overwhelmed]," Johnson says.

WHAT IS BURNOUT?

Burnout is a form of exhaustion that occurs when someone feels overwhelmed and unable to maintain their physical and/or emotional equilibrium. "It can happen to anyone who experiences prolonged emotional,

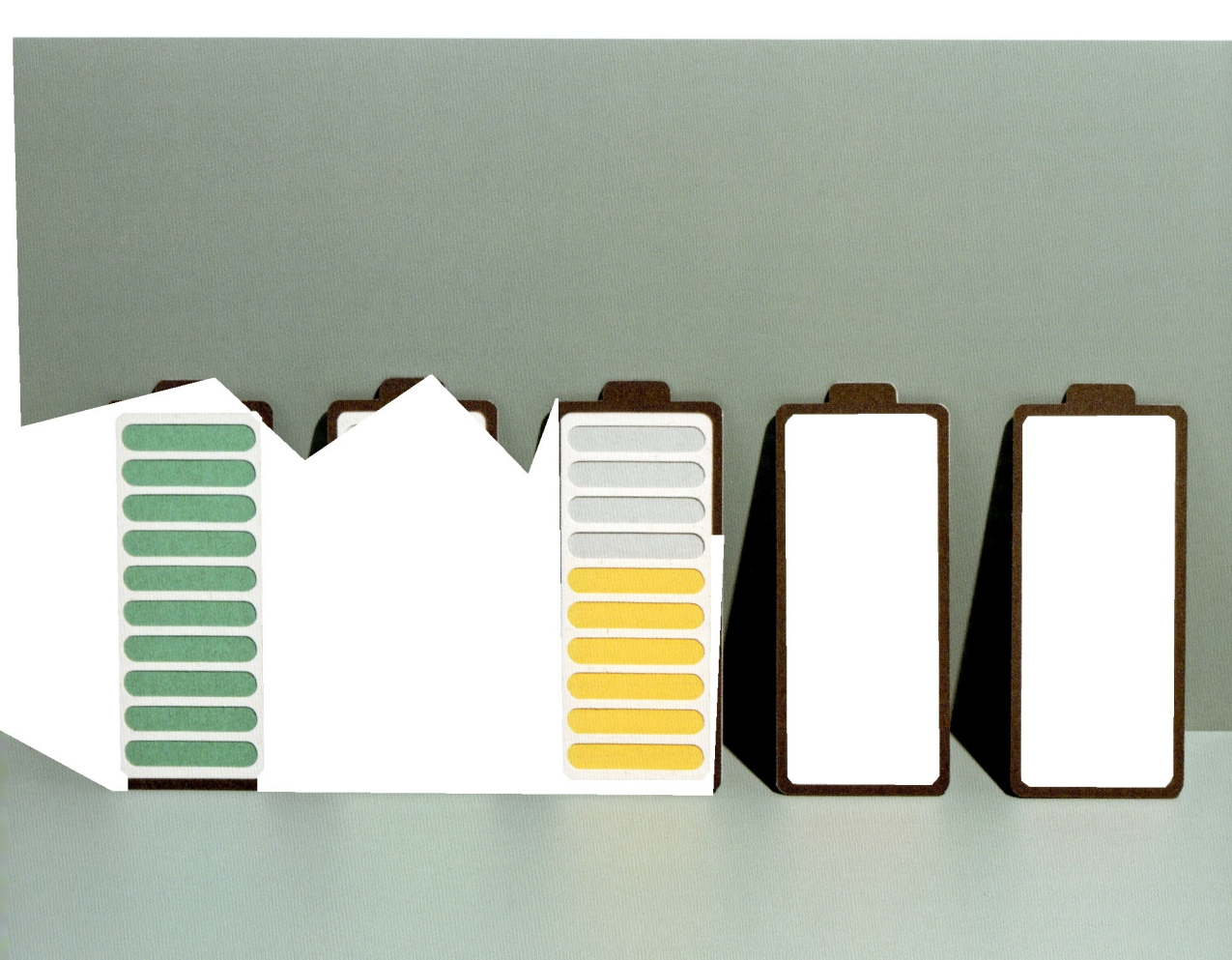

physical, or mental stress," explains Johnson.

It's most common to hear about burnout in the workplace, but home and caregiver burnout are also prevalent, according to Jake Goodman, M.D., mental health expert for the United Brain Association.

Physical Burnout Symptoms

- Headaches
- Changes in appetite
- Gastrointestinal issues
- Difficulty staying focused in conversation
- Difficulty sleeping
- Significant fatigue
- Chronic illness

Mental Burnout Symptoms

- Neglecting your personal needs
- Anxiety or depression
- Irritability or moodiness
- A sense of inner emptiness or hopelessness
- A persistent feeling of inadequacy and fear that you can't meet standards you feel have been set for you

HOW TO PREVENT (AND RECOVER FROM) BURNOUT

Working through burnout isn't easy, but there are some reliable coping mechanisms that can help you begin to feel steady again.

Step 1

Recognize burnout

"Sometimes, I ask myself questions like *Am I feeling so drained that I'm unable to find enjoyment or purpose at work? Am I having more bad days than good ones?*" says Goodman. "If the answer to either of these questions is yes, it can be a sign that I'm heading toward burnout." Goodman adds that it may take someone else to recognize burnout for you. If a friend or loved one has mentioned that you've been more withdrawn or cynical lately, that could be a sign.

Step 2

Establish daily routines

Johnson says prioritizing personal routines like adequate sleep hygiene, exercise, consistent meals, and developing an identity outside of the home, work, or caregiving can make a huge difference. This will also give you a good baseline for knowing when things are going smoothly versus when burnout may be creeping in.

Step 3

Reach out for support

Keep a consistent level of support from friends, loved ones, colleagues, and others in place at all times. "Consistently having open and honest discussions about your stress, followed by action steps toward change, are highly effective ways to keep your head above water," Johnson adds.

Emotions Can Be Contagious

▶ Because people naturally mimic facial expressions and body language, someone else's anxiety could become yours. Protect your emotional boundaries by limiting the time you spend with chronic complainers and excusing yourself from negative conversations.

Step 4

Manage your workload

If you feel overcommitted, have a conversation with the people around you about what's happening. Also, acknowledge to yourself that you can't perform at a quality level in a burned-out state. Try to narrow your responsibilities so you can keep up with your responsibilities and maintain better health.

Step 5

Find what brings you joy

Think about hobbies you enjoy—like gardening, cooking, or yoga—and invest time in these practices. This will help you nurture your mental health, and it will act as a welcome distraction from life's more stressful moments.

Step 6

Seek professional help

If these strategies aren't helping, you may want to find a therapist. If you begin to feel hopeless to the point of suicidal ideation, it's critical that you reach out to a mental health professional or call a crisis line, Goodman says: "In the United States, anyone can call or text the 988 Lifeline 24/7 to receive confidential support in a mental health crisis."

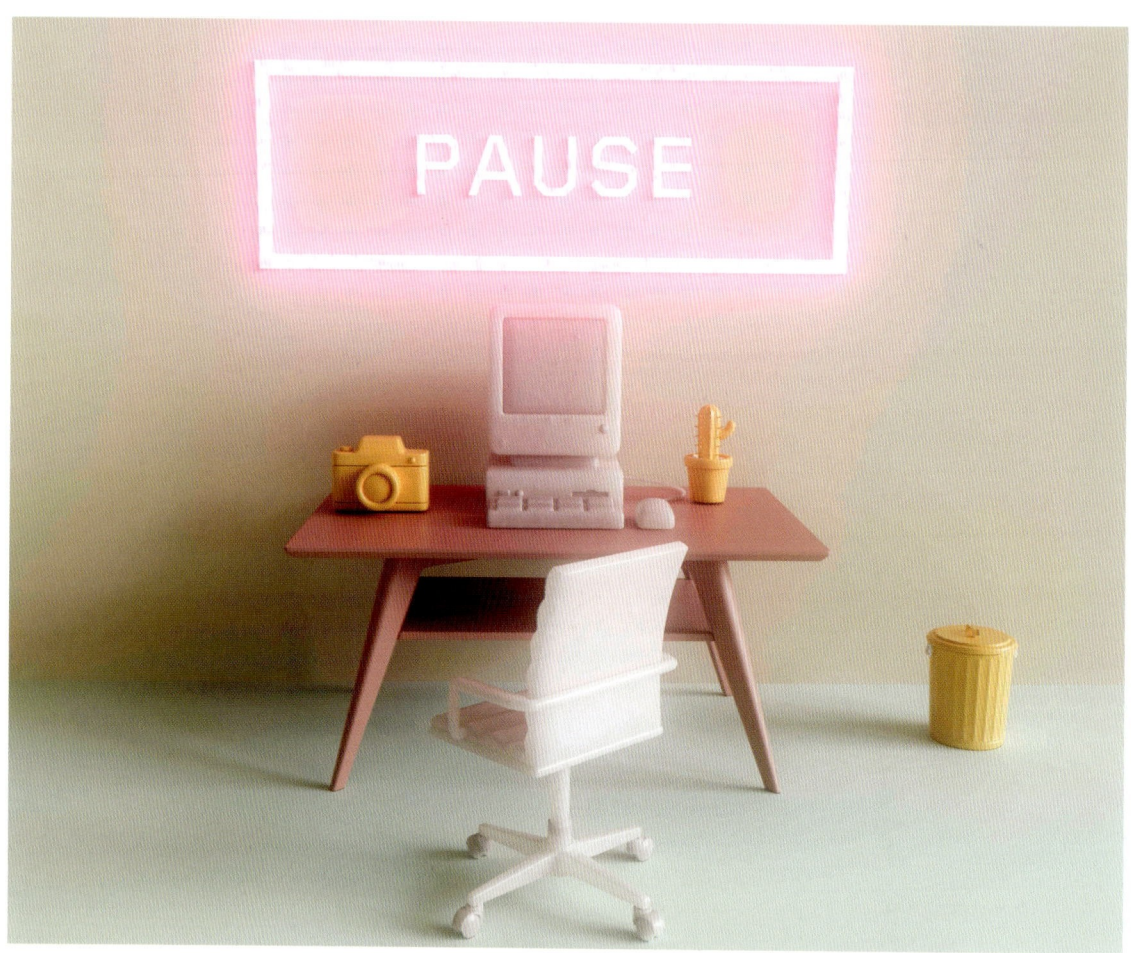

Be Stress-Resistant with Self-Care

IN A NERVE-WRACKING WORLD, THE CHALLENGE IS TO establish a state of inner calm that will help you stand up to stress better and allow you to become less physically and emotionally reactive. You can do that by incorporating stress-relieving forms of self-care into your life on a daily basis. Simply devoting five to ten minutes throughout the day to these measures can help you feel less anxious physically and mentally.

GIVE YOURSELF BREATHING LESSONS

The way you breathe can either calm your body's response to stress—or fuel it. If you breathe shallowly, you can amp up the body's fight-or-flight response, which will make you feel more stressed. To ease stress and calm yourself, practice diaphragmatic breathing: Inhale deeply, allowing your chest and abdomen to rise to a count of four, then exhale slowly to a count of four; repeat four times. Do this several times throughout the day, every day.

PRACTICE MINDFULNESS MEDITATION

You don't need special training or a mantra to meditate. Sit in a quiet, comfortable place with your back straight and your head in line with your spine; as you breathe slowly, focus on your breath or sensations in your body. When thoughts come to mind, it's fine to notice them, as if they're leaves floating on a stream, without judging or engaging them; simply return your attention to your breath and continue.

SCAN YOUR BODY

Stress can be a pain in the neck, the jaw, or just about anywhere else, because when you're under emotional strain, your muscles contract and become tense. That's why it's smart to periodically assess where you're carrying tension in your body and to consciously release it—with a practice called progressive muscle relaxation. Start at your toes and focus on different parts of your body—your feet and legs, hands and arms, shoulders, back, neck, jaw—as you head north; along the way, note any points of tension, then let it go by intentionally relaxing those muscles.

GET MOVING

Even a 10-minute brisk walk can lower anxiety levels, research shows. This makes sense considering that any form of exercise boosts mood-regulating neurochemicals in the brain—including serotonin, which helps induce a feeling of calmness, and dopamine, which activates the brain's reward system. Combine your walk with music you love or a phone conversation with a friend, or make it a group jaunt for an extra mental boost.

TAKE A TEA BREAK

Cradling a cup of tea in your hands can make you feel cozy and peaceful, and being mindful can boost the benefits, says New York City–based meditation instructor Kirat Randhawa. While you're sipping, "notice the color of the tea, the shape of the mug, the scent, the taste, and how it feels in your body," she says. Teas brewed with calming herbs like chamomile, lavender, and cornflower can make an extra-relaxing brew.

STRETCH YOUR MUSCLES

Stretching eases tension and helps relax tight muscles, and there's also evidence that it can ease mental tension: After all, when your body is tense, your mind feels tense as well. A controlled three-month trial showed that stretching for 10 minutes after work made people feel less anxious and burned out. Breathe in a slow and controlled way and focus on the muscles you want to stretch.

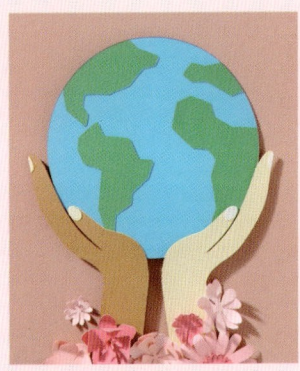

The Power of Taking One Small Action

▶Whether the subject is politics, eco-anxiety, or racial injustice, worry about the state of the world can leave you feeling overwhelmed or powerless. But taking a concrete action every day—such as helping with a campaign, mentoring someone, donating time or money to a cause, or biking instead of driving on errands—moves you one small step closer to a better world. Plus, doing something to help other people or the planet may make you feel more empowered.

You're in Good Company

When work stress or household stress starts getting to him, Paul, a lawyer with two grown kids and two step-kids, often pushes the pause button so he can do a brief mindfulness meditation, using an app. "It's like an enforced time-out that helps me let the stressors go and focus on just being," he explains. "After 5 to 10 minutes, I feel refreshed and lighter—and I appreciate the kindness I've shown myself."

The Value of Sleep

IT'S TIME TO GIVE SLEEP THE RESPECT IT DESERVES. A 2023 study found that up to 8% of deaths from any cause could be attributed to poor sleep patterns, and people who have healthier sleep habits are less likely to die prematurely.

But it's easy to skimp on snooze time to cram more activities into our waking hours, staying up late playing on our phones or binge-watching our favorite shows. When we do that, we don't set ourselves up for a sound night's sleep, which affects our lives in so many ways.

Turns out, many people ruminate about sleep twice a day: at night when they're tired and desperately want to go to sleep but can't, and again in the morning when they're still tired and want to stay in bed. Insufficient sleep can affect the entire day as poor sleepers miss out on emotional regulation. Plus, sleep deprivation affects immune regulation as well as tissue restoration and repair, says Jessica Payne, Ph.D., a sleep and stress neuroscience expert and a psychology professor at the University of Notre Dame.

Good-quality shut-eye is important for short- and long-term health. In the short term, getting enough sleep can help you avoid getting sick, maintain a healthy weight, reduce stress, improve your mood and ability to focus, and even reduce your risk of having motor vehicle accidents. Over time, it can reduce your risk of developing chronic diseases like type 2 diabetes, heart disease, high blood pressure, and stroke.

By contrast, insufficient sleep or poor-quality sleep "sends our bodies into a state of stress in which excessive amounts of the stress hormone cortisol [are] released," says Angela Holliday-Bell, M.D., a board-certified physician, certified sleep specialist, and founder of the Solution Is Sleep. "This increase in baseline cortisol leads to inflammation that can lead to the weakening of the blood vessels and heart disease." People are also significantly more likely to experience anxiety and depression when

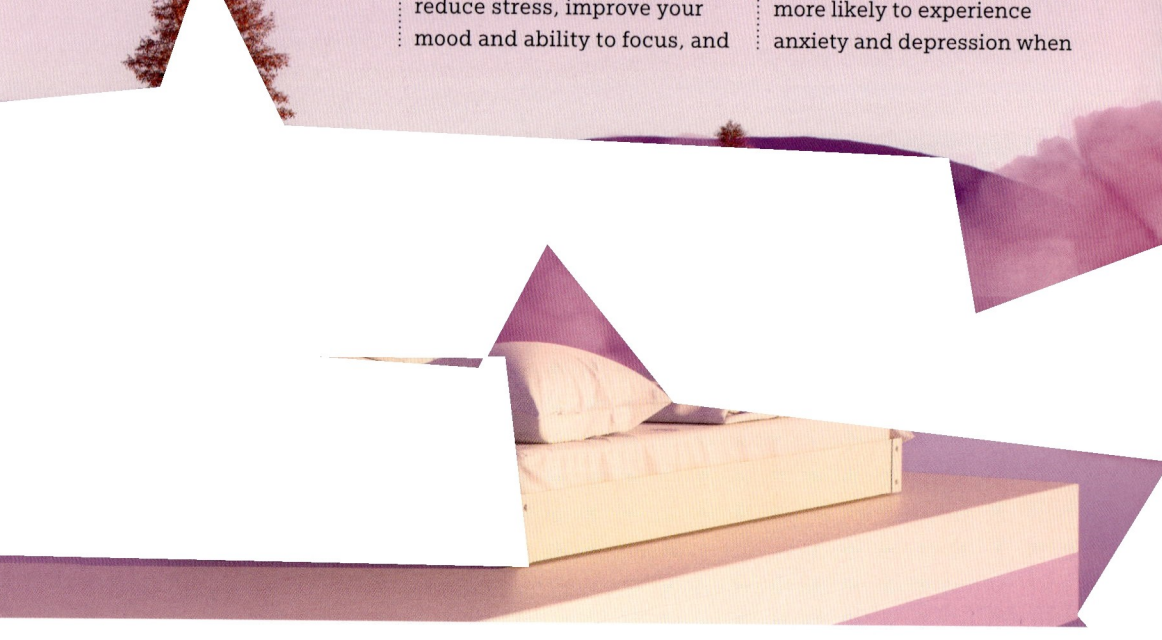

they don't get sufficient sleep, she adds. And it becomes more difficult to exercise regularly and make healthy food choices when you're experiencing sleep scarcity.

While stress may keep you awake at night, insomnia can impair your ability to regulate stress the next day, creating a "sleep-stress snowball," Payne says. Given sleep's ability to wreak havoc on your waking hours, it makes sense that what happens during the day might be causing sleep troubles at night.

Adequate sleep is one of the lifestyle factors that can affect how long you live. But it doesn't happen in a vacuum: The ability to get a good night's sleep depends on having healthy daytime activities to regulate your body's biological clock, or circadian rhythm. "The interplay of sleep and rest, when it's on a schedule, helps signal your brain as to where it is within a 24-hour circadian rhythm," says W. Chris Winter, M.D., a sleep medicine specialist and the author of *The Sleep Solution: Why Your Sleep Is Broken and How to Fix It.*

How Sleep Changes with Age

▶ Everyone has a biological clock that determines when they get tired at night and when their body wakes up in the morning. But starting around age 40, your internal clock begins to shift. Researchers aren't sure exactly why this happens, but the result is that your body will naturally start to wake up earlier, decreasing the amount of sleep you're getting, explains Hans Van Dongen, Ph.D., director of the Sleep and Performance Research Center at Washington State University. By the time you hit your 60s, you could be waking up two hours earlier than you did in your 30s.

In addition, research has found that the amounts and patterns of secretion of sleep-related hormones—such as growth hormone, cortisol, and melatonin—change as people get older, which can affect their ability to fall asleep and stay asleep.

To accommodate your body's shifting sleep patterns, try moving your bedtime earlier so you can get the amount of sleep you need. If you're worried that you'll lie awake because you're going to bed earlier than you're used to, Van Dongen offers reassurance. "You're probably naturally getting tired earlier, but it's easy to ignore or not notice the sleepiness if you're used to staying up late," he says. "Most older people find that when they start getting into bed earlier, they fall asleep easily."

Good-Quality Sleep Is a 24-Hour Endeavor

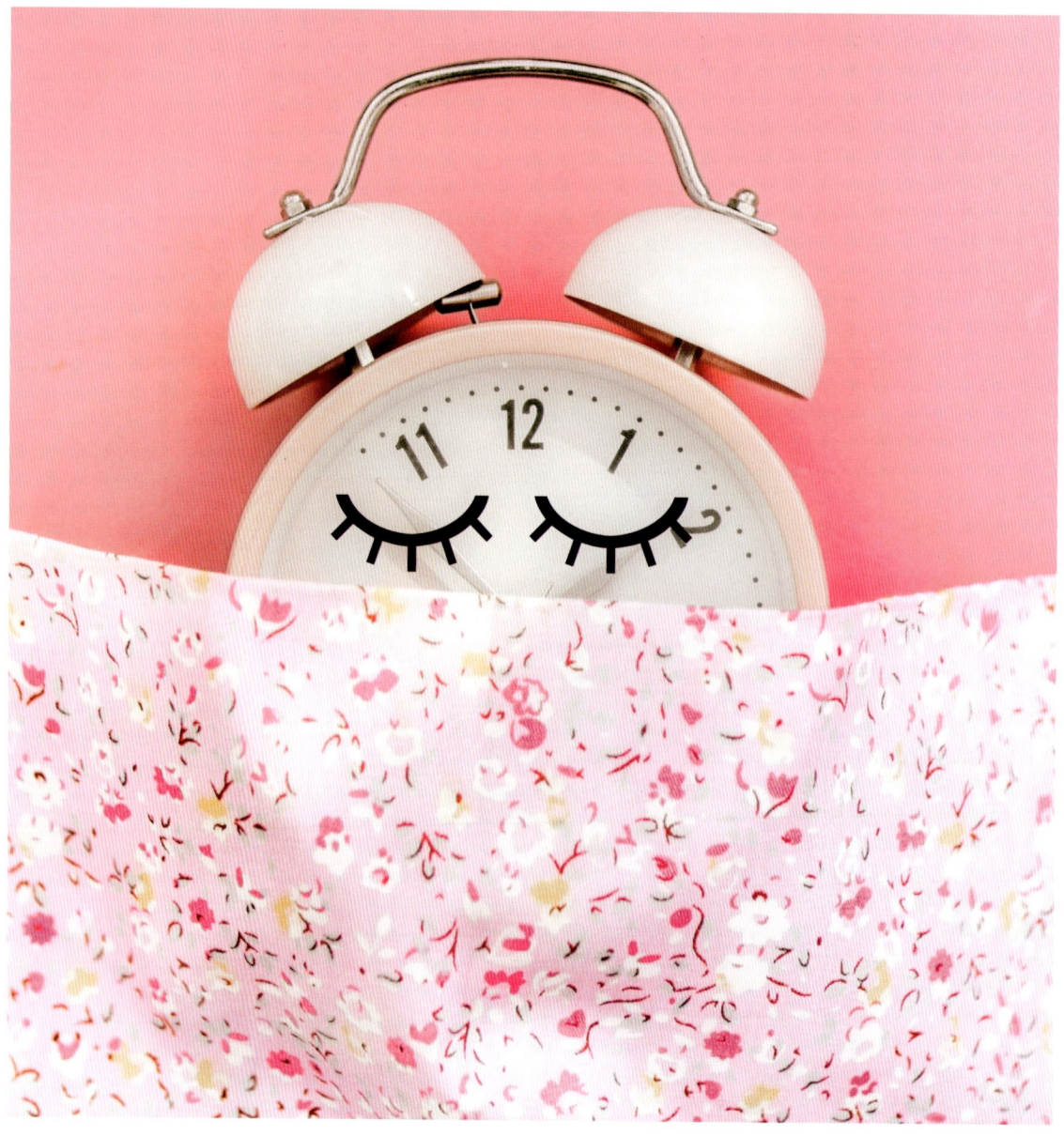

HERES'S AN AROUND-THE-CLOCK GUIDE

to help you sleep better, starting tonight.

MORNING

Quit hitting snooze.

People's greatest sleep mistakes happen in the morning, says sleep medicine specialist W. Chris Winter, M.D. After a bad night, it's tempting to give yourself a pity pass to sleep in or take a sick day. But a regimented response at the start of the day actually helps set your brain's sleep-wake clock. The exception: If you wake up too early, don't try to force a return to sleep—it's smarter to get up then. That reduces the chance of developing a chronic case of insomnia, according to research conducted at Penn Medicine.

Eat breakfast.

Skipping breakfast to bank calories for dinner leads to overeating in the evening, followed by a night of fitful sleep as you try to digest all that food. In the morning, make sure some protein—such as eggs, yogurt, fish, meat, or milk—is on your menu. "In general, protein tends to facilitate the production of dopamine, a wakefulness neurotransmitter," Dr. Winter says.

Step outside early.

Exposure to morning sunlight supports internal clock regulation and suppresses melatonin, especially when combined with exercise like a walk with the dog or even to the bus stop. Even on a cloudy day, a walk provides more light than being indoors with all the lights on. If you can do a workout, even better: According to Dr. Winter, that will increase the release of serotonin, which enhances mood and wakefulness and helps regulate your body's internal clock.

AFTERNOON

Catch 10 minutes of downtime.

Your body temperature naturally drops around lunchtime, causing sleepiness. A short catnap during your lunch break at the same time each day can reboot energy levels, but it isn't necessary to fall asleep. "Resting isn't a failed nap," Dr. Winter says. It's valuable in and of itself. You can use that rest time to practice relaxation techniques that will be useful at night. Let your mind wander and get drowsy for about 10 minutes, then get back to what you were doing, feeling refreshed.

Don't chug coffee to keep you going.

Our bodies produce a chemical called adenosine, which promotes sleepiness, says Reeba Mathew, M.D., a sleep medicine specialist in Houston. A stimulant, caffeine blocks the release of adenosine and inhibits your brain's natural increase in sleepiness as you move toward nighttime. While caffeine can help you stay alert in the afternoon, it could continue to have that effect into the evening, which isn't what you want. Instead stick to herbal tea or water later in the day.

Work out before dark.

Exercising raises body temperature and levels of the hormones epinephrine and adrenaline, which are sleep fighters. You should work out by early evening to provide sufficient time for your body heat and these hormone levels to settle down. "A falling body temperature almost acts like a signal that brings on sleep," Dr. Mathew says.

Do a short meditation.

Decreasing daytime anxiety and worry can help you snooze more deeply at night. During the day, find 5 to 10 minutes to use the "body scan" meditation technique (page 157). You can ease stress on your own or use a guided meditation in an app or on YouTube.

The Scoop on Sleep Disorders

▶ The prevalence of many sleep disorders—including insomnia, obstructive sleep apnea (OSA), and restless legs syndrome— increases with advancing age, and these can have serious consequences for people's daytime health. For example, OSA, a condition in which the sleeper periodically stops breathing for several seconds at a time, increases the risk of high blood pressure, heart disease, and stroke. If your partner tells you that your snoring is really loud or you briefly stop breathing while you're sleeping, or if you have an uncomfortable feeling in your legs or an overwhelming urge to move your legs at night, and it's disrupting your sleep, talk to your doctor. Treatments are available to help both conditions.

Write down what's bugging you.

Jessica Payne, Ph.D., a sleep and stress neuroscience expert, says that without offloading the day's events, your brain will continue to process stressful situations throughout the night. Compartmentalize by writing down your problems or worries in the evening and putting them aside until the morning, when you can swing into problem-solving mode. In the meantime, you're off duty!

Turn off the overhead lights.

After 6 p.m. or so, ditch the overhead lights and rely on table lamps and floor lamps with warm- or orange-hued light bulbs. Electronic devices should be set to night mode to warm the screen color. The reason: Exposure to bright blue light emitted by these devices can reduce melatonin levels by up to 50%, says Satchidananda Panda, Ph.D., a professor at the Salk Institute for Biological Studies in San Diego and the author of *The Circadian Code*. That drop in melatonin could compromise your zzz's.

Stop eating two hours before bed.

Keep dinner on the lighter side. Avoid rich or heavy meals or overdoing it with alcohol in the evening. Your body's digestive and waste functions need rest and downtime and to learn when "the kitchen is closed," Panda says. This will also help prevent midnight snacking.

Create a soothing bedtime ritual.

Any kind of stimulus is problematic—even *Law & Order* reruns—because it can lead to subtle increases in blood pressure, heart rate, and pupil dilation. Instead, take at least 20 minutes to dial down. Try gentle stretching, meditating, listening to soothing music, reading a book, or taking a bath. Think of this as a bookmark at the end of the day, Payne says, one that tells the body and brain that it's OK to sleep.

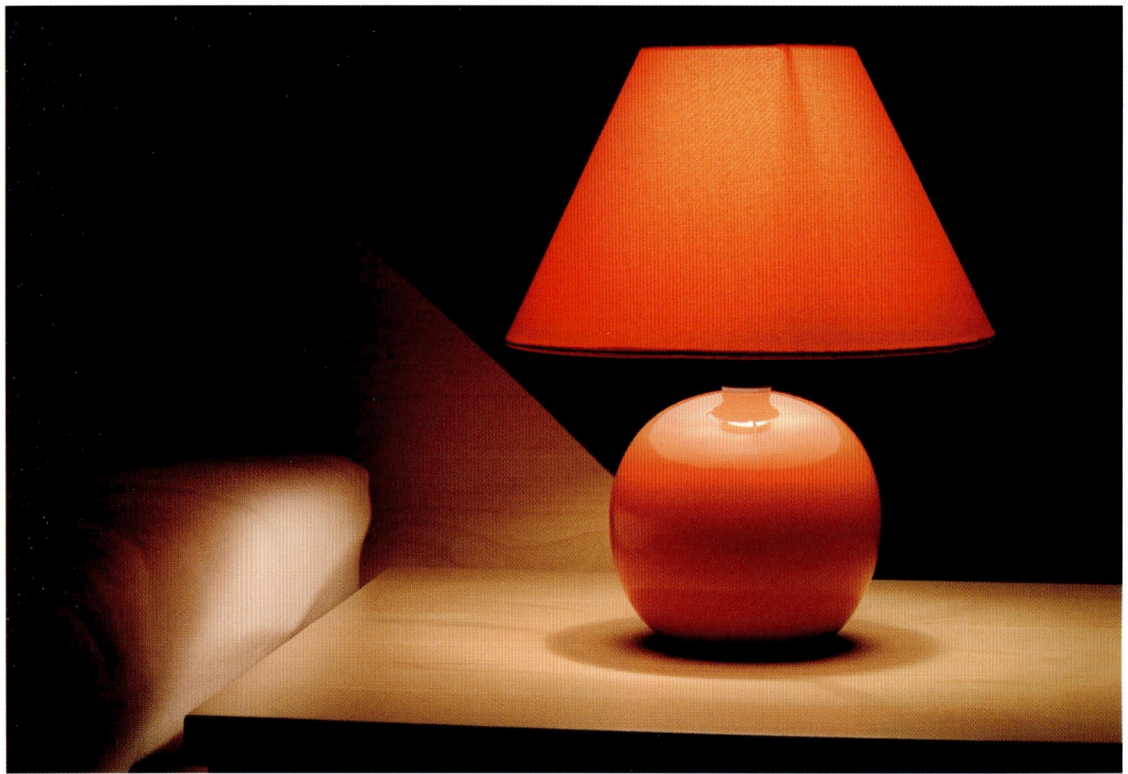

Temperature

Set your thermostat between 60°F and 67°F. Body temperature goes down during sleep, so a cooler room helps that process happen faster and helps you sleep more deeply. Over age 65? Research suggests older adults may benefit from warmer temperatures—between 68°F and 77°F—at night. Experts think warmer might be better because older bodies have a harder time regulating body temperature.

Sound

Your bedroom should be as quiet as a library. You may be able to block noise from neighbors or the street with heavy curtains or shades and a tight seal on bedroom windows. Or, mask it by running a fan or white-noise app.

Bedding

Find the mattress and linens that are comfiest to you. Most people prefer a medium-firm mattress. The right bed linens should allow you to sleep comfortably without sweating.

Darkness

The room should be so dark that you can't see your hand in front of your face. Can't get to peak opacity? An eye mask should do the trick.

Clock position

Turn the clock away from you so you can't see it. Clock-watching during the night triggers anxiety and increases levels of stress hormones, Dr. Mathew says.

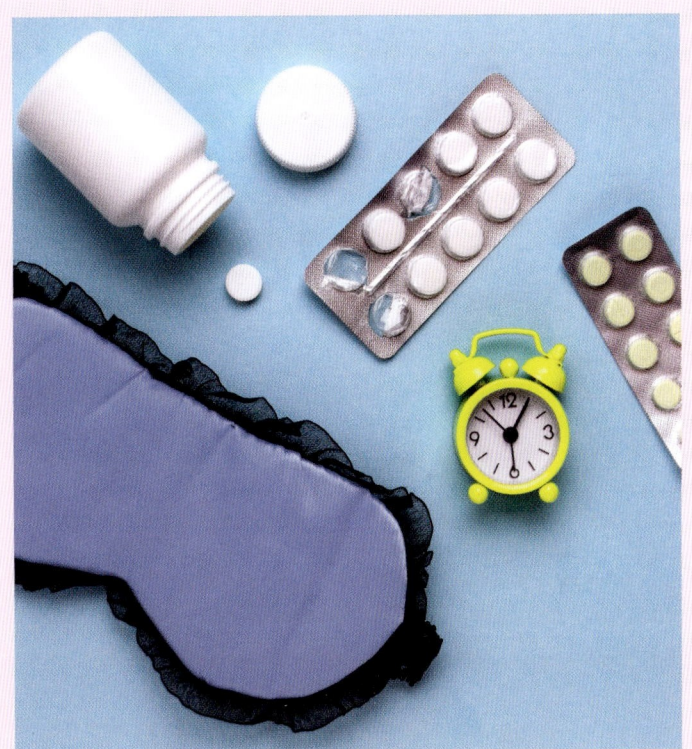

Sleeping Pills May Increase Risk for Dementia

▶ About 4% of adults over the age of 20 use prescription sleeping pills in the U.S., but one small study in 2023 raised eyebrows after linking these common sleep aids to an increased risk for dementia. It tracked sleep data for more than 3,000 people age 70 and older. Of all the participants, 138 white participants and 34 Black participants reported taking sleep medications five or more times a month. Those participants had a significantly higher risk of developing dementia—79% higher, to be exact. However, the link was only found in white participants, and the number of subjects was small.

If you need help getting the sleep you need, talk to your doctor about sleep interventions. Other medications and nondrug remedies may be safer options. If you're struggling with insomnia, you may be referred for cognitive behavioral therapy for insomnia: This brief, skills-based treatment focuses on helping people learn better sleep-related habits and changing their attitude toward sleep. It incorporates elements of mindfulness meditation and relaxation practices to help the mind and body get to a state where sleep is more likely to happen. A sleep expert can also help address your sleep issues.

The Ideal Amount of Sleep in Middle and Older Age

WE'VE BEEN TOLD TIME AND TIME AGAIN THAT adults need seven to nine hours of sleep every night, but new research points to the exact amount of quality zzz's that may support cognitive abilities, ward off early signs of dementia, and even protect mental health.

A study published in the journal *Nature Aging* found that around seven hours of sleep is ideal for middle- and older-aged adults.

The research found anything more or less than seven hours was associated with a reduced ability to remember, learn new things, focus, solve problems, and make decisions. Additionally, more or less sleep was linked to symptoms of anxiety and depression and worse overall well-being.

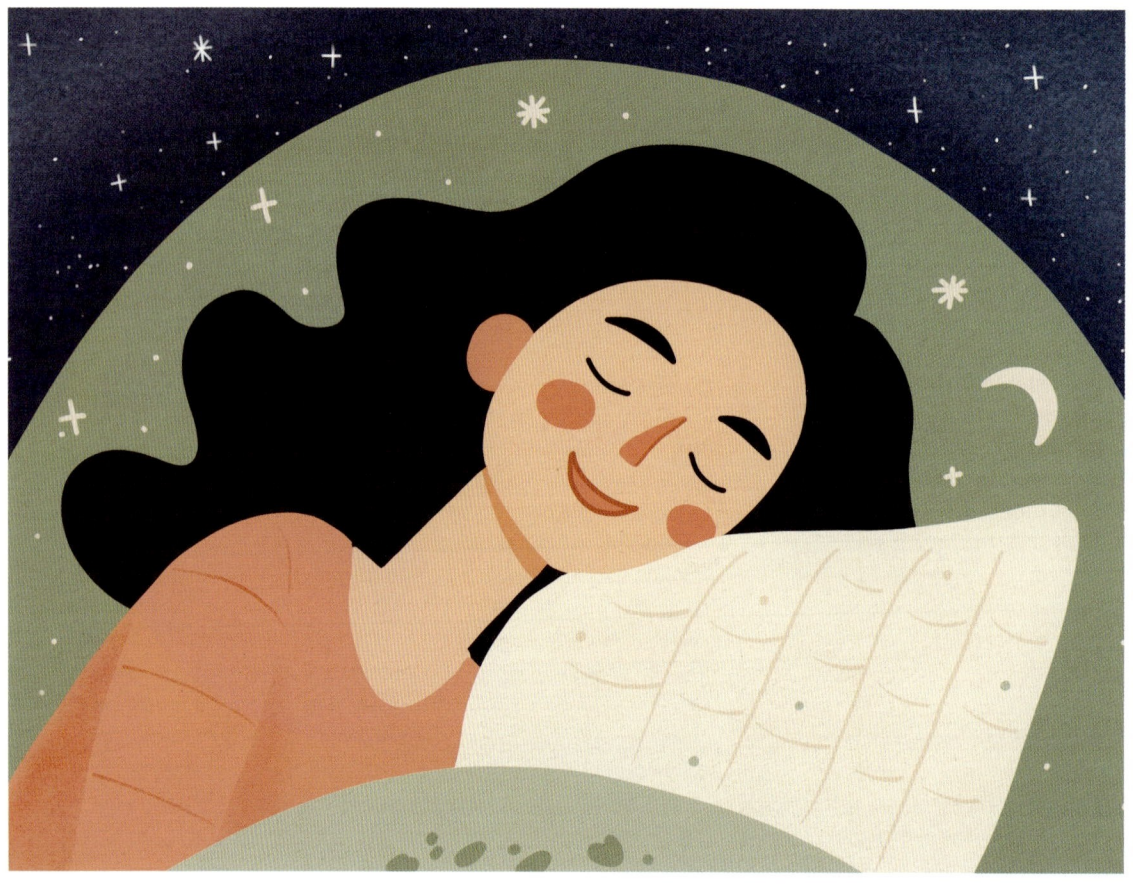

Is a Sleep Divorce Healthy for You and Your Partner?

▶ A sleep divorce means sleeping separately from your partner to get better-quality sleep—whether that's strategically seeking refuge from your partner's snoring or constant tossing and turning or because you have different sleeping preferences (for example, one person likes to sleep in cooler temperatures, while the other is more comfortable with lots of blankets).

The term "sleep divorce" has a negative connotation, but for some couples, sleeping separately can lead to increased closeness and intimacy. In fact, good-quality sleep has been shown to be an important indicator of relationship health: A study from Ohio State University showed that it could improve communication and reduce conflict and irritability over time.

So, if sleeping with your partner is making it hard for you to get seven restful hours per night, it may be worth considering separate sleep spaces.

The key is to have clear conversations about why you'd like to make the switch and whether you see it as a long-term change or a temporary one. Having a shared understanding about the reasons will also help you explain it to your kids or anyone else you decide to tell.

HOW SLEEP IMPACTS YOUR HEALTH

"While we can't say conclusively that too little or too much sleep causes cognitive problems, our analysis looking at individuals over a long period of time appears to support this idea," Jianfeng Feng, M.Sc. and Ph.D., a corresponding author of the study and a professor from Fudan University in China said in a statement. "But the reasons why older people have poorer sleep appear to be complex, influenced by a combination of our genetic makeup and the structure of our brains."

The team found the amount of sleep someone gets can impact the structure of some brain regions that are involved in cognitive processing and memory. The greatest negative changes were found in people who got more or less than seven hours of sleep regularly.

Additionally, the researchers said one possible reason for cognitive decline due to less than optimal sleep may be because of a disruption in deep sleep. This disruption has previously been shown to impact memory. Getting enough deep sleep may be more important than the actual hours spent in bed.

"Getting a good night's sleep is important at all stages of life, but particularly as we age. Finding ways to improve sleep for older people could be crucial to helping maintain good mental health and well-being and avoiding cognitive decline, particularly for patients with psychiatric disorders and dementias," Barbara Sahakian, F.MedSci, D.Sc., an author of the study and a professor in the department of psychiatry at the University of Cambridge, said in a statement.

You're in Good Company

Jenny, a now 75-year-old retired educator, had always slept well. But after losing her husband four years ago, she found herself lying awake at night, her mind whirring through worst-case scenarios. While she'd eventually fall asleep, she woke exhausted and found herself groggy and brain-fogged throughout the day. She finally spoke to her doctor, who prescribed an anti-anxiety medication. Jenny also began attending daily exercise classes at a local senior center and making an effort to socialize several times a week. Slowly, her sleep returned to normal. While she still occasionally has insomnia, more often than not, she gets a full night's sleep.

Your Three-Week Longevity Challenge

IN THIS BOOK YOU'VE **DISCOVERED YOUR PHYSICAL AND** mental health are equally important to achieving an optimal health span— and that it's never too late to start something new. Throughout, we've provided tips and tools for staying healthy and engaged for many years.

This three-week health challenge is designed to accommodate you wherever you are starting and to inspire you to build a long lifetime of happiness and health. The actions listed below include small measures that you can add to your daily routine, as well as one-time or annual actions to add to your calendar as reminders to maintain your well-being. New habits that you can add each day are denoted with a ⭐ symbol.

Week 1

As you begin you'll undertake a few bigger efforts to establish building blocks for healthful habits. Each day you'll add at least one small, super doable action from each category: Nutrition, Physical Health, Mental Health, and Exercise.

Day 1
- ☐ Drink a glass of water as soon as you wake up. It's good to start your day hydrated and supports your digestion. ⭐
- ☐ Meditate for 1 minute. Before you start your day, set your timer and your intentions. ⭐
- ☐ Take a 5-minute walk. Don't think about it, just walk out the door and take a stroll around the block. ⭐
- ☐ Add a weekly reminder to check your blood pressure. You can use home equipment or visit a local pharmacy or fire station without an appointment.

Day 2
- ☐ Add an antioxidant to your daily meals, such as berries, many beans, and leafy greens. ⭐
- ☐ Text an old friend just to say hi.
- ☐ Stand up from your chair and walk around the room at least once an hour throughout the day. ⭐

- ☐ Make an appointment with your primary doctor for a physical.

Day 3
- ☐ Drink your tea or coffee with half the sugar you normally add, or none at all. ⭐
- ☐ Write down 3 things you are grateful for. ⭐
- ☐ Try the strength and balance tests (pages 132 and 136, respectively).
- ☐ Add a minimum 30-SPF sunscreen to your daily skincare regimen. ⭐

Day 4
- ☐ When buying or looking for a snack today, find one that is not ultra processed— 5 ingredients or fewer is a good gauge.
- ☐ Try 2X breathing, when your exhale is twice the length of your inhale. It helps regulate the nervous system. ⭐
- ☐ Add exercise to your daily routine: Take the stairs, get off the bus a stop early, or walk the dog at lunch. ⭐
- ☐ Make a vision appointment.

Day 5
- ☐ Drink water instead of soda or a sugary coffee drink. ⭐
- ☐ Sign up for a class to learn something new—could be knitting, a language, or cooking.

- ☐ Have a one-song dance party: Cue up your favorite tune, dance like crazy, and then get back to your day.
- ☐ Bicycling is a fabulous and low-impact exercise and even a mode of transportation. If riding outside, always wear a helmet.

Day 6

- ☐ Eat a salad made with dark, leafy greens—these brain- and heart-healthy plants are loaded with nutrients. ⭐
- ☐ Smile or wave to someone you know but don't usually talk to.
- ☐ Sit, stand, and sit back down again 10 times without using your hands (for tips see page 136). ⭐
- ☐ If you use tobacco in any form, make an appointment with your doctor to talk about quitting.

Day 7

- ☐ Check your pee (yes, really!). If it's dark, you need to drink more water. ⭐
- ☐ Sit or walk in nature for 30 minutes without your phone or other distractions. You can experience nature wherever you are— in a local park or by walking around the block taking in the birds, bugs, and tiny plants you see.
- ☐ Put light weights wherever you watch TV and do 2 sets of 10 bicep curls while watching your shows. (See other strength-training exercises beginning on page 136.)
- ☐ Do a full body exam (and ask a friend to look at your back and scalp), looking for asymmetrical moles and other signs of skin cancer.

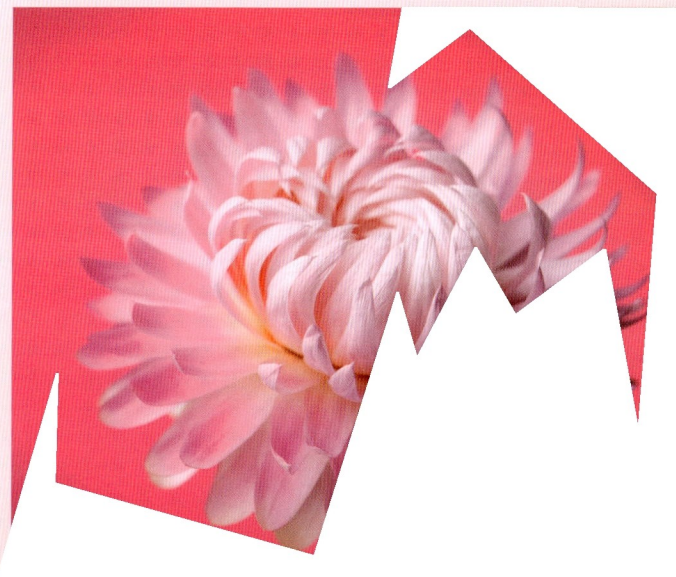

Week 2

It's time to double-down on the healthy habits you began last week.

Day 1

- ☐ Introduce one no-meat day per week, starting today.
- ☐ Meet a friend for a meal, coffee, or a walk.
- ☐ Take a 20-minute walk. ⭐
- ☐ Make an appointment for dental cleaning.

Day 2

- ☐ Set a weekly reminder to go through your fridge and use or freeze anything close to expiring.
- ☐ Find out the birthdays of your closest friends and family and enter them in your calendar (then use these as a reminder to wish them a happy birthday).
- ☐ Stretch for 10 minutes using the exercises on page 129. ⭐
- ☐ Check your first-aid kit; restock anything that's low.

Day 3

- ☐ Eat oatmeal for breakfast (or add a serving of fiber to your day; see some options on page 66). ⭐
- ☐ Clean and organize your bedroom—having an uncluttered space to go to sleep and wake up in will help you rest and will clear your mind.
- ☐ When waiting for your coffee to brew or water to boil, do two sets of 10 squats. ⭐

☐ If you find yourself struggling to hear conversations, make an appointment to check your hearing. There are less expensive and more discreet hearing aids that can improve your quality of life.

Day 4

☐ Add a whole grain to your diet. Bulgur, black rice, and quinoa can be fun alternatives to oatmeal and brown rice. ⭐

☐ Attend a yoga class (almost all yoga centers have beginners' class).

☐ Balance on each leg for 10 seconds at a time when you are brushing your teeth. ⭐

☐ Go through your old medications and throw out any that are expired.

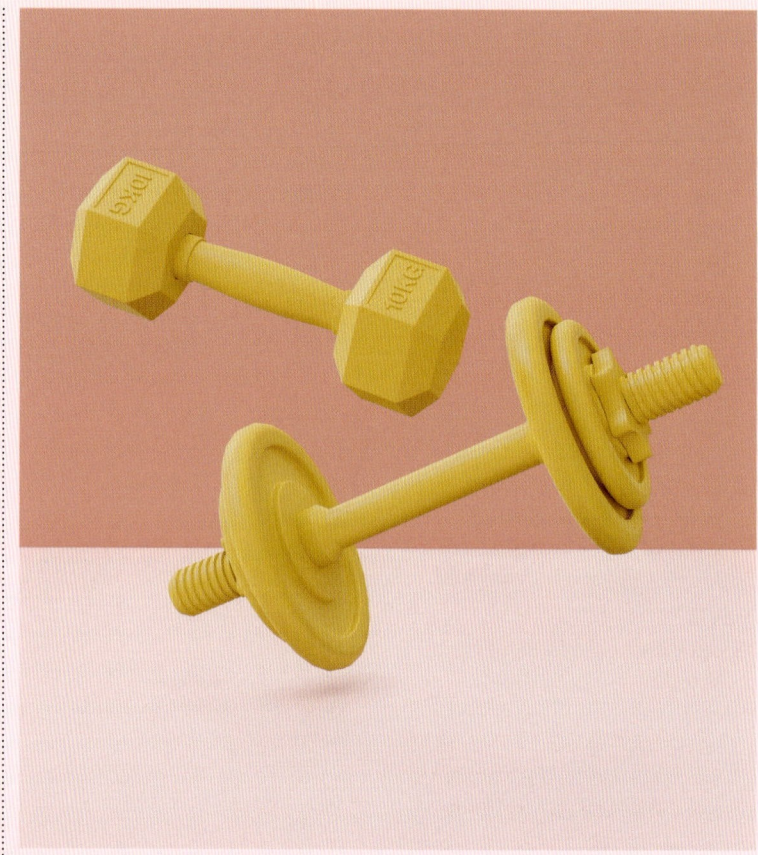

Day 5

☐ Try a new recipe using simple whole ingredients. If you like it, add it to your meal rotation. (There are tons of great recipes at Prevention.com!)

☐ Declutter your email inbox and set an alarm to clean out your inbox daily. ⭐

☐ Do something active that you loved as a child: jump rope, roller-skate, swim, or try out a hula hoop. Exercise can be fun. ⭐

☐ To reduce digital eyestrain, take breaks from the computer or tablet. Set your computer at 20–30 inches from your eyes, and consider blue-blocking or computer-specific glasses.

Day 6

☐ For healthy bones, add calcium and vitamin D to your daily diet. Dairy products are one source, and so are beans, sweet potatoes, tofu, nuts, and dried figs and dates. ⭐

☐ Meet a friend for a coffee date.

☐ Trip-proof your home. Go through each room looking for possible trip hazards. Replace slippery rugs, clear clutter, and add lighting to dark staircases.

☐ Start a skincare routine. Every morning and night, wash your face, try a serum, and moisturize. In the morning, add SPF too. ⭐

Day 7

☐ If you drink alcohol, cut your intake to no more than one drink per day. ⭐

☐ Write in a journal for 5 minutes. It can just be passing thoughts, a summary of your day, or intentions for the future. ⭐

☐ Take a 30-minute walk. ⭐

☐ Make your yearly mammogram appointment and check to see when you are due for a pap test. ⭐

Week 3

Now that you're developing some good healthy habits, commit to an ongoing practice.

Day 1
- [ ] Meal prep 2 or 3 healthy meals for the upcoming week.
- [ ] Change up your walking route today—the shift will give your brain a boost.
- [ ] Do 5 minutes of yoga. ⭐
- [ ] Find out whether you are due for any vaccine boosters or flu shots and make an appointment.

Day 2
- [ ] Eat mindfully. Instead of scrolling on your phone or eating on the run, sit down and focus on each bite. ⭐
- [ ] Sign up to volunteer at an animal shelter, food bank, school, or other organization on a weekly basis.
- [ ] Buy a pair of good-fitting running or walking shoes. Your feet will thank you for it.
- [ ] Buy a houseplant. They increase indoor air quality, and caring for them can provide mental health benefits.

Day 3
- [ ] Pause before snacking today. When you crave a snack, have a cup of herbal tea or do a few stretches. Notice when and what you like to snack on. The point isn't not to snack but to snack mindfully.
- [ ] Try not to complain today. If you catch yourself starting to grumble, write down

one thing to be grateful for instead. ⭐
- [ ] Go to a trial exercise class. Moving in a new way will shake up your routine, and maybe you'll love it.
- [ ] Find 30 minutes in your day to rest—maybe it's a bath or a nap or just lying down without distractions for a half hour. ⭐

Day 4
- [ ] Today, try to only eat foods from the Mediterranean Diet (see page 112). What appeals to you? What can you add to your daily diet?
- [ ] Look for laughter. Find opportunities to giggle through videos, books, or talking with a friend who always makes you crack up. ⭐
- [ ] Find an exercise buddy—knowing your friend is waiting will help you hold yourself accountable.
- [ ] Cut out caffeine after noon. It will help you sleep better and may help with anxiety. ⭐

Day 5
- [ ] Make a dish using one of these spices: ginger, turmeric, cayenne, or cinnamon. They have many healthful benefits including reducing inflammation and sharpening memory.
- [ ] Spend 5 to 30 minutes alone. Disconnect from your phone and everyone else. Let your thoughts wander. ⭐
- [ ] If you are struggling to exercise due to arthritis or other chronic pain issues, schedule a time to swim or

join a Pilates or low-impact yoga class. All three can provide low-impact strength and aerobic exercise. ⭐
- [ ] Limit the time on your smartphone—tech neck is real and leads to neck and shoulder strains and hunching. ⭐

Day 6
- [ ] Hydrate mindfully. Ask yourself if you are thirsty. If the answer is yes, drink a glass of water. ⭐
- [ ] Take a class: cooking, a college course in American history, or ceramic painting—the topic doesn't matter. It will boost your brain, social connections, and mental health.
- [ ] Take the strength and balance tests to see what's changed in 3 weeks. Still not hitting your goal? No problem; just keep working at it.
- [ ] Follow up and confirm your upcoming physicals.

Day 7
- [ ] Set a regular calendar for meatless days, no-alcohol days, and Mediterranean Diet days.
- [ ] Take stock. How do you feel mentally 21 days later? Write it down.
- [ ] Commit to exercising in some way for 30 minutes every day. Walking, dancing, gardening, roller-skating, swimming—they all count. ⭐
- [ ] Do a 20-minute body scan. Lie down and tune in to your body. Notice your feelings. Listen to what your body is telling you.

Index

A

A1C test, 65, 71
Abate, Ejigayehu, 78
acupuncture, 97
Adedinsewo, Demilade, 64
adenosine, 161
Adimoolam, Deena, 7
adrenaline, 150, 161
Agbai, Oma, 107
Aggarwal, Rashi, 150, 153
aging
    advances in field of, 4, 5
    advantages of, 5, 14
    attitudes toward, 22–23
    biological age and, 12–13
    feeling better longer, 10–11
    future self and, 22–27
    heart disease and, 63
    longevity myths and, 16–17
    mental health benefits of, 42–43
    perceptions of, 14–15, 17, 21
    Prevention Medical Review
        Board Members on, 6–7
    superagers, 18–19
aging mindset, 14–15
AI interventions, 18
air quality, 76
alcohol consumption
    brain health and, 37
    cancer and, 72, 73, 76–77
    heart health and, 67
    inflammation and, 69
    libido and, 84, 87
    life expectancy and, 121
    longevity and, 17
Ali, Sherrie D., 32–33, 34
allostatic load, 150
alopecia, 106
Alzheimer's disease
    cardiovascular health and, 37
    dementia distinguished from, 40
    inflammation and, 68
    loneliness linked to, 52
    MIND diet and, 115
    physical activity and, 124
    prevention of, 33, 34
    statistics on, 36
American Heart Association,
    Essential 8, 13
anchor activities, 56–57
andropause, 53
antidepressants, 85, 97, 109
anti-interleukin-11 drug, 18
anxiety
    anxiety or depression quiz,
        44–45
    cognitive abilities and, 38
    deep breathing and, 152
    inflammation and, 68
    libido and, 85
    lifestyle factors and, 51
    loneliness and, 55
    menopause and, 89, 93, 97
    myths about, 46–48
    physical activity and, 43
    prevalence of, 42
    sleep habits and, 158–159, 164,
        165
appetite changes, 45, 47, 48, 155
arthritis, 53, 69, 79, 85, 124
asbestos, 77
autoimmune disorders, 48, 63, 68, 70
Awkar-Lazo, Nelly, 72, 73

B

Bailey, Cynthia, 89
balance, 126, 127, 132–135
Barbach, Lonnie, 80, 81
Barzilai, Nir, 18, 19
Benzo, Roberto, 152
Berman, Laura, 82
Be-Your-Best-Self Checklist, 21
biological age, 12–13
Bird Dog, 144
blood clots, 94
blood glucose levels, 70, 71
blood pressure management
    deep breathing and, 152
    Essential 8 and, 13
    exercise and, 139
    heart health and, 64–65
    Mediterranean diet and, 114
    sodium intake and, 67
    stress management and, 150
    superfoods for, 118
    walking and, 148
blood sugar management, 13, 65,
    70–71, 117
body weight. <u>See</u> weight
    management
bone density, 78–79, 136, 137
Bonney, Seema, 125
bowling, 147
brain fog, 38, 39, 89, 92
brain health. <u>See also</u> memory
    diet and, 33, 37, 38–39, 112,
        113–115
    games and, 34–35
    neuroplasticity and, 32–33
    physical activity and, 33, 37, 38
    sleep habits and, 34, 38
    social connections and, 35–36
    water intake and, 121
Braunstein, Glenn D., 83
breathing techniques, 34, 97, 152,
    156–157
Brotto, Marco, 127
Bryant, Cedric, 125
Buehler, Stephanie, 87
burnout, 154–155

C

Caccappolo, Elise, 37, 38, 39
caffeine, 161
calcium supplements, 79, 97
Caldwell, Jessica, 39
cancer
    diet and, 72, 73, 112, 113, 114
    family history of, 75, 89
    inflammation and, 68
    physical activity and, 72, 73, 75,
        124
    risk factors for, 72–73, 74, 75–77
    strength training and, 137
    superfoods for, 119
    treatments for, 63
cancer screenings, 72, 73, 74
cardiac stiffness, 20
cardio training, 133, 135, 146–147
cardiovascular disease. <u>See</u> heart
    disease
cardiovascular fitness, 37, 127
cardiovascular health. <u>See</u> heart
    health
Carstensen, Laura, 5, 22–23, 28–29,
    53
Carter, Christine, 51
Carter, Jocelyn Smith, 47, 48
cellular aging process, 11, 12
cellular dysfunction, 11
cellular senescence, 19
Cen, Putao, 75, 76
Cha, Ann, 96
Chan, Julie T., 29
Chang, Claire, 103, 105
chemical peels, 102–103
chemical sunscreens, 103, 105
chemotherapy, 109
Chen, Cheng-Han, 13
cholesterol
    diabetes and, 71
    diet and, 67
    Essential 8 and, 13
    heart disease and, 63, 64
    high-density lipoprotein (HDL),
        64, 65
    low-density lipoprotein (LDL), 64,
        65, 95, 117, 119
    menopause and, 89
    superfoods for, 117
    triglycerides and, 64, 65
chronic pain, 85, 150
circadian rhythm, 159, 161
cognitive abilities. <u>See also</u> memory
    age-related cognitive decline, 40
    diet and, 38–39
    exercise and, 33, 37, 124

improvement in, 21, 32–34
learning new things and, 33–34
meditation and, 34, 35
retirement and, 28
sleep habits and, 34, 39, 164, 165
social isolation and, 34, 35
walking and, 148
cognitive behavioral therapy (CBT),
50, 97, 163
cognitive tasks, 37
Cole, Steve, 53
collagen production, 99, 100, 103
colonoscopy, 74, 77
colorectal cancer screening, 77
community. See also social
connections
sense of, 7, 13
concentration ability, 45, 47
Cording, Jessica, 115
core strength, 136
Core Toe Taps, 143
cortisol levels, 124, 150, 159
CRISPR/Cas9, 18–19
Curl, Angela, 26
Cutler, David, 120

D

DASH diet, 112, 113, 114–115
dating, 58–59
dating apps, 58–59
Davis, Melanie, 80
dehydration, 120–121
dementia
diagnosis of, 40
Mediterranean diet and, 114
memory and, 36–37
menopause and, 94, 97
physical activity and, 124
risk factors and, 19, 34
sleep habits and, 34, 36, 164
sleeping pills and, 163
dental health, 63
depression
anxiety or depression quiz,
44–45
functional fitness and, 127
heart disease and, 63
inflammation and, 48, 68
libido and, 85
lifestyle factors and, 51
loneliness linked to, 52
menopause and, 89, 93, 97
myths about, 46–48
physical activity and, 43
prevalence of, 15, 42
sleep habits and, 158–159, 164
stress management and, 150, 151
treatment for, 38, 45, 48, 49
Devi, Gayatri, 39
DEXA scan, 79
DHEA, 92

diabetes
gestational diabetes, 63, 71
gut microbiome and, 122
inflammation and, 68
Mediterranean diet and, 33, 112
prevention of, 11, 70–71
strength training and, 137
symptoms of, 70–71
type 1 diabetes, 48, 70
type 2 diabetes, 70, 71, 112
diastolic blood pressure, 65
Diaz, Natasha, 91
diet
brain health and, 33, 37, 38–39,
112, 113–115
cancer and, 72, 73, 112, 113, 114
DASH diet, 112, 113, 114–115
Essential 8 and, 13
fiber intake and, 21
gray hair and, 106, 107
hair loss and, 109
heart health and, 65, 66–67
improvements in, 5, 6, 7
inflammation and, 68–69, 112
libido and, 85
longevity and, 17
Mediterranean diet, 33, 68–69,
112–114
menopause and, 93, 95
mental health and, 43, 51, 112
osteoporosis and, 78
plant-based diets, 67, 73, 113,
114, 116
premature aging and, 4
probiotics and, 122, 123
sexual activity and, 80
sleep habits and, 161, 162
superfoods for longevity,
116–119
divorce, 35, 53, 58
Dmitrieva, Natalia, 121
DNA, 17, 72, 77, 127
Dog Aging Project, 11
dopamine, 86, 157, 161
Doraiswamy, Murali, 37
Dueñas, Michael, 107
dysthymia, 47

E

elastin, 103
Elinav, Eran, 122
Ellor, James, 54, 55
emotional boundaries, 155
endorphins, 87, 124, 151
environment
adaptability to, 15, 39
cancer risk and, 76, 77
cellular aging process and, 11
DNA damage and, 72
gut microbiome and, 122
longevity and, 17

risk factors of, 19
stress management and, 109
Epel, Elissa, 150
epigenetic changes, 19
epinephrine, 161
erectile dysfunction, 63, 80, 85, 87
Essential 8, 13
estrogen, 82–83, 88, 89, 91, 92, 93,
101
estrogen therapy, 95
eustress, 152
executive-functioning skills, 35
exercise. See also physical activity;
strength training
aerobic exercise, 87, 125, 127
blood pressure management
and, 139
cancer and, 72, 73
cognitive abilities and, 33, 37, 124
functional fitness, 126–127
inflammation and, 69
mental health and, 43, 51
resistance training and, 15, 79,
127
timing of, 161
exposure therapy, 46
Extended Cat, 131

F

facial massage, 100
falls, 79, 124, 136
fasting blood glucose, 65, 71
Faubion, Stephanie S., 86, 87, 93
Feng, Jianfeng, 165
fermented foods, 69, 123
ferulic acid, 100
fiber intake, 21, 73, 123
fight-or-flight response, 46, 150
financial resources, 26–27
Fisher, Helen, 58
flexibility, 127, 128, 129–131
flexible sigmoidoscopy, 77
follicle-stimulating hormone, 89
Foot Towel Stretch, 131
Ford, Michele Patterson, 24, 25
forgetfulness, 89
friendships, 56–57
frontotemporal dementia (FTD), 40
Front Plank Body Saw to Pike, 138
Fruge, Danine, 124
fruits and vegetables, 66, 73, 112–
114, 116
full-body skin exam, 77
Fulop, Judy, 117, 118
Fusco, Francesca, 108
future self, 22–27

G

Gallaher, Daniel, 117, 119
games, brain-training games, 34–35
Garlapati, Ramya, 100

Garshick, Marisa, 107
Gazzaley, Adam, 34–35
gene therapy, 19
genetic mutations, 18, 75
genetics, 11, 13, 17, 18, 75, 107, 109
genetic testing, 75
Genie Twist, 129
genitourinary syndrome of
    menopause (GSM), 93, 94
gerotherapeutics, 18
gestational diabetes, 63, 71
glucose tolerance test, 71
Gohara, Mona A., 6
Goodman, Jake, 155
Goodman, Whitney, 56
Gould, Neda, 153
gratitude practice, 6, 55, 153
growth factors, 100
growth hormone, 159
gut microbiome, 69, 73, 122–123

H

hair, 92, 106–109
hair dyes, 77
Harris-Jackson, Tameca, 85
Hawkley, Louise, 54, 55
Healthcare.gov, 27
health insurance, 27
health screenings, 16, 17, 72–74, 77
health span, 5, 10–11, 166
hearing loss, 39
heart attacks, 63, 65
heart disease
    diabetes and, 63, 70
    high blood pressure linked to, 63,
        64–65
    loneliness linked to, 52
    menopause and, 63, 89, 93, 94,
        95, 97
    prevention of, 11, 37, 62, 124, 139
    sleep habits and, 158
    strength training and, 137
    stress management and, 150
    treatment of, 7
heart health
    biological age and, 12–13
    blood pressure management
        and, 64–65
    chronic conditions and, 62
    DASH diet and, 115
    dental health and, 63
    lifestyle factors for, 37, 62, 66–67
    Mediterranean diet and, 33, 112,
        113–114
    strength training and, 136
    stress management and, 63, 65
    walking and, 148
heart palpitations, 92, 95
Helicobacter (H. pylori), 76
hemoglobin Alc, 65
hepatitis B, 76

hepatitis B vaccine, 76
hepatitis C, 76
high blood pressure
    DASH diet and, 114–115
    diabetes and, 71
    diet and, 112
    heart disease linked to, 63, 64–65
    hot flashes and, 95
    loneliness linked to, 52
    stress management and, 150
high-density lipoprotein (HDL), 64,
    65
HIIT (high-intensity interval training),
    33, 140, 145
Holland, Thomas, 37, 38–39
Holliday-Bell, Angela, 158
Holt-Lunstad, Julianne, 52
Hope, Marisa, 146, 147
hormone replacement therapy (HRT),
    91, 93, 94–95
HPV (human papilloma virus), 76
Hui, Jessica, 6
hyaluronic acid, 101
hyperpigmentation, 100
hypertension. See high blood
    pressure
hypoactive sexual desire disorder
    (HSDD), 87

I

Iadecola, Constantino, 37
immunotherapy, 4
incontinence, 85
infections, superfoods for, 117
inflammation
    bone density and, 79
    depression and, 48, 68
    diet and, 68–69, 112
    heart health and, 67, 68, 69
    hot flashes and, 95
    meditation and, 19, 69
    Mediterranean diet and, 114
    physical activity and, 146
    sleep habits and, 68, 69, 158
    stress management and, 69, 150,
        151
    superfoods for, 119
injury prevention, 127, 128, 136
insomnia, 161, 163
insulin, 70, 146
insulin resistance, 70
insulin sensitivity, 115
intellectual ability and performance,
    15
intellectual engagement, 7, 16
intergenerational connection, 53
isoflavones (phytoestrogens), 95
Iyengar, Neil, 73

J

Jampolis, Melina B., 148
Jeste, Dilip, 52
Johnson, Catherine, 17
Johnson, Charryse, 154–155
Johnson, Erica L., 68, 69

K

Kaeberlein, Matt, 10–11, 18
Kanji, Aleem, 71
Karras, Tula, 29
Kelaher, Hope, 57
Khan, Sadiya, 69
kidney disease, 68, 70
Klosk, Melissa, 57
Kopecky, Stephen, 10
Krishnamurthy, Smitha, 74–75, 76, 77
Kumar, Rekha B., 6

L

Lal, Karan, 99, 100, 101
laser and light therapy treatments,
    109
Leary, Mark, 24
Levy, Becca, 5, 14
Lewy body dementia (LBD), 40
libido, 80, 82–83, 84, 85, 86–87, 89, 91
life expectancy, 4, 17, 22–23, 37, 121
lifespan, increase in, 5, 10, 22–23,
    26, 28
lifestyle factors. See also diet;
        exercise; sleep habits;
        social connections; stress
        management
    anxiety and depression, 51
    brain health and, 37, 38
    cancer and, 72, 73
    cellular aging process and, 11
    Essential 8 and, 13
    genetic testing and, 75
    hair loss and, 109
    heart health and, 37, 62, 66–67
    improvements in, 4, 5
    inflammation and, 68–69
    life expectancy and, 17, 37
    longevity and, 5, 17
    menopause and, 91, 96, 97
    osteoporosis and, 78, 79
Litzy, Karen, 6
liver, 64, 118
liver disease, 67, 94
Live to 100 and Love It Challenge, 5
loneliness, 4, 52, 53, 54–55, 69
longevity
    balance and, 132
    flexibility and, 128
    lifelong vitality and, 18–19
    lifestyle factors and, 5, 17
    Mediterranean diet and, 113
    myths about, 16–17

physical activity and, 17, 20, 124, 125
superfoods for, 116–119
Three-Week Challenge for Longevity, 166–169
Longevity Project study, 16
longevity science, 18–19
loss of interest, 45
low-density lipoprotein (LDL), 64, 65
Luke, Janiene, 107

M

MacDowell, Andie, 107
male pattern baldness, 109
mammograms, 74
Manson, JoAnn E., 91
Markowitz, Orit, 103
Marques, Luana, 150, 151
Mashimo, Hiroshi, 7
masturbation, 83
matchmakers, 59
Matheny, Albert, 149
Mathew, Reeba, 161, 163
Mead, Margaret, 97
Medicare, 27
medications
    avoiding falls and, 79
    brain fog and, 39
    cognitive abilities and, 38
    depression and, 48
    gerotherapeutics, 18
    hair loss and, 109
    for hypertension, 65
    libido and, 85
    for menopause, 91, 96–97
    sexual activity and, 80
    for sleep, 163
meditation
    body scan meditation, 157, 161
    cognitive abilities and, 34, 35
    inflammation and, 19, 69
    libido and, 86–87
    mental health and, 51
    sleep habits and, 161, 163
    stress management and, 157
Mediterranean diet, 33, 68–69, 112–114
melatonin, 91, 93, 159, 161, 162
memory. See also Alzheimer's disease; brain health; cognitive abilities; dementia
    causes of memory loss, 36, 37, 38–39
    long-term memory, 37
    recall quiz, 41
    short-term memory, 15, 33, 37
    sleep and, 34
    working memory, 32, 35, 37
memory loss, 15
men, 4, 85, 109
menopausal zest, 97

menopause
    average age of, 89, 90
    bladder issues and, 91, 93, 94
    bone density and, 78, 79
    brain fog and, 39, 89, 92
    estrogen levels and, 82–83, 88, 89, 91, 92, 93, 101
    fat distribution and, 93, 123
    heart disease and, 63, 89, 93, 94, 95, 97
    hormone replacement therapy (HRT), 91, 93, 94–95
    hot flashes and, 88, 89, 91, 92–93, 94, 95, 97
    management of, 91, 96–97
    menstrual cycle and, 88–89, 97
    mood changes and, 93, 97
    natural remedies for, 91
    perimenopause and, 83, 88–89, 93, 95, 97, 109
    postmenopause, 89, 92, 95
    progesterone and, 82, 83, 88, 91
    sexual activity and, 80, 83, 91
    sleep habits and, 39, 89, 91, 93, 97
    social connection and, 53
    symptoms of, 89, 91, 92–93, 94, 95, 96–97
    vaginal dryness and, 20–21, 85, 89, 91, 92, 93, 97
mental health. See also anxiety; depression; stress management
    benefits of aging and, 42–43
    burnout and, 155
    diet and, 43, 51, 112
    in-person interactions and, 55
    interactions with physical health, 5
    memory and, 38
    myths about, 46–48
metabolic syndrome, 33
metabolism, 123
metformin, 19
Metz, Oona, 7
microdermabrasion, 103
microneedling, for skincare, 102, 103
Mikhail, Alexa, 18
mild cognitive impairment (MCI), 40
Millheiser, Leah, 87
Mills, Adam, 148
Milstein, Marc, 56, 57
mind-body practices, 43, 51, 89
MIND Diet, 115
mindfulness
    cognitive abilities and, 34, 35
    libido and, 86–87
    menopause and, 96, 97
    mental health and, 51
    sleep habits and, 163

stress management and, 7, 152, 157
mineral sunscreens, 103
Minkin, Mary Jane, 91
Mirren, Helen, 107
Mitchell, Latreal, 146
mitochondrial function, 19
moderation, 7
monounsaturated fats, 67
mood, 38, 43, 46, 48, 93, 97, 136
mood-regulating chemicals, 48
morbidity, compression in, 4
multiple sclerosis, 48
multitasking, 39, 151–152
muscle mass, 15, 124, 137
muscle memory, 125

N

nails, 99
Neidich, Haley, 46–47
Nelson, Marissa, 58
neurodegenerative diseases, 112
neuropeptides, 39
neuroplasticity, 32–33
Newman, Cory, 47, 48
New Map of Life, 23
new old age, 4–5
niacinamide, 101
norepinephrine, 86
nostalgia, 46
Nutrafol, 109

O

obesity, 63, 71, 73, 83
obstructive sleep apnea (OSA), 161
octisalate, 103
"old age," as social construct, 15
omega-3 fatty acids, 66–67
One Arm, One Leg Dumbbell Row, 145
One-foot Hop, 134
Oratz, Ruth, 7
orexin, 39
orgasms, 80–81, 83, 85, 87
ospemifene, 92
osteopenia, 79
osteoporosis, 78–79, 89, 94, 97, 127
O'Toole, Mary, 88, 89
Overhead Triceps, 142
oxybutynin, 95
oxytocin, 80, 86

P

Panda, Satchidananda, 162
pap test, 76
Pardel, Paula, 59
Paroxetine (Brisdelle), 95
Payne, Jessica, 158, 159, 162
peptides, 101
perimenopause, 83, 88–89, 93, 95, 97, 109

personality, consistency of, 15
pets, 55
Pew Research Center, 52
phenotypic age, 12–13
Phillips, Adrienne, 75, 77
physical activity. See also exercise; sedentary habits
    brain health and, 33, 37, 38
    cancer and, 72, 73, 75, 124
    daily activities, 133
    developing habit of, 135
    diabetes and, 71, 75
    Essential 8 and, 13
    heart health and, 65, 67, 75
    importance of, 6, 7, 124–125
    inflammation and, 146
    libido and, 83, 87
    longevity and, 17, 20, 124, 125
    menopause and, 93, 95, 97
    mental health and, 43
    metabolism and, 123
    osteoporosis and, 79
    sexual activity and, 80
    stress management and, 124, 151
    telomerase produced by, 19
physical intimacy. See sexual activity
Pilates, 137–139
Pilates Hundred, 138
Pillow Stance, 134
Planells, Angel, 116
Plank Singles, 139
plaque, 34, 64, 68
pneumonia/influenza, 68
polycystic ovary syndrome, 71
polyphenols, 114
Pontzer, Herman, 123
postbiotics, 123
postmenopause, 89
postpartum preeclampsia, 65
prebiotics, 122–123
precision medicine, 18
prediabetes, 63, 71
preeclampsia, 63, 65
prefrontal cortex, 33
premature aging, 4
premature ejaculation, 85
Prestipino, Melissa, 132
preventive care, 4, 7, 16, 17
probiotics, 122, 123
processed foods, 66, 73, 113, 114
processed meats, 73, 113
progesterone, 82, 83, 88, 91
progressive muscle relaxation, 51, 157, 161
prolactin, 83
proprioception, 132
prostate cancer, 115
PTSD, 48
purpose, sense of, 16, 26, 43
Push-Up with Reach Out, 143

R
race, 71, 163
racing or ruminative thoughts, 45
Rajagopal, Usha, 109
Randhawa, Kirat, 157
rapamycin, 19
recall quiz, 41
red meat, 73, 113
regenerative procedures, 4
Reinagel, Monica, 123
relaxation techniques, 97
Renn, Brenna, 33, 40
resilience, 16, 18
resistance training, 15, 79, 127
restless legs syndrome, 161
resveratrol, 19
retinoids, 99, 102
retinol, 99, 101
retirement, 15, 26–29, 43
rheumatoid arthritis, 69, 150
ROAR Forward, 29
Roberts, Sally, 128
Roizen, Michael F., 26–27
The Roll Down, 130
roller skating, 147
Ross, Alison, 45
Ross, Sherry, 87, 91, 94
Routhenstein, Michelle, 21
Rowen, Tami, 85

S
Sabgir, David, 124
sadness, 45
Saedi, Nazanin, 98, 99, 100, 101
Sahakian, Barbara, 165
Sahlgren, Gabriel H., 26
salt intake, 67, 85, 114, 121
Santoro, Nanette, 93
Savage, Teddy, 147
sedentary habits, 4, 20, 73
selective serotonin reuptake inhibitors (SSRIs), 95, 97
self-care, 51, 156–157
self-concept, 24–25
Semicircle Sweeps, 135
senolytics, 19
sensory processes, 15, 152
serotonin, 48, 151, 157, 161
sex hormones, 82–83
sexual activity
    communication and, 80, 81, 83, 85
    erectile dysfunction and, 80, 85, 87
    foreplay and, 81, 87
    improvement in sexual enjoyment, 20–21, 80–83
    libido and, 80, 82–83, 84, 85, 86–87, 91
    lubricants and, 21, 83, 87, 91, 92, 93, 97
    menopause and, 80, 83, 91
    orgasms and, 80–81, 83, 85, 87
    prevalence of, 15
    in your 40s, 82–83
    in your 50s, 60s, and beyond, 83
sexually transmitted infections (STIs), 85
Sheehy, Gail, 83
Shirazi, Azadeh, 106, 107
short-term memory, 15, 33, 37
Side Plank Hip Drop, 137
simple starches, 112
Single-Leg Dead Lift, 133
sit-to-stand test, 136
Skater Taps, 133
skin cancer, 77, 103
skincare
    menopause and, 89
    resilient skin, 102–103, 105
    strategies for, 97–98
    sunscreen use, 17, 76, 99, 103, 105
    in your 40s, 99–100
    in your 50s, 100
    in your 60s and beyond, 101
sleep apnea, 39, 161
sleep habits
    alcohol consumption and, 121
    bedroom setup and, 163
    bedtime ritual and, 162
    brain fog and, 39, 165
    brain health and, 34, 38
    changes in, 159
    cognitive abilities and, 34, 39, 164, 165
    emotional regulation and, 158
    Essential 8 and, 13
    heart health and, 63
    improvements in, 5
    inflammation and, 68, 69, 158
    libido and, 85
    lighting and, 162
    menopause and, 39, 89, 91, 93, 97
    mental health and, 43, 51
    morning, afternoon, evening and, 161–162
    naps and, 34, 161
    premature aging and, 4
    prioritizing of, 7, 165
    sleep divorce, 165
    value of, 158–159
sleeping pills, 163
Sloane, Laurie, 58–59
Small, Gary, 33, 35
smoking
    brain health and, 37, 38
    cancer and, 72, 73
    Essential 8 and, 13

gray hair and, 107
heart disease and, 63
heart health and, 67
inflammation and, 69
longevity and, 17
social isolation compared to, 52
tools for quitting smoking, 77
Snyder, Michael, 19
social connections. See also
    community; loneliness
    bowling and, 147
    brain health and, 35–36
    dating after 50, 58–59
    fostering of, 54
    friendships and, 53, 56–57
    importance of, 6, 7, 13, 16, 34–35
    inflammation and, 69
    mental health and, 43, 51
social isolation, 34, 35, 43, 52, 53, 63
social media, 52, 54, 55, 57, 151
SPF (sun protection factor), 103, 105
Squat Toe Tap Jumps, 145
Squat to Lunge, 142
Stagger Biceps, 144
stem cell therapy, 4, 107
Stockwell, Tim, 121
stool DNA test, 77
Streicher, Lauren, 20–21, 92
strength training
    bone health and, 79, 137
    cardio training and, 135
    functional fitness and, 127
    longevity and, 137
    memory improvement and, 37
    mixed exercise routine and, 7
    mood and, 43, 136
    9 moves for strength and health,
        140–145
    recommendations on, 125, 137,
        143
    strength test, 136
    tips on, 143, 166
stress management
    anxiety and, 45
    brain recharge and, 150–151
    burnout and, 154–155
    getting outdoors and, 55
    gray hair and, 106
    hair loss and, 109
    heart health and, 63, 65
    improvements in, 5
    inflammation and, 69, 150, 151
    libido and, 84, 85, 86
    memory and, 35
    mindfulness and, 7, 152, 157
    physical activity and, 124, 151
    premature aging and, 4
    reframing thinking and, 152–153
    self-care and, 51, 156–157
    sleep habits and, 39, 159
    social isolation and, 53

stretching, 157
stroke, 21, 33, 52, 65, 68, 95
substance abuse, 47, 48, 55, 153
sugars, 66, 85, 112, 113, 114
suicidal ideation, 47, 155
suicide prevention, 49
Sumo Squat With Drag, 141
sun exposure, 72, 76
sunglasses, 105
sunprotective clothing, 105
sunscreens, 17, 76, 103, 105
superagers, 18–19
superfoods, 116–119
Surowiec, Karen, 46
systolic blood pressure, 65

T

Tadwalkar, Rigved V., 7
tai chi, 43, 79
taurine, 19
Taylor, Richard, 55
tea break, 157
Telnes, Aaron, 46
telogen effluvium, 109
telomerase, 19
telomeres, 11, 19, 140
testosterone, 82–83, 85, 97
therapy
    for anxiety, 46
    for burnout, 155
    for depression, 38, 45, 48, 49
    forms of, 50
    for mental health, 43
Thigh and Hip Stretch, 130
thyroid conditions, 63, 109
titanium dioxide, 103
toxic exposures, 77
trampolines, 146–147
trauma, 50, 63, 109
triglycerides, 64, 65, 115
Twigge, Lauren, 117

U

ultra-processed foods, 66, 73
urinary tract infections (UTIs), 93, 97
U-shaped happiness curve, 42

V

vaginal dryness, 20–21, 85, 89, 91,
    92, 93, 97
vaginal estrogen, 91, 92, 97
Van Dongen, Hans, 159
van Praag, Henriette, 32
vaping, 67
vascular dementia, 40
Veozah (fezolinetant), 93, 95
Viagra, 81
vision loss, 70
vitamin A deficiency, 109
vitamin C products, for skincare,
    100, 101

vitamin D deficiency, 76, 79, 97, 109
vitamin E, 100
Viviscal, 109
Vizthum, Diane, 118, 119
volunteering, 26, 55, 56

W

Waldman, Abigail, 102, 103
walking, 124, 129, 146, 148–149, 151,
    157
water, benefits of, 120–121
Watson, Karol, 6
wearable medical devices, 4
Wegman, Shelly, 117
weight management
    brain health and, 38
    cancer and, 72, 73, 75
    diabetes and, 71
    Essential 8 and, 13
    heart disease and, 63
    inflammation and, 68, 69
    longevity and, 17
    menopause and, 95, 97
    metabolism and, 123
Weinberg, Nicole, 13, 146, 147
Whitbourne, Susan Krauss, 25
Wider, Jennifer, 96, 97
Williams, Brooke, 7
Winter, W. Christopher, 7, 34, 159,
    161
wisdom, 5, 14, 33, 83, 97
women, 4, 24–25, 63, 109, 128. See
    also menopause
Women's Health Initiative (WHI)
    study, 94
working habits, 16, 26, 28–29
working memory, 32, 35, 37
World Health Organization, 42, 67,
    114
worry, 10, 45, 46, 157, 161
Wu, Rachel, 21

Y

yoga practice, 33, 43, 69, 79, 127
Youdim, Adrienne, 118
Your Three-Week Longevity
    Challenge, 166–169

Z

Zak, Tami, 57
Zeichner, Joshua, 100
zinc oxide, 103

Prevention

EXECUTIVE EDITOR
Stephanie Dolgoff

CREATIVE DIRECTOR
Jarred Ford

RESEARCH DIRECTOR
Sonya Maynard

EDITORIAL DIRECTOR,
HEARST LIFESTYLE
GROUP
Jane Francisco

VICE PRESIDENT,
CONTENT OPERATIONS
Kim Cheney

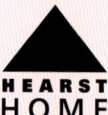

HEARST HOME

VICE PRESIDENT,
PUBLISHER,
HEARST BOOKS
Jacqueline Deval

DEPUTY DIRECTOR,
HEARST BOOKS
Nicole Fisher

DEPUTY MANAGING
EDITOR, HEARST
BOOKS
Maria Ramroop

SENIOR PHOTO EDITOR
Cinzia Reale-Castello

HEARST

HEARST MAGAZINE
MEDIA INC

PRESIDENT
Debi Chirichella

GENERAL MANAGER,
LIFESTYLE BRANDS
Ronak Patel

GLOBAL CHIEF
REVENUE OFFICER
Lisa Ryan Howard

EDITORIAL DIRECTOR
Lucy Kaylin

CHIEF FINANCIAL AND
STRATEGY OFFICER
Regina Buckley

CONSUMER GROWTH
OFFICER
Lindsey Horrigan

CHIEF PRODUCT &
TECHNOLOGY OFFICER
Daniel Bernard

PRESIDENT, HEARST
MAGAZINES
INTERNATIONAL
Jonathan Wright

SECRETARY
Catherine A. Bostron

PUBLISHING
CONSULTANTS
**Gilbert C. Maurer,
Mark F. Miller**

PUBLISHED BY HEARST

PRESIDENT & CHIEF
EXECUTIVE OFFICER
Steven R. Swartz

CHAIRMAN
William R. Hearst III

EXECUTIVE VICE
CHAIRMAN
Frank A. Bennack, Jr.

PRODUCED BY
ONE+ONE BOOKS

CONTRIBUTING
WRITER
AND EDITOR
Stacey Colino

COPYEDITOR
Laura Whittemore

PROOFREADER
Phyllis DeBlanche

PHOTO RESEARCHER
Micah Schmidt

INDEXER
Kay Banning

DESIGN BY **Nicole Tereza**
PRODUCTION DESIGN BY **Gillian MacLeod**

Library of Congress Cataloging-in-Publication Data available on request

10 9 8 7 6 5 4 3 2 1

Published by Hearst Home, an imprint of Hearst Books/Hearst Communications, Inc.
300 W 57th Street New York, NY 10019

Prevention and the Prevention logo are registered trademarks of Hearst Magazines, Inc. Hearst Home, the Hearst Home logo, and Hearst Books are registered trademarks of Hearst Communications, Inc.

For information about custom editions, special sales, premium and corporate purchases: hearst.com/magazines/hearst-books

Printed in China

978-1-958395-58-5

Photography Credits

AS: Adobe Stock, GI: Getty Images, SU: Stocksy United

Cover, Mike Garten; 2, Yagya Parajuli/GI; 4, NEW/AS; 8-9, Giada Canu/SU; 10-11, Marc Tran/SU; 12-13, Jennifer A Smith/GI; 15, pinstock/GI; 16, Ruth Black/SU; 17, Ruth Black/SU; 18, Eugene Mymrin/GI; 20 (top), Mikhail Bogdanov/GI; 20 (bottom), Mouse family/AS; 21 (top) Tara Moore/GI; 21 (bottom), Cavan Images/GI; 22-23, J. Anthony/SU; 24-25, 101cats/GI; 27, kritiyakorn Srikum/GI; 28, Naypong/GI; 30-31, AUDSHULE/SU; 32-33, Peter Dazeley/GI; 35, Malte Mueller/GI; 36, Dan Saelinger; 38, Dan Saelinger; 39, Dan Saelinger; 40, Lucidio Studio, Inc./GI; 42-43, Sadik Demiroz/GI; 43, Natalia Vetrova/GI; 44, Iryna Auhustsinovich/SU; 45, Iryna Auhustsinovich/SU; 47, Juan Moyano/SU; 48, Juan Moyano/SU; 49, PhotographerOlympus/GI; 50, Eugene Mymrin/GI; 51, goir/GI; 52, mitay20/GI; 54, Vera Lair/SU; 56, Olga Nikiforova/GI; 57, Aliaksandr/AS; 58, Yaroslav Danylchenko/SU; 59, Yaroslav Danylchenko/SU; 60-61, Giada Canu/SU; 62-63, jiray/AS; 64, Malte Mueller/GI; 66, antonbelo/GI; 67 (left), ollo/GI; 67 (right), Daniel Megias/500px/GI; 68 (both), The Voorhes;70-71, Andriy Onufriyenko/GI; 72, Rawf8/GI; 74, Mary Long/GI; 75-77 (all), Anastasia Usenko/GI; 78, Lew Robertson, Brand X Pictures/GI; 80-81, Yaroslav Danylchenko/SU; 82, Yaroslav Danylchenko/SU; 84, Raimund Linke/GI; 86, imageBROKER/AVTG/GI; 88, Yaroslav Danylchenko/SU; 90, AntonioSolano/GI; 92, Yaroslav Danylchenko/SU; 94-95, Ani Dimi/SU; 96, Yaroslav Danylchenko/SU; 98-99, Iryna Veklich/GI; 100-101, Rodica Cojocaru/500px/GI; 102-103, Westend61/GI; 104, Marianna Massey/GI; 105, Igishevamaria/GI; 106, Andreas Kuehn/GI; 107, Andreas Kuehn/GI; 108, Peter Dazeley/GI; 110-111, Yaroslav Danylchenko/SU; 112, Danielle Occhiogrosso Daly; 113, Mike Garten; 114, JulPo/GI; 116, Emily Kate Roemer; 117 (left to right), mariusFM77/GI; Science Photo Library/GI; Sorin Banica/500px/GI; 118 (left), Matt Rainey; 118 (right), Image Source/GI; 118-119, Mike Garten; 119, Burazin/GI; 120-121, Marc Tran/SU; 122, Hiroshi Watanabe/GI; 124-125, French Anderson Ltd/SU; 126, mixetto/GI; 128, MirageC/GI; 129-131 (all); Philip Friedman/Studio D; 132, Cagkan/AS; 133-135, Lauren Perlstein/Studio D; 135 (bottom), FreshSplash/GI; 136, Iryna Veklich/GI; 137-139 (all), Tyler Joe; 140, PM Images/GI; 141-145 (all), Terry Doyle/Laura Hinds; 146, mariakray/GI; 148-149, Kseniya Ovchinnikova/GI; 150-151, AUDSHULE/SU; 152, Pepino de Mar studio/SU; 153, Serbogachuk/SU; 154, MirageC/GI; 156, Giada Canu/SU; 157, Marc Tran/SU; 158, Juanjo McLittle/SU; 160, Carol Yepes/GI; 162, LianeM/GI; 163, Siarhei Khaletski/GI; 164, juanma hache/GI; 167, karandaev/GI; 168, Stephen Davies/AS